Mechanical Circulatory Support

Editors

PALAK SHAH
JENNIFER A. COWGER

CARDIOLOGY CLINICS

www.cardiology.theclinics.com

November 2018 • Volume 36 • Number 4

ELSEVIER

1600 John F. Kennedy Boulevard • Suite 1800 • Philadelphia, Pennsylvania, 19103-2899

http://www.theclinics.com

CARDIOLOGY CLINICS Volume 36, Number 4
November 2018 ISSN 0733-8651, ISBN-13: 978-0-323-64159-3

Editor: Stacy Eastman
Developmental Editor: Sara Watkins

Cardiology Clinics (ISSN 0733-8651) is published quarterly by Elsevier Inc., 360 Park Avenue South, New York, NY 10010-1710. Months of issue are February, May, August, and November. Business and Editorial Offices: 1600 John F. Kennedy Blvd., Ste. 1800, Philadelphia, PA 19103-2899. Customer Service Office: 3251 Riverport Lane, Maryland Heights, MO 63043. Periodicals postage paid at New York, NY and additional mailing offices. Subscription prices are $339.00 per year for US individuals, $640.00 per year for US institutions, $100.00 per year for US students and residents, $430.00 per year for Canadian individuals, $804.00 per year for Canadian institutions, $464.00 per year for international individuals, $804.00 per year for international institutions and $220.00 per year for Canadian and international students/residents. To receive student/resident rate, orders must be accompanied by name of affiliated institution, data of term, and the *signature* of program/residency coordinator on institution letterhead. Orders will be billed at individual rate until proof of status is received. Foreign air speed delivery is included in all *Clinics* subscription prices. All prices are subject to change without notice. **POSTMASTER:** Send address changes to *Cardiology Clinics*, Elsevier Health Sciences Division, Subscription Customer Service, 3251 Riverport Lane, Maryland Heights, MO 63043. **Customer Service: 1-800-654-2452 (U.S. and Canada); 314-447-8871 (outside U.S. and Canada). Fax: 314-447-8029. E-mail: journalscustomerservice-usa@ elsevier.com (for print support); journalsonlinesupport-usa@elsevier.com (for online support).**

Reprints. For copies of 100 or more, of articles in this publication, please contact the Commercial Reprints Department, Elsevier Inc., 360 Park Avenue South, New York, NY 10010-1710. Tel.: 212-633-3874; Fax: 212-633-3820; E-mail: reprints@elsevier.com.

Cardiology Clinics is also published in Spanish by McGraw-Hill Interamericana Editores S. A., P.O. Box 5-237, 06500, Mexico D. F., Mexico; in Portuguese by Reichmann and Alfonso Editores Rio de Janeiro, Brazil; and in Greek by Dimitrios P. Lagos, 8 Pondon Street, GR115-28 Ilissia, Greece.

Cardiology Clinics is covered in *MEDLINE/PubMed (Index Medicus), Excerpta Medica, The Cumulative Index to Nursing and Allied Health Literature* (CINAHL).

Contributors

AUTHORS

SAIMA ASLAM, MD, MS
Associate Professor, Medical Director, Division
of Infectious Diseases and Global Public
Health, University of California, San Diego,
San Diego, California, USA

PAVAN ATLURI, MD
Assistant Professor of Surgery, Director of Heart
Transplantation and Mechanical Circulatory
Support Program, Division of Cardiovascular
Surgery, Hospital of the University of
Pennsylvania, Philadelphia, Pennsylvania, USA

DONALD F. BROPHY, PharmD, MSc
Department of Pharmacotherapy and
Outcomes Science, Virginia Commonwealth
University School of Pharmacy, Richmond,
Virginia, USA

JENNIFER A. COWGER, MD, MS, FACC
Medical Director, Mechanical Circulatory
Support, Section of Heart Failure and
Transplantation, Department of Cardiology,
Henry Ford Hospital, Detroit, Michigan, USA

TODD F. DARDAS, MD, MS
Assistant Professor, Department of Medicine,
University of Washington, Seattle, Washington,
USA

SHASHANK DESAI, MD
Heart Failure and Transplantation, Inova Heart
and Vascular Institute, Falls Church, Virginia, USA

LORI G. EDWARDS, MSN, RN
Lead VAD Coordinator, Advanced Heart
Failure/Mechanical Circulatory Support, Inova
Fairfax Hospital, Falls Church, Virginia, USA

ALY EL BANAYOSY, MD
Director of ECMO Program, Department of
Heart Failure Cardiology, Integris Baptist
Medical Center, Oklahoma City, Oklahoma,
USA

KIMBER ELEUTERI, MSN, ACNP
Medical Affairs Manager, Mechanical
Circulatory Support, Medtronic, Framingham,
Massachusetts, USA

TONYA ELLIOTT, MSN, RN, CCTC, CHFN
Program Development Specialist, MCS
Program, MedStar Heart & Vascular Institute,
Washington, DC, USA

JERRY D. ESTEP, MD
Department of Cardiovascular Medicine, Heart
and Vascular Institute, Kaufman Center for
Heart Failure, Cleveland Clinic, Cleveland,
Ohio, USA

GILLIAN GRAFTON, DO
Department of Cardiology, Henry Ford
Hospital, Detroit, Michigan, USA

PAUL A. GURBEL, MD, FACC
Director, Interventional Cardiology and
Cardiovascular Medicine Research, Inova
Center for Thrombosis Research and Drug
Development, Inova Heart and Vascular
Institute, Falls Church, Virginia, USA

BASHAR HANNAWI, MD
Department of Cardiology, Houston Methodist
Hospital, Houston, Texas, USA

DOUGLAS HORSTMANSHOF, MD
Director of Heart Failure Program, Department
of Heart Failure Cardiology, Integris Baptist
Medical Center, Oklahoma City, Oklahoma,
USA

AJAY KADAKKAL, MD
Advanced Heart Failure Program, MedStar
Heart & Vascular Institute, MedStar
Washington Hospital Center, Washington,
DC, USA

JU H. KIM, MD
Department of Heart Failure and
Transplantation, Methodist DeBakey
Cardiology Associates, Houston Methodist
Hospital, Houston, Texas, USA

MICHAEL MATHIAS KOERNER, MD, PhD
Cardiovascular Intensive Care, Director of
Critical Care, Integris Baptist Medical Center,
Oklahoma City, Oklahoma, USA

BRENT C. LAMPERT, DO, FACC
Associate Professor of Clinical Medicine,
Division of Cardiovascular Medicine,
The Ohio State University Wexner Medical
Center, Columbus, Ohio, USA

SAMER S. NAJJAR, MD
Advanced Heart Failure Program, MedStar
Heart & Vascular Institute, MedStar
Washington Hospital Center, Washington,
DC, USA

NIKHIL NARANG, MD
Section of Cardiology, Department of
Medicine, The University of Chicago,
Chicago, Illinois, USA

FRANCIS D. PAGANI, MD, PhD
Professor, Department of Cardiac Surgery,
University of Michigan Frankel Cardiovascular
Center, Ann Arbor, Michigan, USA

COLLEEN PIETRAS, MD
Heart and Lung Transplantation, Mechanical
Circulatory Support Fellow, Division of
Cardiovascular Surgery, Hospital of the
University of Pennsylvania, Philadelphia,
Pennsylvania, USA

JAYANT RAIKHELKAR, MD
Section of Cardiology, Department of
Medicine, The University of Chicago,
Chicago, Illinois, USA

DIYAR SAEED, MD, PhD
Clinic for Cardiovascular Surgery,
Heinrich-Heine University Düsseldorf,
Düsseldorf, Germany

GABRIEL SAYER, MD
Section of Cardiology, Department of
Medicine, The University of Chicago,
Chicago, Illinois, USA

KEYUR B. SHAH, MD
Advanced Heart Failure and Transplant,
Pauley Heart Center, Virginia Commonwealth
University, Richmond, Virginia, USA

PALAK SHAH, MD, MS, FACC, FHFSA
Director, Heart Failure Research, Department of Heart Failure and Transplantation, Assistant Professor of Medicine, The George Washington University, Inova Heart and Vascular Institute, Falls Church, Virginia, USA

PAUL C. TANG, MD, PhD
Assistant Professor, Department of Cardiac Surgery, University of Michigan Frankel Cardiovascular Center, Ann Arbor, Michigan, USA

UDAYA S. TANTRY, PhD
Inova Center for Thrombosis Research and Drug Development, Inova Heart and Vascular Institute, Falls Church, Virginia, USA

NIR URIEL, MD, MSc
Section of Cardiology, Department of Medicine, The University of Chicago, Chicago, Illinois, USA

Contents

The field of mechanical circulatory support (MCS) has evolved from earlier-generation pulsatile-flow devices that were primarily used to support critically ill patients in the hospital to newer-generation continuous-flow devices that permit hospital discharge and resumption of normal life activities. The technology is used to bridge transplant-eligible patients and can be used for long-term support of patients who are transplant ineligible. Left ventricular assist devices are proved to improve long-term survival and quality of life for patients with advanced heart failure. Adverse events associated with MCS therapy remain the Achilles heel of the field and strategies to improve biocompatibility are ongoing.

This article on continuous-flow device technology engages in an in-depth discussion on the engineering aspects of continuous-flow devices. The authors examine the energy transfer mechanics of centrifugal versus axial devices, and the impact of novel noncontact pump bearings. Furthermore, this article reviews the relationship between continuous-flow pump speed, flow, and pressure gradients across the device. Potential future advances in pump design with greater algorithmic responses to changes in patient physiology are also considered.

Surgical maneuvers for implantation of a continuous-flow ventricular assist device are revolutionary concepts that have been associated with a reduction in pump-related complications. With the advancement of technology, surgical implant strategy continues to evolve, incorporating less-invasive approaches into the armamentarium of the experienced surgeon.

Cardiogenic shock (CS) refractory to conventional therapies continues to be a challenging medical syndrome, with poor prognosis and high complication and mortality rates. The application and use of temporary mechanical circulatory support (MCS) is a component in the treatment of CS patients and should be applied early in the presentation. Crucial to the success of their application, temporary MCS devices should be chosen based on degree of patient acuity and etiology of CS. Not all temporary MCS devices deliver the same degree of hemodynamic support and range from minimal support to systemic support via veno-arterial extracorporeal membrane oxygenation.

the incidence/prevalence of both ischemic and hemorrhagic stroke in patients with continuous-flow LVADs, compare axial and centrifugal devices, and discuss the major risk factors for neurologic events that have been identified.

Antithrombotic Strategies and Device Thrombosis

Paul A. Gurbel, Palak Shah, Shashank Desai, and Udaya S. Tantry

Despite improvements in left ventricular assist device (LVAD) technology, bleeding and thrombotic complications are major concerns that adversely influence morbidity and mortality. Current antithrombotic therapy recommendations for LVAD thrombosis prophylaxis are largely derived from clinical device trials that implement a one-size-fits-all strategy. Objective serial laboratory-based assessment of thrombogenicity is needed to balance the risk of bleeding and thrombotic complications. Finally, the newest-generation device, the HeartMate 3, has been associated with lower levels of shear and reduced hemolysis that may mitigate thrombotic event occurrences.

Impact of Mechanical Circulatory Support on Posttransplant Outcomes

Todd F. Dardas

Mechanical circulatory support (MCS) has markedly improved the likelihood of transplant among patients with advanced heart failure. Transplant survival following MCS is similar for supported and unsupported recipients. Transplant survival is only reduced following left ventricle assist device (LVAD) support complicated by infection, total artificial heart support, and extracorporeal life support. Despite allosensitization and a higher incidence of vasoplegia syndrome, posttransplant survival for durable LVADs is similar to patients with inotropes alone at the time of transplant. MCS as a bridge to transplant offers significant benefits over waiting without support.

Hemodynamic Pump-Patient Interactions and Left Ventricular Assist Device Imaging

Nikhil Narang, Jayant Raikhelkar, Gabriel Sayer, and Nir Uriel

Left ventricular assist devices (LVAD) provide a durable option for patients with advanced hear failure. Axial and centrifugal pump physiology differs with regard to the relationship between pump inflow-outflow cannula pressure differential and flow, which results in device behavior that can vary drastically under different loading conditions. Ramp studies can aid the clinician in choosing the optimal speed to adequately unload the left ventricle. Advances in 3-dimensional echocardiography enhance the understanding of chamber geometry for both types of LVADs. Novel outflow graft imaging techniques have been developed to better characterize aortic insufficiency, which may be underestimated with current standard methods.

Ambulatory Ventricular Assist Device Patient Management

Tonya Elliott and Lori G. Edwards

Understanding the ventricular assist device (VAD) patient pump interface and developing expertise in monitoring patients with a VAD are the goals of care in the ambulatory setting. The objective is to improve long-term outcomes. The purpose of expert, focused, routine outpatient surveillance is to facilitate the integration of pulseless, electrically dependent VAD patients into the community. Other goals of outpatient care include maximizing quality of life, maintaining equipment integrity, treating heart failure symptoms, monitoring for common VAD-related complications, ensuring viability as a heart transplant candidate, consideration for patients implanted to become transplantable, and monitoring for possible cardiac recovery.

Recent advances in mechanical circulatory support have allowed patients with end-stage heart failure to be successfully bridged to heart transplantation or live for many years on continuous-flow left ventricular assist devices (CF-LVADs) as destination therapy. As survival and quality of life continue to improve and the number of patients supported by CF-LVADs continues to grow, utilization of different imaging modalities in the care for these patients has become an integral part of many heart failure centers. We review currently available imaging modalities, with a focus on echocardiography, that aid to diagnose and manage common adverse events associated with CF-LVADs.

Some degree of right ventricular (RV) dysfunction can be observed in most patients with advanced heart failure assed for left ventricular assist device (LVAD) implantation. This article describes critical factors that need to be considered in the assessment of the RV before LVAD surgery. Further, detailed description of the most important perioperative management strategies to prevent (RV) dysfunction is included. Finally, the most commonly used temporary and permeant RV support strategies are discussed, including anatomic and physiologic challenges and barriers associated with the off-label use of continuous-flow LVAD pumps for the right-sided circulation.

CARDIOLOGY CLINICS

SERIES OF RELATED INTEREST

Cardiac Electrophysiology Clinics
Heart Failure Clinics
Interventional Cardiology Clinics

THE CLINICS ARE AVAILABLE ONLINE!
Access your subscription at:
www.theclinics.com

Preface

Defining a Decade of Experience with Continuous-Flow Left Ventricular Assist Devices

In the past decade, there has been tremendous growth in the use of durable mechanical circulatory support (MCS) to treat patients with advanced heart failure and cardiogenic shock. Through the advent of continuous-flow left ventricular assist devices (LVADs), the MCS field has greatly improved the durability, applicability, and mortality of LVAD therapy for the end-stage patient population. Nevertheless, the therapy is associated with significant morbidity, and continued research is needed to improve the safety profile of the treatment before it can be applied more broadly and to the less-sick patient population.

To better understand and highlight the most salient features of LVAD therapy, we have invited multiple experts in the MCS field to provide a systematic review of the critical elements needed to evaluate and manage this complex and growing patient population. Importantly, critical gaps in the field and areas of future research are highlighted. This text should serve as a comprehensive overview for new faculty or trainees or for those established clinicians looking to refresh fundamental MCS concepts in a specific domain. We hope you enjoy reading this as much as we enjoyed putting it together!

Sincerely,

Palak Shah, MD, MS, FACC, FHFSA
Inova Heart and Vascular Institute
3300 Gallows Road
Falls Church, VA 22042, USA

Jennifer A. Cowger, MD, MS, FACC
Henry Ford Hospital
2799 West Grand Boulevard
Detroit, MI 48202, USA

E-mail addresses:
Palak.shah@inova.org (P. Shah)
jennifercowger@gmail.com (J.A. Cowger)

Cardiol Clin 36 (2018) xiii
https://doi.org/10.1016/j.ccl.2018.07.001
0733-8651/18/© 2018 Published by Elsevier Inc.

The Evolution of Mechanical Circulatory Support

Ju H. Kim, MD[a], Jennifer A. Cowger, MD, MS[b],
Palak Shah, MD, MS[c],*

KEYWORDS

- Ventricular assist device • Heart failure • Cardiac transplantation • Mechanical circulatory support
- Total artificial heart

KEY POINTS

- Mechanical circulatory support was developed by early pioneers in the field of heart failure, cardiac surgery, and transplantation.
- Mechanical circulation is used to support the heart at the time of open heart surgery.
- Initial devices were large, extracorporeal, pulsatile-flow devices that eventually developed into smaller, intracorporeal, continuous-flow devices, termed *left ventricular assist devices (LVADs)*, which are less prone to mechanical wear with longer support durations.
- Patients receive LVADs as a bridge to transplant (BTT) or as destination therapy (DT) for patients who are ineligible for transplant. Due to insufficient organ supply, more patients globally receive an LVAD as opposed to a cardiac transplant.
- The future application of this therapy will continue to grow as best practices in patient management and device design are identified to mitigate adverse events associated with LVAD therapy.

INTRODUCTION

Heart failure (HF) currently affects an estimated 6.5 million people in the United States. As the population ages, diabetes prevalence grows, and more individuals survive myocardial infarction, the prevalence of HF is expected to increase to greater than 8 million individuals by 2030.[1] Advanced HF recalcitrant to medical therapy (American College of Cardiology/American Heart Association stage D HF) has an estimated prevalence of 250,000 to 300,000 individuals in the United States.[2] Although hospice and/or palliative care with or without intravenous inotrope support may be the most appropriate management for some patients with stage D HF, carefully selected individuals may achieve improved quality of life and survival with advanced HF therapies, including long-term mechanical circulatory support (MCS) or cardiac transplantation.

With an average survival of 50% at 13 years, the gold standard for the treatment of advanced HF remains heart transplantation. Although cardiac

Disclosure Statement: J.H. Kim—no disclosures; J.A. Cowger—reports institutional research and speaking for Abbott, institutional research, steering committee, and paid speaking for HeartWare; P. Shah reports grant support from Merck, Haemonetics, and an AHA Scientist Development Award cofunded by the Enduring Hearts Foundation (17SDG33660431).
[a] Department of Heart Failure and Transplantation, Houston Methodist Hospital, 6565 Fannin Street, Houston, TX 77030, USA; [b] Section of Heart Failure and Transplantation, Henry Ford Hospital, 2799 West Grand Boulevard, Detroit, MI 48202, USA; [c] Department of Heart Failure and Transplantation, Inova Heart and Vascular Institute, 3300 Gallows Road, Falls Church, VA 22042, USA
* Corresponding author.
E-mail address: palak.shah@inova.org

cardiology.theclinics.com

Abbreviations	
BTT	Bridge to transplant
DT	Destination therapy
FDA	Food and Drug Administration
HF	Heart failure
INTERMACS	Interagency Registry for Mechanically Assisted Circulatory Support
IVAD	Implantable ventricular assist device
LVAD	Left ventricular assist device
LVAS	Left ventricular assist system
MCS	Mechanical circulatory support
NHLBI	National Heart, Lung and Blood Institute
PVAD	Paracorporeal ventricular assist device
REMATCH	Randomized Evaluation of Mechanical Assistance for the Treatment of Congestive Heart Failure
TAH	Total artificial heart
VAD	Ventricular assist device

transplantation has historically been offered to only approximately 2200 individuals annually in the United States since 2010, the number of patients receiving a cardiac transplant has gradually increased and is currently approximately 3300 patients a year.[3,4] Each year, approximately 10% of patients on the heart transplant wait list die awaiting a suitable organ.[3]

Continued advancements in durable MCS have significantly altered the landscape of advanced HF by improving survival and quality of life for both those awaiting heart transplantation (ie, bridge to transplant [BTT]) as well as those who may not qualify for transplantation (ie, destination therapy [DT]). In the United States, only 22,000 total ventricular assist device (VAD) implants have been reported to the Interagency Registry for Mechanically Assisted Circulatory Support (INTERMACS) since 2006.[5] To contrast outcomes with current-generation continuous-flow LVADs, the Risk Assessment and Comparative Effectiveness of Left Ventricular Assist Device and Medical Management in Ambulatory Heart Failure Patients (ROADMAP) study compared survival of HF patients who were not inotrope dependent but had advanced HF symptoms (New York Heart Association class III or IV) to a similarly matched cohort of patients who elected to receive a VAD.[6] The medical therapy patients had significantly worse event-free survival. At 1-year and 2-year event-free survival, rates in the medical management group were 63% and 41%, respectively,

compared with average survivals of 80% and 70%, respectively, in VAD recipients.[5–7] Furthermore, patients on LVAD support had greater improvements in 6-minute walk distance and quality of life. The ROADMAP data suggest that carefully selected, non–inotrope-dependent patients with advanced HF symptoms may gain benefit from MCS therapy. The Randomized Evaluation of VAD InterVEntion before Inotropic Therapy pilot trial attempted to investigate this hypothesis through randomized study. Unfortunately, the trial was terminated due to a high number of adverse events (especially device thrombosis) in the MCS arm.[8] The Multicenter Study of MagLev Technology in Patients Undergoing Mechanical Circulatory Support Therapy with HeartMate3 trial included patients with non–inotrope-dependent systolic HF and a cardiac index less than 2.2 L/min/m^2 but this subgroup only comprised approximately 2200 15% of the cohort and long-term outcomes are not yet available.[9] As adverse event burdens improve with each evolution of device therapy, further study in non–inotrope-dependent patients with advanced HF can be anticipated.

HISTORY OF DURABLE MECHANICAL CIRCULATORY SUPPORT

The field of MCS has matured significantly since the development of the first cardiopulmonary bypass device—the Gibbon-IBM heart-lung machine. The Gibbon-IBM heart-lung machine was first used in 1953 by Dr John Gibbon during an atrial septal defect closure in an 18-year-old woman.[10] The first VAD was implanted in 1963 by Drs Michael DeBakey and Domingo Liotta.[11–13] A patient named George Washington, who suffered cardiac arrest after aortic valve replacement, received the first such device in 1963. The inflow of the VAD was attached to the left atrium and the outflow to the descending thoracic aorta, providing pump flows of 1.8 L/min to 2.5 L/min[14] The patient survived with improvement in pulmonary edema until his death on the fourth postoperative day, attributed to brain damage from the cardiac arrest. In 1966, DeBakey[11,14] implanted another version of an extracorporeal left ventricular bypass pump, the Liotta-DeBakey LVAD, with the inflow attached to the left atrium and outflow attached to the right axillary artery in Esperanza del Valle Vasquez, a woman unable to be weaned from the heart-lung machine after aortic and mitral valve replacements. With pump flows of 1.2 L/min, the patient was successfully weaned from the heart-lung machine. By postoperative day 10, the

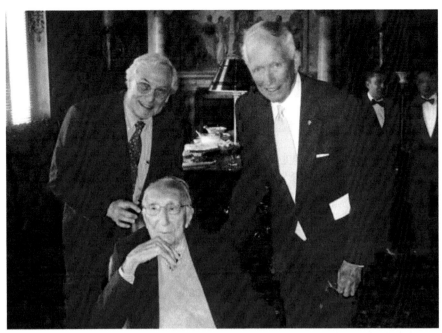

Fig. 1. Pioneers in the field of MCS. (*left to right*) Dr O.H. "Bud" Frazier, Dr Michael E. DeBakey, and Dr Denton A. Cooley. (*Courtesy of* O.H. Frazier, MD, Houston, TX.)

VAD was also able to be removed with myocardial recovery and the patient survived to discharge.

The first total artificial heart (TAH) was implanted as a BTT by Dr Denton Cooley with Dr Liotta in 1969 in Haskell Karp, a 47-year-old man with ischemic cardiomyopathy awaiting heart transplantation at St. Luke's Episcopal Hospital in Houston, Texas (**Fig. 1**). After undergoing ventricular aneurysmectomy, the patient could not be weaned from the heart-lung machine. Cooley and Liotta implanted the Liotta TAH, a pneumatically powered pump with Dacron-lined grafts and mechanical valves. He survived on TAH support for 64 hours until he received a heart transplant. Unfortunately, Karp died 32 hours after his transplant due to a *Pseudomonas* pneumonia.[15,16] These pioneers sparked the development of a field dedicated to providing long-term MCS for patients with end-stage HF awaiting heart transplantation.

The development of the TAH continued into the 1970s with the Akutsu III designed by Dr Tetsuzo Akutsu.[15] This device was implanted by Cooley and colleagues[17] in 1981 as a BTT in a patient with postcardiotomy shock after coronary bypass surgery. In 1982, the first TAH implant for DT support was performed by Dr William DeVries using the Jarvik 7, designed by Dr Robert Jarvik under the direction of Dr Willem Kolff at the University of Utah.[18] The patient was Dr Barney Clark, then 61 years old with a nonischemic cardiomyopathy, who survived for 112 days until his death after

numerous complications, including renal failure, epistaxis, gastrointestinal bleeding, aspiration pneumonia, and pseudomembranous colitis. The longest duration of support using the Jarvik 7 was 620 days and was complicated by multiple strokes and infections.[19]

In 1984, the first successful implant of an isolated left VAD (LVAD) occurred with the Novacor left ventricular assist system (LVAS) (World Heart, Oakland, California) as BTT.[20] The Novacor LVAS was an electric, dual pusher-plate device that was constructed of a polyurethane pump sac with gelatin-sealed inflow and outflow grafts containing porcine bioprosthetic valves that facilitated unidirectional flow.[21] It was not until 1994 that the first patient implanted with a pulsatile-flow LVAD by Dr O. H. Frazier was able to be discharged from the hospital, representing 3 decades of work that began with announcement of the National Heart, Lung, and Blood Institute (NHLBI) Artificial Heart Program in 1964 (see **Fig. 1**; **Table 1**).[22,23] First-generation pulsatile LVADs, such as the Novacor LVAS, HeartMate XVE (Thoratec, Pleasanton, California), Thoratec IVAD (Thoratec, Pleasanton, California), Thoratec PVAD (Thoratec), and LionHeart LVAD (Arrow International, Reading, Pennsylvania) were volume-displacement pumps designed to mimic the systolic and diastolic flow of the native heart (**Fig. 2**). These devices, however, were large and noisy and durability was problematic due to

Table 1 Early milestones in the development of mechanical circulatory support	
Year	**Milestone**
1963	First VAD implantation
1964	NHLBI founds the Artificial Heart Program
1969	First TAH implantation
1972	NHLBI initiates an LVAD program
1975	NHLBI sponsors clinical trials of pneumatic LVADs
1980	Request for proposals for untethered, electric, portable LVADs
1991	First implantation of electric, portable LVAD
1994	First patient discharge from hospital with portable LVAD
2001	REMATCH trial demonstrates superiority of LVAD over optimal medical therapy in New York Heart Association class IV patients[25]

Courtesy of O.H. Frazier, MD, Houston, TX.

multiple mechanical parts that were subject to wear and tear (eg, pusher plates and porcine tissue valves to ensure unidirectional flow).[24] For example, the HeartMate XVE used in the landmark Randomized Evaluation of Mechanical Assistance for the Treatment of Congestive Heart Failure (REMATCH) trial weighed 1255 g and the probability of device failure was 35% at 2 years.[25]

To overcome the limitations of pulsatile-flow devices with respect to mechanical wear and to permit application to smaller recipients, the field focused on development of continuous-flow pumps. Continuous-flow LVAD technologies, including the HeartMate II (Abbott Laboratories, Abbott Park, Illinois), DuraHeart LVAD (Terumo Heart, Ann Arbor, Michigan), MicroMed DeBakey VAD (MicroMed Technology, Houston), HVAD (Medtronic, St. Paul, Minnesota), HeartAssist5 (ReliantHeart, Houston, Texas), Evaheart

(Evaheart, Houston, Texas), Jarvik 2000 (Jarvik Heart, New York, New York), VentrAssist (Ventracor, Sydney, Australia), and Levacor (WorldHeart, Salt Lake City, Utah), are of a smaller profile with a single moving part—the impeller/rotor—significantly improving durability with reduced noise emission (see **Fig. 2**). Continuous-flow devices presently offer 2 flow configurations—axial flow or centrifugal flow—and each device has its own response to filling pressure, afterload (the pressure (H) versus flow (Q) curve), and speed augmentation, as presented in Paul C. Tang and Francis D. Pagani's article, "Continuous-Flow Device Engineering and Pump Technology," in this issue.

Clinical Trials of Continuous-Flow Left Ventricular Assist Device Technologies

Continuous-flow LVADs were studied in the early 2000s,[26] but wide-scale clinical application of continuous-flow LVAD therapy effectively began in 2008 with Food and Drug Administration (FDA) approval for BTT therapy after the presentation of the HeartMate II BTT clinical trial.[27] This was a prospective, multicenter study of 133 patients listed for cardiac transplant with New York Heart Association class IV systolic HF and inotrope dependence or need for intra-aortic balloon pump support. With a median support of 126 days, overall survival was 75% at 6 months and 68% at 1 year, with improved functional status and quality of life.[27] The superiority of the continuous-flow device for DT support was later shown in a randomized trial comparing the HeartMate XVE and the HeartMate II.[28] This trial reported a 2-year actuarial survival of 24% in the HeartMate XVE versus 58% in the HeartMate II as well as almost one-eighth the incidence of device failure compared with the pulsatile device. This led to HeartMate II gaining FDA approval for DT in 2010.

Centrifugal flow technology provides continuous-flow by use of a bearingless, magnetically levitated rotor with intrapericardial placement. Currently, the HVAD and the HeartMate 3

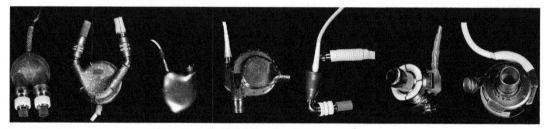

Fig. 2. Evolution of durable LVADs. (*Left to right*) The first 2 pumps represent older-generation pulsatile-flow pumps and are followed by continuous-flow pumps with older-generation to newer-generation devices.

are primary centrifugal flow technologies used within the United States. The HVAD received FDA approval for BTT in 2012 after the Advanced Heart Failure Bridge to Transplant trial showed a 91% survival (to transplant or on the original pump) at 6 months.[29] The Clinical Trial to Evaluate the HeartWare Ventricular Assist System (ENDURANCE) studied the efficacy of the HVAD in 446 DT patients.[30] Compared with the HeartMate II, the HVAD was found noninferior with respect to survival free from disabling stroke or reoperation for device malfunction at 2 years. More patients who received the HVAD suffered strokes (29.7% vs 12.1%), however, compared with the HeartMate II recipients.[30] Analysis of the ENDURANCE data found multiple possibilities for the stroke association on HVAD support, including pump inflow design (absence of sintering on early pumps), lower international normalized ratios in HVAD patients, lower-dose aspirin use, and elevated mean arterial pressures.

Therefore, the ENDURANCE Supplemental Trial was designed to study the effectiveness of a blood pressure management strategy on the incidence of neurologic injury at 12 months. Patients were instructed to record their blood pressure twice per day for the first 3 months and continued close monitoring throughout the study period to maintain a mean arterial pressure less than or equal to 85 mm Hg using an automated cuff or less than or equal to 90 mm Hg using a Doppler method. Results from the ENDURANCE Supplemental Trial presented at the International Society of Heart and Lung Transplantation annual meeting in 2017 showed that intense blood pressure management led to a nonsignificant reduction in the rate of overall stroke at 12 months, from 22.3% in ENDURANCE to 16.9% in the Supplemental Trial , with the greatest impact reflected in a 50% reduction in the rate of hemorrhagic stroke.[31] With a combination of data from the original ENDURANCE and the Supplemental Trial , the HVAD gained FDA approval for DT support in 2017.

The HeartMate 3 is a newer-generation, fully magnetically levitated, centrifugal continuous-flow pump designed to improve hemocompatibility by means of wider blood flow paths as well as

Table 2
Clinical trial design and milestones in US regulatory approval of continuous-flow left ventricular assist devices

Device	Clinical Trial Design	Primary Endpoint	Seminal Publication and Food and Drug Administration Approval
HeartMate II BTT[27]	BTT patients, no control arm	Survival at 6 mo, noninferiority to expected survival of 65% for BTT patients	2007/2008
HeartMate II DT[28]	Randomization of DT patients 2:1 for HeartMate II vs HeartMate XVE	Survival at 2 y, free of disabling stroke (MRS >3) or device failure	2010
HVAD BTT[29]	Control arm was chosen from INTERMACS registry	Noninferior survival at 6 mo	2012
HVAD DT[30]	Randomization of DT patients in 2:1 for HVAD vs HeartMate II	Noninferior survival at 2 y free of disabling stroke (MRS $\geq$ 4) or device failure[a]	2017
HeartMate 3 BTT[9]	Randomization of both BTT and DT patients in 1:1 ratio to HeartMate 3 vs HeartMate II	Noninferior survival at 6 mo free of disabling stroke (MRS >3) or device failure	2017
HeartMate 3 DT	Nested within the same trial as the BTT study	Noninferior survival at 2 y free of disabling stroke (MRS >3) or device failure	2018

Abbreviation: MRS, modified Rankin scale.
  [a] Despite meeting the primary noninferiority endpoint, there was a concern for a higher incidence of stroke in the HVAD group. As a result, the FDA mandated a supplemental trial that tested efficacy of tight blood pressure control to reduce the incidence of strokes with HVAD. Based on a combination of data from the original and supplemental trial, the device was then FDA approved for DT.

an artificial intrinsic pulse generated through modulation of the rotor speed. The Multicenter Study of MagLev Technology in Patients Undergoing Mechanical Circulatory Support Therapy with HeartMate 3 (MOMENTUM 3) is a multicenter, nonblinded, randomized trial designed to show noninferiority of the HeartMate 3 compared with the HeartMate II with respect to survival free of disabling stroke or survival free of reoperation to replace or remove the device at 6 months.[9] Analysis of the short-term cohort at 6 months after implant demonstrated an event-free survival of 86.2% in HeartMate 3 recipients versus 76.8% in those on the HeartMate II (HR 0.55, $P = .037$).[9] The HeartMate 3 was approved for short-term support (BTT indication) in 2017 but DT approval is pending at the time of this article.

Remarkably, the HeartMate 3 cohort had no cases of suspected or confirmed pump thrombosis compared with the 10% seen in the HeartMate II cohort ($P<.0001$). Lower rates of hemolysis, reduced shear stress and increased pulsatility with the HeartMate 3 are certainly steps forward in the development of hemocompatible pumps. Although early data suggest increased preservation of high-molecular-weight von Willebrand multimers with the HeartMate 3, functional improvement in hemocompatibility has not yet been demonstrated.[32] In the MOMENTUM 3 study, no significant differences were noted in frequencies of stroke (7% vs 10%, $P = .39$) or gastrointestinal bleeding (15% vs 15%, $P = .87$),[9] highlighting the ongoing limitations of current device technology and the complexity of designing a fully hemocompatible pump.

Between clinical trials and with approved devices, more than 30,000 adults have been implanted with continuous-flow LVADs and the field's knowledge with respect to patient selection, device management, and diagnosis and management of device complications has blossomed. An overview of the major milestones with respect to the FDA regulatory approval of continuous-flow LVADs is presented (**Table 2**).

Clinical Trials of Total Artificial Heart Support

Initial TAH development was driven by poor survival after cardiac transplantation. With the advent of cyclosporine in the early 1980s,[33] transplant survival improved dramatically and eclipsed the development of the TAH. The modern version of the Jarvik 7, currently marketed as the Syncardia TAH (SynCardia Systems, Tucson, Arizona) gained FDA approval for use in end-stage biventricular HF as BTT in 2004 and is commercially available in the United States.[34] Data cited for approval include that of a nonrandomized study of 120 patients listed for cardiac transplant, of whom 81 underwent TAH implant. One-year survival in the TAH group was 70% versus 31% in controls.[35] A DT trial is now under way as are trials investigating a newer, smaller, 50-cm^3 device, compared with the original 70-cm^3 model. The device also has a new portable driver that allows for added patient mobility and discharge from the hospital in appropriately selected patients. Despite these advances, the TAH implantation constitutes only 2% of the total number of MCS devices implanted between June 2006 and December 2016.[5] Other TAH devices, such as BiVACOR (BiVACOR, Houston, Texas), SmartHeart (Cleveland Heart, Cleveland, Ohio), and CARMAT (Vélizy-Villacoublay, France) are in development.[36]

SUMMARY

With more than 50 years of experience with durable MCS, there has been tremendous growth and development within the field to generate the currently available continuous-flow VADs. This technology is vital for bridging transplant-eligible patients and for those ineligible for transplant to improve long-term survival and quality of life. Adverse events associated with MCS therapy remain the Achilles heel of the field. Further advances in the hemocompatibility of devices, as well as the development of fully implantable pumps, are imperative for widespread application of the therapy in stage D HF and for subsequent use in the less sick HF population. Well-designed and well-executed basic science research and translational clinical trials are critical to spur advances in this exciting field.

REFERENCES

1. Benjamin EJ, Blaha MJ, Chiuve SE, et al. Heart disease and stroke statistics-2017 update: a report from the American heart association. Circulation 2017;135(10):e146–603.
2. Miller LW. Left ventricular assist devices are underutilized. Circulation 2011;123(14):1552–8 [discussion: 1558].
3. Colvin M, Smith JM, Skeans MA, et al. OPTN/SRTR 2015 annual data report: heart. Am J Transplant 2017;17(Suppl 1):286–356.
4. Lund LH, Khush KK, Cherikh WS, et al. The registry of the international society for heart and lung transplantation: thirty-fourth adult heart transplantation report-2017; focus theme: allograft ischemic time. J Heart Lung Transplant 2017;36(10):1037–46.
5. Kirklin JK, Pagani FD, Kormos RL, et al. Eighth annual INTERMACS report: special focus on framing

the impact of adverse events. J Heart Lung Transplant 2017;36(10):1080–6.

6. Estep JD, Starling RC, Horstmanshof DA, et al. Risk assessment and comparative effectiveness of left ventricular assist device and medical management in ambulatory heart failure patients: results from the ROADMAP study. J Am Coll Cardiol 2015; 66(16):1747–61.

7. Starling RC, Estep JD, Horstmanshof DA, et al. Risk assessment and comparative effectiveness of left ventricular assist device and medical management in ambulatory heart failure patients: the ROADMAP study 2-year results. JACC Heart Fail 2017;5(7): 518–27.

8. Pagani FD, Aaronson KD, Kormos R, et al. The NHLBI REVIVE-IT study: understanding its discontinuation in the context of current left ventricular assist device therapy. J Heart Lung Transplant 2016; 35(11):1277–83.

9. Mehra MR, Naka Y, Uriel N, et al. A fully magnetically levitated circulatory pump for advanced heart failure. N Engl J Med 2017;376(5):440–50.

10. Gibbon JH Jr. Application of a mechanical heart and lung apparatus to cardiac surgery. Minn Med 1954; 37(3):171–85. passim.

11. DeBakey ME. Left ventricular bypass pump for cardiac assistance. Clinical experience. Am J Cardiol 1971;27(1):3–11.

12. Liotta D, Hall CW, Henly WS, et al. Prolonged assisted circulation during and after cardiac or aortic surgery. prolonged partial left ventricular bypass by means of intracorporeal circulation. Am J Cardiol 1963;12:399–405.

13. Hall CW, Liotta D, Henly WS, et al. Development of artificial intrathoracic circulatory pumps. Am J Surg 1964;108:685–92.

14. DeBakey ME. Development of mechanical heart devices. Ann Thorac Surg 2005;79(6):S2228–31.

15. Cooley DA. The total artificial heart. Nat Med 2003; 9(1):108–11.

16. Cooley DA, Liotta D, Hallman GL, et al. Orthotopic cardiac prosthesis for two-staged cardiac replacement. Am J Cardiol 1969;24(5):723–30.

17. Cooley DA, Akutsu T, Norman JC, et al. Total artificial heart in two-staged cardiac transplantation. Cardiovasc Dis 1981;8(3):305–19.

18. DeVries WC, Anderson JL, Joyce LD, et al. Clinical use of the total artificial heart. N Engl J Med 1984; 310(5):273–8.

19. DeVries WC. The permanent artificial heart. Four case reports. JAMA 1988;259(6):849–59.

20. Portner PM, Oyer PE, Pennington DG, et al. Implantable electrical left ventricular assist system: bridge to transplantation and the future. Ann Thorac Surg 1989;47(1):142–50.

21. Oyer PE, Stinson EB, Portner PM, et al. Development of a totally implantable, electrically actuated left ventricular assist system. Am J Surg 1980;140(1): 17–25.

22. Frazier OH, Delgado RM. Mechanical circulatory support for advanced heart failure: where does it stand in 2003? Circulation 2003;108(25):3064–8.

23. Frazier OH. First use of an untethered, vented electric left ventricular assist device for long-term support. Circulation 1994;89(6):2908–14.

24. Giridharan GA, Lee TJ, Ising M, et al. Miniaturization of mechanical circulatory support systems. Artif Organs 2012;36(8):731–9.

25. Rose EA, Gelijns AC, Moskowitz AJ, et al. Long-term use of a left ventricular assist device for end-stage heart failure. N Engl J Med 2001;345(20):1435–43.

26. El-Banayosy A, Arusoglu L, Morshuis M, et al. Initial human experience with the Terumo DuraHeart - a magnetically levitated centrifugal left ventricular assist system. J Heart Lung Transplant 2005;24(2):S57–8.

27. Miller LW, Pagani FD, Russell SD, et al. Use of a continuous-flow device in patients awaiting heart transplantation. N Engl J Med 2007;357(9):885–96.

28. Slaughter MS, Rogers JG, Milano CA, et al. Advanced heart failure treated with continuous-flow left ventricular assist device. N Engl J Med 2009; 361(23):2241–51.

29. Aaronson KD, Slaughter MS, Miller LW, et al. Use of an intrapericardial, continuous-flow, centrifugal pump in patients awaiting heart transplantation. Circulation 2012;125(25):3191–200.

30. Rogers JG, Pagani FD, Tatooles AJ, et al. Intrapericardial left ventricular assist device for advanced heart failure. N Engl J Med 2017;376(5):451–60.

31. Milano CA, Rogers JG, Tatooles AJ, et al. The treatment of patients with advanced heart failure ineligible for cardiac transplantation with the heartware ventricular assist device: results of the ENDURANCE supplement trial. J Heart Lung Transplant 2017; 36(4):S10.

32. Netuka I, Kvasnicka T, Kvasnicka J, et al. Evaluation of von Willebrand factor with a fully magnetically levitated centrifugal continuous-flow left ventricular assist device in advanced heart failure. J Heart Lung Transplant 2016;35(7):860–7.

33. Pennock JL, Oyer PE, Reitz BA, et al. Cardiac transplantation in perspective for the future. Survival, complications, rehabilitation, and cost. J Thorac Cardiovasc Surg 1982;83(2):168–77.

34. Cook JA, Shah KB, Quader MA, et al. The total artificial heart. J Thorac Dis 2015;7(12):2172–80.

35. Copeland JG, Smith RG, Arabia FA, et al. Cardiac replacement with a total artificial heart as a bridge to transplantation. N Engl J Med 2004;351(9): 859–67.

36. Goerlich CE, Frazier OH, Cohn WE. Previous challenges and current progress-the use of total artificial hearts in patients with end-stage heart failure. Expert Rev Cardiovasc Ther 2016;14(10):1095–8.

Continuous-Flow Device Engineering and Pump Technology

Paul C. Tang, MD, PhD*, Francis D. Pagani, MD, PhD

KEYWORDS

- Heart failure • Right ventricular failure • Mechanical circulatory support
- Left ventricular assist device • Centrifugal pump • Axial pump

KEY POINTS

- Continuous-flow rotary pumps now clinically dominate the field of mechanical circulatory support due to greater reliability, smaller size, quieter operation, and reduced incidence of adverse events.
- Continuous-flow pumps are differentiated by flow design; axial or centrifugal, and by the design of the impeller levitation.
- Flow through a continuous-flow rotary pump is proportional to pump speed and inversely proportional to the pressure difference across the inlet and outlet orifices of the pump.
- The relationship between flow and pressure or "head curve" characterizes a pump's response to changes in flow in pressure.
- Flow through a continuous-flow pump is variable due to the interactions with the contractions of the native heart. Flow is higher in systole and less in diastole.

HISTORICAL PERSPECTIVE

Despite the controversies surrounding the issues of maintaining pulsatile or nonpulsatile circulation, the field of mechanical circulatory support (MCS) has significantly evolved from the use of volume displacement pulsatile pumps to continuous-flow (CF) rotary blood pumps.[1–5] CF rotary pumps now dominate the field of MCS with nearly all left ventricular assist device (LVAD) implants in the United States representing CF rotary pump technology.[6,7] This trend has continued for both short term (ie, nonimplantable temporary devices) and implantable, durable MCS device designs.[6,8] CF rotary pumps offer several advantages over pulsatile, volume displacement pumps. These advantages include the following: (1) a smaller pump size (because of the elimination of the displacement chamber required for a pulsatile pump); (2)

fewer moving parts (limited to a single internal rotating impeller) resulting in greater durability and reliability; (3) limited blood contacting surfaces; (4) lower noise; and (5) reduced energy requirements that have translated into significantly improved clinical outcomes.[4,5] The small size of implantable CF rotary pumps has facilitated expansion of the therapy into children or patients with small body habitus[9,10] and has promoted applications including implantable durable biventricular support,[11] total artificial heart support,[12] and minimally invasive surgical approaches.[13,14]

GENERAL PUMP DESIGN

A CF rotary pump consists of blood inlet and outlet ports and a single internal rotating element, that is, rotor or impeller that is suspended within a pump housing that propels blood forward by spinning

Disclosure Statement: The authors have nothing to disclose.
Department of Cardiac Surgery, University of Michigan Frankel Cardiovascular Center, 5158 Cardiovascular Center, 1500 East Medical Center Drive, Ann Arbor, MI 48109-5864, USA
* Corresponding author.
E-mail address: tangpaul@med.umich.edu

Abbreviations	
BTT	Bridge to transplant
CF	Continuous flow
CI	Confidence interval
DT	Destination therapy
HVAD	HeartWare ventricular assist device
LV	Left ventricular
LVAD	Left ventricular assist device
MCS	Mechanical circulatory support

the impeller at high speeds, imparting significant kinetic energy to the blood that overcomes outflow resistance to the pump. The spinning of the impeller is accomplished by sequentially actuating an electrical current and creating a magnetic field that is coupled to the internal magnets within the impeller.[15,16] CF rotary pumps in clinical use today are powered by a brushless direct current motor and currently require an external power source (most often provided by rechargeable batteries or an alternating current power cord) that is transmitted to the internal pump through a percutaneous cable or driveline. In the near future, wireless energy transfer systems should eliminate the need for the percutaneous lead to power implantable pumps.[15,16]

CONTINUOUS-FLOW ROTARY PUMP DESIGN: AXIAL VERSUS CENTRIFUGAL PUMPS

There are essentially 2 types of CF rotary pumps in clinical use today: a centrifugal flow pump and axial flow pump[15,16] (**Fig. 1**). The primary difference between centrifugal flow and axial flow

pumps lies in the design of their rotating element. In a centrifugal pump, the outlet path is positioned 90° relative to the axis of rotation or centerline of the impeller, and the rotating element acts as a spinning disk with blades that capture fluid and propels the blood from impeller blades to the outflow cannula along a tangential course.[15,16] In an axial flow pump, the inlet and outlet blood paths are positioned parallel relative to the axis of rotation or centerline of the impeller, and the rotating element operates like a propeller in a pipe that pushes fluid forward. In both cases, blood exits opposite to the direction of thrust generated by the pump motor.

The rate at which a pump adds energy to a fluid is[17]

$$\dot{W} = \frac{dV}{dt} \times \Delta P = Q \times \Delta P$$

where $Q = dV/dt$ is the flow and ΔP is difference in pressure between inlet and outlet orifices of the pump. The efficiency of a pump is defined as the ratio of the useful power output to the required power input:

$$\eta_{pump} = \frac{Q \times \Delta P}{W_{input}}$$

Centrifugal devices generally have greater hydraulic efficiency at energy transfer and provide CF at rotational speeds that are much slower, approximately 2000 to 6000 rpm compared with 8000 to 15,000 rpm for pumps with axial flow designs.[15,16] Slower rotation speeds means a lower shear stress is exerted on the blood elements and that there is a lower risk of hemolysis.[18] The hydraulic efficiency, defined above as the ratio of power imparted to the fluid divided by the power

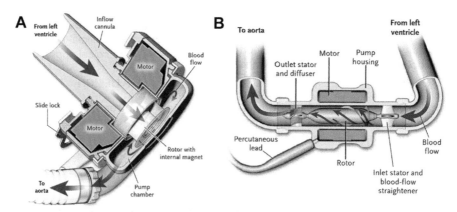

Fig. 1. (A) Diagram of a centrifugal blood pump where blood enters the pump inlet cannula along the axis of rotation or centerline of the impeller and is driven outward, tangentially to the outlet of the pump. (B) Diagram of the axial-flow pump. Blood enters at the inlet end of the rotor and is driven along the axis of rotation or centerline of the rotor to the outflow end of the pump. (*From* Mehra MR, Naka Y, Uriel N, et al. A fully magnetically levitated circulatory pump for advanced heart failure. N Eng J Med 2017;376:443; with permission.)

input to the impeller, is related to the ability of a pump to transport fluid with minimal power loss over the blood flow path. Hydraulic efficiency is an important, but not sole determinant of overall LVAD system efficiency. LVAD systems require power supplies and controllers that have unique methods of operating the pump. It is the sum of the efficiency of the motors and controllers and the hydraulic efficiency that contribute to the overall system efficiency.

BEARING DESIGN/IMPELLER SUSPENSION

CF rotary pump designs can be further distinguished by the mechanism of impeller suspension or levitation and include use of (1) mechanical bearings (**Fig. 2**); (2) hydrodynamic bearings (fluid forces); (3) hydrodynamic bearings working in synergy with magnetic suspension (**Fig. 3**); or (4) variations of active and/or passive magnetic suspension[15–19] (**Fig. 4**).

Mechanical Bearing

A mechanical pivot design or contact bearing uses mechanical bearings on spherical surfaces rotating in sockets (see **Fig. 2**). These bearings are made of ceramic components with low friction coefficient (ie, ceramic or ruby) and have long durability attributed to, in part, boundary lubrication from blood immersion.[15–20] Although

simplistic in design, a major limitation of this mechanism of impeller support is that the point of contact of the mechanical bearings is a point of friction and heat generation that represents potential sites for fibrin deposition with thrombus formation.[21] Washing of these points by blood or fluid is necessary to provide adequate dissipation of heat. In addition, the concentration of hydrodynamic loads on these bearings, especially at stress concentration points, makes these contact points theoretically susceptible to wear and fatigue.

Non-Contact-Bearing Designs

Non-contact-bearing designs incorporate either hydrodynamic or magnetic forces or a combination of both to achieve suspension of the internal impeller without the use of mechanical contact supports.[15–19] Without the need for mechanical contacts, these suspension systems do not have points of friction and theoretically have an infinite or limitless lifespan. These levitation systems must control for 6 degrees of freedom of the impeller: 3 rotational movements (rotation around "x," "y," and "z" axis) and 3 translational movements (displacement without rotation). Rotation around the axis of rotation or centerline of the pump is achieved by electromagnetic coupling of the motor stator and internal magnet of the impeller.

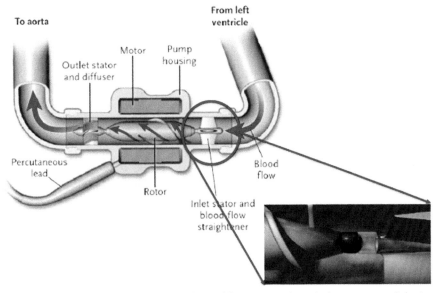

Fig. 2. A CF rotary pump (axial pump) using a mechanical bearing or pivot design to suspend the internal rotor. (*insert*) Lower left-hand corner of the figure demonstrates a "ball-and-socket" mechanical bearing design. The surfaces of the bearing are interspersed with a thin film of fluid to reduction friction and wear of the bearing. (*Adapted from* Mehra MR, Naka Y, Uriel N, et al. A fully magnetically levitated circulatory pump for advanced heart failure. N Eng J Med 2017;376:443; with permission.)

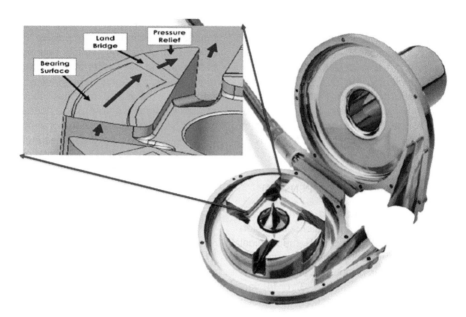

Fig. 3. A CF rotary pump (HVAD; Medtronic Inc, Minneapolis, MN) using a combination of magnetic and hydrodynamic suspension of the internal rotor. The insert in the upper left-hand corner of the picture details the hydrodynamic surface of the impeller that uses fluid forces to oppose magnetic forces generated from opposing magnets within the center post and impeller. (*Courtesy of* Medtronic Inc, Minneapolis, MN; with permission.)

Hydrodynamic Bearing

Hydrodynamic bearings use pressure generated from a fluid film that acts to separate the rotating surfaces of the impeller from the stationary base of the pump[15–19,22] (see **Fig. 4**). However, in order to generate a hydrodynamic force, the surface of the impeller must be moving. When the impeller is stationary (for example, at pump startup or stop), the impeller and stationary surfaces including the pump housing, will come into contact. Contact between these components could result in damage to the surfaces of the impeller or pump housing resulting in potential niduses for thrombus formation. Contact can also occur if rotating impeller speeds are not sufficient to

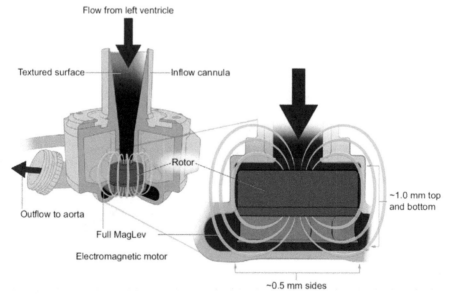

Fig. 4. A CF rotary pump with total magnetic levitation of the internal impeller. (*From* Netuka I, Sood P, Pya Y, et al. A fully magnetically levitated left ventricular assist system for treating advanced HF: a multicenter study. J Am Coll Cardiol 2015;66(23):2582; with permission.)

overcome outflow pressures resulting in impeller contact with the housing or, in the absence of contact, cause a significant decrease in the distance between impeller and pump housing, resulting in increased shear and friction of blood elements passing between impeller and pump housing. Importantly, hydrodynamic forces dissipate quickly as a function of distance; thus, this limits the distances between the stationary base (pump housing) and rotating impeller. As a result, the load-bearing fluid film is prone to higher shear stresses that theoretically can result in more damage to blood elements with hemolysis. Hydrodynamic suspension systems do not use position sensors, resulting in a less complicated electronic design that enhance the ability to miniaturize pump sizes.

Magnet Bearing

Magnetic forces may be passive without the consumption of power (permanent magnet) or active (induction of magnetic field with electricity) in design[15–19] (**Fig. 5**). Passive magnets use rare earth magnets such as neodymium boron–iron magnets within the rotor and along the housing to achieve suspension of the impeller. Permanent magnet bearings allow for a larger gap between the static motor armature and the rotor, while eliminating the need for mechanical bearings, lubrication, sealing, or purging fluid. However, the magnetic forces are dependent on the instantaneous position of the rotor (ie, magnetic forces are greater when magnets, impeller and pump housing, are at closer distances). Magnetic bearings are often used in conjunction with hydrodynamic or electromagnetic bearings. Control of any axis can be active or passive. In active mode, the repelling force is adjusted by changing the supplied current to the electromagnets based on the instantaneous position or other feedback. In a passive mode, the supplied current to the electromagnets is constant. The electromagnetic force adjusts automatically based on the position itself, that is, as the impeller approaches the magnet in the pump housing, the repelling forces increase. However, electromagnetic systems are complex, requiring position sensors, electromagnets and extra conductors, connector pins, and electronics to execute the dedicated position control algorithm. If, for example, there is an electrical contact failure in a connector pin, or momentary instability encountered in the control algorithm, pump failure can occur. To make the system failsafe, electromagnetic bearing elements frequently use hydrodynamic bearings as a fail-safe, which require no control. Distances between impeller

and pump housing maintained by magnetic fields are a function of the strength of the magnetic field, and hence, a function of the size of the magnet. Thus, overall pump size and degree of miniaturization are functions of the size of the magnet needed to maintain the desired gap between impeller and pump housing. Overall efficiencies of the pump are also determined, in part, by magnet strength. The major advantages of magnetic bearings are that distances between impeller and pump housing are generally larger and the degree of shear stresses on blood elements is less compared with mechanical contact bearings or hydrodynamic suspension systems.

HYDRODYNAMIC PERFORMANCE OF CONTINUOUS-FLOW PUMPS

Blood flow through CF pumps, both axial and centrifugal, is directly proportional to pump speed and inversely proportional to the pressure difference across the inlet (eg, left ventricular [LV] pressure) and outlet (eg, aortic pressure) orifices of the pump.[15–19] This pressure differential across the pump is referred to as the "ΔP" or "head pressure" and represents the work performed by the pump on the blood. A combination of torque and velocity allows the impeller to transfer energy to the blood and generate flow and pressure to overcome head pressure.

The relationship between ΔP and flow can be displayed in a series of curves reflecting blood flow over varying pressure gradients at differing pump speeds, that is, the pressure-flow relationship or "head curve" (see **Fig. 5**; **Fig. 6**). This relationship between ΔP and flow is unique to each CF rotary pump, analogous to an individual's fingerprint. Generally speaking, most axial flow rotary pumps in clinical use to date have been designed with steeper pressure-flow relationships compared with centrifugal flow rotary pumps, but the generalizations do not hold for every pump design. A steep relationship between ΔP and flow is often represented by an almost linear relationship. A shallow or "flat" head curve represents greater sensitivity between the pressure-flow relationship such that small changes in pressure elicit greater changes in flow with any given change in pressure.

For a CF rotary pump with a flat head curve, the same ΔP will elicit a larger change in flow during systole relative to diastole compared with a CF rotary pump with a steep head curve. There are several important advantages of a flat head curve compared with a steep head curve. The more responsive pressure-flow relationship in CF rotary pumps with a flat head curve results in a greater

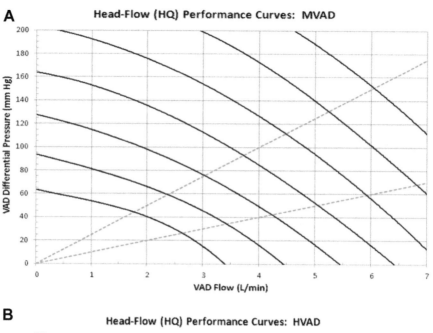

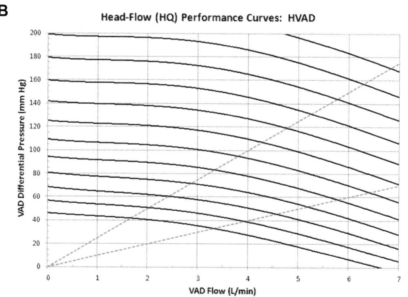

Fig. 5. (*A*) A pressure-flow relationship or "head curve" for an axial flow rotary blood pump. The relationship between pressure and flow is nearly linear and represents a blood pump with a "steep" pressure-flow relationship. Each line on the graph represents differing pump speeds. (*B*) A pressure-flow relationship or "head curve" for a centrifugal flow rotary blood pump. The relationship between pressure and flow is flat and represents a blood pump with greater sensitivity to changes in pressure. Each line on the graph represents differing pump speeds. HQ, head-flow; VAD, ventricular assist device. (*Courtesy of* Medtronic Inc, Minneapolis, MN; with permission.)

degree of flow variability across the cardiac cycle (less flow in diastole and more flow in systole). In theory, the benefits of a rotary pump with a flat head curve versus that with a steep head curve are greater aortic pulse pressure. Furthermore, because ΔP increases in settings of lower preload, flow in a rotary pump with a flat head curve will decrease substantially more than a rotary pump with a steep head curve. Thus, there is theoretically less propensity to create ventricular collapse or a "suction event" resulting from the greater drop in pump flow as LV diastolic pressures decrease. Ventricular collapse or "suction" events elicited by a CF rotary pump may cause ventricular arrhythmias or increase the propensity for thrombus formation on bearings as a result of low flow or on

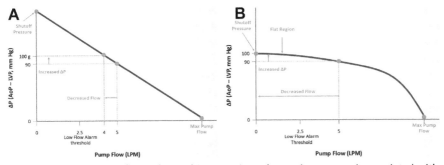

Fig. 6. (*A*) With a "steep" pressure-flow relationship, any given change in pressure is associated with a relatively small change in flow. (*B*) In a "flat" pressure-flow relationship, a small change in pressure is associated with a relatively larger change in flow. Pumps with a "flat" pressure-flow relationship are more sensitive to changes in preload and afterload conditions, and in general, impart a greater degree of pulsatility to the systemic circulation. AoP, aortic pressure; LPM, liters per minute; LVP, left ventricular pressure. (*Courtesy of* Abbott Laboratories, Chicago, IL; with permission.)

the endocardium owing to trauma or increase the risk of damage to blood elements through generation of high negative pressures.

Interaction of the Continuous-Flow Rotary Pump and Native Heart

CF rotary pumps do not generate pulsation. However, CF rotary pumps operate in conjunction with the native ventricles that influence both hemodynamics and mechanical interactions with changes in ventricular function and systemic pulsatility. Flow through a CF rotary pump is continuous throughout the cardiac cycle but has superimposed phasic changes in pump flow caused by the interaction of the heart with the CF rotary pump.[15–19] Depending on hemodynamic conditions, contractile state of the LV, pump speed, and hydrodynamic properties of the pump, flow through a CF rotary pump may be more or less pulsatile. The hydrodynamic properties of the steepness of the head curve have important effects on the flow pattern of the CF rotary pump and its interaction with the native cardiac contraction. During the cardiac cycle, pump flow is greater during native cardiac systole because the native LV contraction raises intracardiac pressure, thereby lowering the ΔP (eg, the difference between aortic and LV pressures) the pump must overcome to generate forward flow. During diastole, the difference between LV pressure and aortic pressure is increased (ie, ΔP is greater), and thus, pump flow is less relative to systole (**Fig. 7**). These phasic changes in blood flow with a CF rotary pump impart a pulse to the native circulation. The magnitude of pulse pressure typically is diminished compared with the pulse pressure that is generated with a native heart contraction or a pulsatile flow pump. The magnitude of a pulse generated with a CF rotary

pump is dependent on the relative differences in pressure changes during the cardiac cycle and contributions of the native heart to the total cardiac output. Thus, conditions that create greater LV pressure generation (ie, greater preload [Frank-Starling mechanism], inotrope therapy, native LV recovery) will create a greater pulse pressure. Under normal circumstances (ie, pump working in conjunction with the native heart contraction), the aortic flow pattern with a CF rotary pump is more accurately described as being continuous, rather than using the description of nonpulsatile flow. In circumstances in which there is absence of native heart contraction (eg, ventricular fibrillation), the flow through a CF rotary pump is nonpulsatile. Importantly, CF rotary blood pumps do not contain unidirectional valves. In circumstances wherein afterload exceeds pressure generated by the pump and or if pump speed is inadequate, backflow through the pump may occur during portions of the cardiac cycle or throughout the entire cardiac cycle.

PARALLEL AND SERIES CIRCULATION

Depending on pump design and hemodynamic conditions, CF rotary pumps can either provide full support (pump responsible for all cardiac output) or partial support (pump supplies a portion of the total cardiac output). In circumstances of full pump support, the circulation is described as in "series" (**Fig. 8**). Conversely, in circumstances of partial pump support, the circulation is described as in "parallel." The presence of series or parallel circulations can vary during support. For example, a series circulation may exist early following pump implantation, but as native LV function recovers, a parallel circulation may be created. Changes in a patient's preload caused by changes in volume status or activity could impart moment to moment

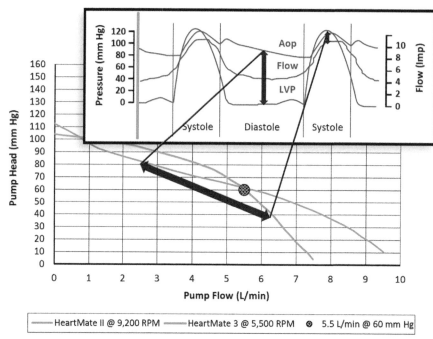

Fig. 7. Flow through a CF rotary pump varies with the cardiac cycle owing to the changes in head pressure during diastole and systole. During diastole, ΔP is greater and flow through the pump is less relative to systole, where the difference in pressure between the left ventricle and aorta is less and ΔP is smaller. This flow variation across the cardiac cycle imparts a pulse to the systemic circulation. The size of the pulse imparted to the systemic circulation is dependent on the degree of flow variation during the cardiac cycle and on contributions of the native heart to total cardiac output. The diagram shows 2 head curves, one for the HeartMate II pump (axial) and one for the HeartMate 3 pump (centrifugal). Imp, liters per minute. (*Courtesy of* Abbott Laboratories, Chicago, IL; with permission.)

cycling between series and parallel circulations (**Fig. 9**). With a series circulation, the aortic valve is continuously closed during the cardiac cycle and has been associated with development of physiologic important aortic insufficiency during pump support. Thus, there may be relative benefits of a parallel circulation compared with a series circulation.

FLOW ESTIMATION

Flow through a rotary blood pump is proportional to motor current or pump power, thus permitting motor current to be used as a sensorless index of pump flow and virtual index of LV pressure during the cardiac cycle. However, the relationship between motor current and pump flow is not linear

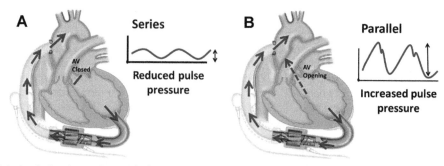

Fig. 8. (*A*) A circulation in "series" with the rotary pump. All cardiac output is delivered by the rotary pump, and there is no native LV ejection. In this circumstance, the systemic pulse pressure is significantly reduced compared with the native circulation. (*B*) A circulation in "parallel" with the rotary blood pump. In this circumstance, both rotary pump and native heart contractions contribute to total cardiac output. The systemic pulse pressure in these circumstances is generally greater owing to the contribution of the native heart ejection. AV, aortic valve.

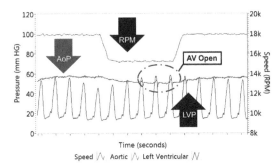

Fig. 9. Cycling between series and parallel circulations. As LV pressure exceeds aortic pressure, native ejection occurs, imparting contributions of the native heart to total cardiac output and a greater pulse pressure to the systemic circulation. Native heart ejection depends on hemodynamic conditions, preload and afterload, state of contractility of the native heart, and pump speed. (*Courtesy of* Medtronic Inc, Minneapolis, MN; with permission.)

throughout the entire range of flows, and the relationship between motor current and flow differs between axial and centrifugal pumps. In addition, the point of power measurement may differ between different pump designs. Power output for centrifugal pumps tends to be more linear in the operating range of the pump compared with axial flow pumps, particularly at low flow rates. Thus, estimation of pump flow for centrifugal pumps tends to be more accurate as compared with axial flow pumps[15–19] (**Figs. 10** and **11**). In addition, viscosity has important effects on pump flow and power, with increasing hematocrit increasing motor current at any given flow. Incorporation of the hematocrit into the flow estimation thus increases the accuracy of the flow estimate.

LIMITATIONS IN FLOW CONTROL WITH CONTINUOUS-FLOW ROTARY PUMPS

LVAD support with CF rotary pumps is associated with adverse physiologic sequelae that, in large part, represent the limitations of the current design of clinical LVADs operating in a "fixed speed" mode algorithm that causes diminished arterial pulse pressure.[23–26] Furthermore, this operating algorithm requires frequent provider interaction and assessment with clinical, echocardiographic, or right heart catheterization data to determine appropriate pump speeds necessary for clinical optimization. Changes in pump flow in CF rotary pumps can occur without changes in pump speed ("fixed speed" mode; reliance on the Starling mechanism to alter pump output) or occur as a consequence of changes in pump speed based on an algorithm-based adjustment from a

signal input (physiologic flow adjustments).[12] The absence of autonomous speed control in LVADs eliminates the potential for creating pulsatility, matching that of the normal physiologic state, or significantly hinders the ability of current LVADs to respond to widely varying changes in preload and afterload conditions. Although current clinical LVADs possess hydrodynamic properties (Starling mechanism) that permit changes in pump output to altering preload and afterload conditions, this response, under some circumstances, is not appropriate because the hydrodynamic properties of CF rotary pumps are less sensitive to changes in preload (ie, small changes in pump output relative to large changes in preload) and more sensitive to changes in afterload (ie, large changes in pump flow relative to small changes in afterload) as compared with the native heart.[27] Thus, more appropriate changes in pump output are limited without alteration of pump speed. This "uninformed" mode of speed operation limits CF rotary pumps from autonomously and appropriately responding to widely varying changes in loading conditions and precludes the following: (1) optimizing preload in the setting of increased physiologic demand; (2) maintenance of adequate pump flows in times of high afterload (ie, hypertension); (3) maintenance of adequate LV volumes in times of low preload (ie, prevention of "suction events"); and (4) appropriate flow balancing in applications with biventricular assist devices. Incorporation of physiologic pump speed adjustments based on physiologic input (eg, left atrial or LV pressure) to increase the safety of CF rotary pumps or to induce greater pulsatility to the systemic circulation has proved challenging.[23–27] Although CF rotary pumps in use today do not have speed algorithms to adjust flow to physiologic demand, systems do have speed adjustment algorithms to respond to "suction events" that use power assessments and the relationship between pump power and flow.

CURRENT DURABLE CONTINUOUS-FLOW LEFT VENTRICULAR ASSIST DEVICES
HeartMate II

The HeartMate II LVAD (Abbott, Inc, Abbott Park, IL, USA)[4,5,28–30] is a CF rotary pump with axial design and mechanical bearing support of the internal impeller. The HeartMate II was approved for bridge to transplant (BTT) therapy in 2008 and for destination therapy (DT) in 2010, following 2 pivotal safety and efficacy trials, and is the most utilized and studied LVAD pump to date. In a prospective, multicenter, controlled study of HeartMate II as BTT, 133 patients with end-stage

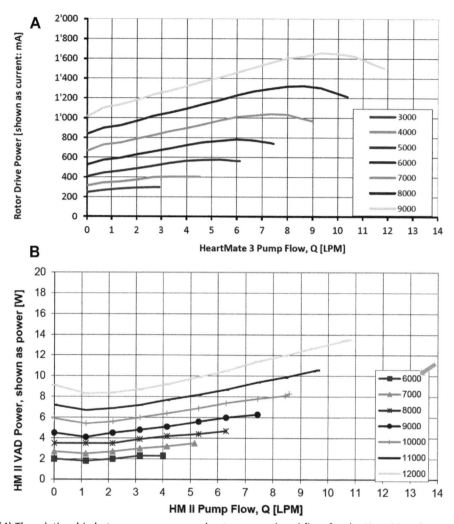

Fig. 10. (*A*) The relationship between pump power (motor current) and flow for the HeartMate 3 pump (centrifugal). The relationship between power (motor current) and flow is nearly linear over the operating range of the pump. (*B*) Diagram of the relationship between pump power and flow for the HeartMate II pump (axial). The relationship between power and flow is not as linear over the operating range of the pump as compared with the HeartMate 3 pump (centrifugal), particularly at the lower ranges of flow. (*Courtesy of* Abbott Laboratories, Chicago, IL; with permission.)

heart failure while on the waiting list for heart transplantation underwent implantation of the LVAD. Overall actuarial survival for patients continuing to receive LVAD support was 89% at 1 month, 75% at 6 months, and 68% at 12 months.[29] A follow-up report of the initial 133 patients in addition to 148 patients entered through the Continuous Access Protocol[4] reveals that at 18-month follow-up, 157 (55.8%) patients had received a heart transplant, 58 (20.6%) remained alive with ongoing LVAD support, 56 (19.9%) patients died, 7 (2.5%) patients recovered cardiac function and underwent device explantation, and 3 (1%) patients were withdrawn from the study after device explantation and exchange for another type of LVAD. Overall survival for the patients who continued on LVAD support was 82% (95% confidence interval [CI]: 77% to 87%) at 6 months, 73% (95% CI: 66% to 80%) at 1 year, and 72% (95% CI: 65% to 79%) at 18 months. The most common adverse effects were bleeding, stroke, infection, and neurocognitive dysfunction, whereas sepsis and stroke were the primary causes of mortality.

HeartMate 3

The HeartMate 3 LVAD (Abbott, Inc) is a new compact intrapericardial-positioned CF rotary pump with centrifugal design.[31] The unique feature of the HeartMate 3 is the full magnetic levitation of

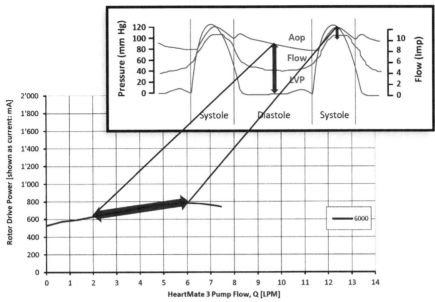

Fig. 11. Relationship between power (motor current) and flow over the operating ranges for the HeartMate 3 pump (centrifugal) is nearly linear. With correction for viscosity (hematocrit adjustment), flow estimation for the HeartMate 3 pump (centrifugal) is significantly more reliable as compared with the HeartMate II pump (axial). (*Courtesy of* Abbott Laboratories, Chicago, IL; with permission.)

the internal rotor as previous mentioned. The design differs from previous devices due to active control of rotation and levitation of the rotor that permits impellor movement further away from the outer housing, creating larger gaps for blood flow within the device. The larger gaps may reduce blood component trauma and improve biocompatibility. The HeartMate 3 is currently under clinical investigation in the United States.

Following the first-in-man implantation at Hannover Medical School in Germany, the device underwent a clinical investigation in Europe and Canada through the Conformite Europeene Mark clinical trial, which enrolled 50 patients with end-stage heart failure. The MOMENTUM 3 trials in the United States show that the HeartMate 3 LVAD is reliable with a very low rate of pump thrombosis or malfunction.[32] Indeed, the 2-year outcomes with the HeartMate 3 showed superior outcomes when compared with the HeartMate 2, which is a mechanical-bearing axial-flow pump. This improvement in outcomes was driven mainly by less need for pump exchange due to device malfunction as well as a lower overall rate of stroke. Reoperation for pump malfunction over 2 years was 1.6% in the HeartMate 3 group versus 17% in the HeartMate 2 population. Actuarial event-free survival in the intention-to-treat population was also higher in the HeartMate 3 arm (77.9% vs 56.4%, *P*<.001).[32]

Heartware Ventricular Assist Device

The Heartware Ventricular Assist Device (HVAD; Medtronic, Inc, Minneapolis, MN, USA) is a small CF rotary pump with centrifugal and non-contact-bearing design. The unique feature of the HVAD is its small design size.[33–35] It has a displacement volume of 45 cc and weighs 145 g with a flow capacity of up to 10 L/min. The device is small enough to place within the pericardial cavity without the need for dissection and creation of a pre–peritoneal pocket. The impellor of the HVAD is suspended in place by a combination of passive magnetic and hydrodynamic (ie, fluid) bearing systems.

The HVAD is approved for use in the United States for BTT and DT indication. The ADVANCE trial was a prospective, multicenter evaluation of the HVAD for BTT indication in the United States using a comparator group implanted contemporaneously with a commercially available device in the INTERMACS registry.[33,35] A total of 140 patients received the investigational pump, and 499 patients received a commercially available pump implanted contemporaneously. Success occurred in 90.7% of investigational pump patients and 90.1% of controls, establishing the noninferiority of the investigational pump (*P*<.001; 15% noninferiority margin). Kaplan-Meier survival estimates at 30, 60, 180, and 360 days were 99%, 96%,

94%, and 86% for the investigational device group and 97%, 95%, 90%, and 85% for the INTER-MACS control group.

SUMMARY

MCS with CF rotary blood pumps has demonstrated the feasibility of extended survival. Although current designs are associated with significant device-related adverse events, new technology has already overcome some of the major obstacles to date. Given the improvement in clinical outcomes with new device designs[32,36] and persistent limitations in heart transplantation as an alternative therapy, MCS with CF rotary pumps is likely to remain the dominant surgical treatment strategy for patients with advanced heart failure.

REFERENCES

1. Wesolowski SA, Fisher JH, Welch CS. Perfusion of the pulmonary circulation by nonpulsatile flow. Surgery 1953;33(3):370–5.
2. Nose Y. Is a pulsatile cardiac prosthesis a dying dinosaur? Artif Organs 1992;16(3):233–4.
3. Hindman BJ, Dexter F, Ryu KH, et al. Pulsatile versus nonpulsatile cardiopulmonary bypass. No difference in brain blood flow or metabolism at 27 degrees C. Anesthesiology 1994;80(5):1137–47.
4. Pagani FD, Miller LW, Russell SD, et al. Extended mechanical circulatory support with a continuous-flow rotary left ventricular assist device. J Am Coll Cardiol 2009;54(4):312–21.
5. Slaughter MS, Rogers JG, Milano CA, et al. Advanced heart failure treated with continuous-flow left ventricular assist device. N Engl J Med 2009;361(23):2241–51.
6. Kirklin JK, Naftel DC, Pagani FD, et al. Seventh INTERMACS annual report: 15,000 patients and counting. J Heart Lung Transplant 2015;34(12):1495–504.
7. Schumer EM, Black MC, Monreal G, et al. Left ventricular assist devices: current controversies and future directions. Eur Heart J 2016;37(46):3434–9.
8. Stretch R, Sauer CM, Yuh DD, et al. National trends in the utilization of short-term mechanical circulatory support: incidence, outcomes, and cost analysis. J Am Coll Cardiol 2014;64(14):1407–15.
9. Baldwin JT, Adachi I, Teal J, et al. Closing in on the PumpKIN trial of the Jarvik 2015 ventricular assist device. Semin Thorac Cardiovasc Surg Pediatr Card Surg Annu 2017;20:9–15.
10. Rogers JG, Pagani FD, Tatooles AJ, et al. Intrapericardial left ventricular assist device for advanced heart failure. N Engl J Med 2017;376(5):451–60.
11. Krabatsch T, Potapov E, Stepanenko A, et al. Biventricular circulatory support with two miniaturized implantable assist devices. Circulation 2011;124(11 Suppl):S179–86.
12. Strueber M, Schmitto JD, Kutschka I, et al. Placement of 2 implantable centrifugal pumps to serve as a total artificial heart after cardiectomy. J Thorac Cardiovasc Surg 2012;143(2):507–9.
13. Maltais S, Davis ME, Haglund N. Minimally invasive and alternative approaches for long-term LVAD placement: the Vanderbilt strategy. Ann Cardiothorac Surg 2014;3(6):563–9.
14. Schmitto JD, Mokashi SA, Cohn LH. Minimally-invasive valve surgery. J Am Coll Cardiol 2010;56(6):455–62.
15. Pagani FD. Continuous-flow rotary left ventricular assist devices with "3rd generation" design. Semin Thorac Cardiovasc Surg 2008;20(3):255–63.
16. Moazami N, Fukamachi K, Kobayashi M, et al. Axial and centrifugal continuous-flow rotary pumps: a translation from pump mechanics to clinical practice. J Heart Lung Transpl 2013;32(1):1–11.
17. Capoccia M. Mechanical circulatory support for advanced heart failure: are we about to witness a new "gold standard"? J Cardiovasc Dev Dis 2016;3(4) [pii:E35].
18. Bottrell S, Bennett M, Augustin S, et al. A comparison study of haemolysis production in three contemporary centrifugal pumps. Perfusion 2014;29(5):411–6.
19. Hosseinipour M, Gupta R, Bonnell M, et al. Rotary mechanical circulatory support systems. J Rehab Ass Technol Eng 2017;4:1–24.
20. Sundareswaran KS, Reichenbach SH, Masterson KB, et al. Low bearing wear in explanted HeartMate II left ventricular assist devices after chronic clinical support. ASAIO J 2013;59(1):41–5.
21. Starling RC, Moazami N, Silvestry SC, et al. Unexpected abrupt increase in left ventricular assist device thrombosis. N Engl J Med 2014;370(1):33–40.
22. Larose JA, Tamez D, Ashenuga M, et al. Design concepts and principle of operation of the HeartWare ventricular assist system. ASAIO J 2010;56(4):285–9.
23. Salamonsen RF, Mason DG, Ayre PJ. Response of rotary blood pumps to changes in preload and afterload at a fixed speed setting are unphysiological when compared with the natural heart. Artif Organs 2011;35(3):E47–53.
24. Salamonsen RF, Pellegrino V, Fraser JF, et al. Exercise studies in patients with rotary blood pumps: cause, effects, and implications for starling-like control of changes in pump flow. Artif Organs 2013;37(8):695–703.
25. Saeed O, Jermyn R, Kargoli F, et al. Blood pressure and adverse events during continuous flow left ventricular assist device support. Circ Heart Fail 2015;8(3):551–6.

26. Ising MS, Sobieski MA, Slaughter MS, et al. Feasibility of pump speed modulation for restoring vascular pulsatility with rotary blood pumps. ASAIO J 2015;61(5):526–32.

27. Tchantchaleishvili V, Luc JGY, Cohan CM, et al. Clinical implications of physiologic flow adjustment in continuous-flow left ventricular assist devices. ASAIO J 2017;63(3):241–50.

28. Jorde UP, Kushwaha SS, Tatooles AJ, et al. Results of the destination therapy post-food and drug administration approval study with a continuous flow left ventricular assist device: a prospective study using the INTERMACS registry (Interagency Registry for Mechanically Assisted Circulatory Support). J Am Coll Cardiol 2014;63(17):1751–7.

29. Miller LW, Pagani FD, Russell SD, et al. Use of a continuous-flow device in patients awaiting heart transplantation. N Engl J Med 2007;357(9): 885–96.

30. Park SJ, Milano CA, Tatooles AJ, et al. Outcomes in advanced heart failure patients with left ventricular assist devices for destination therapy. Circ Heart Fail 2012;5(2):241–8.

31. Schmitto JD, Hanke JS, Rojas SV, et al. First implantation in man of a new magnetically levitated left ventricular assist device (HeartMate III). J Heart Lung Transpl 2015;34(6):858–60.

32. Mehra MR, Goldstein DJ, Uriel N, et al. Two-year outcomes with a magnetically levitated cardiac pump in heart failure. N Engl J Med 2018;378(15):1386–95.

33. Aaronson KD, Slaughter MS, Miller LW, et al. Use of an intrapericardial, continuous-flow, centrifugal pump in patients awaiting heart transplantation. Circulation 2012;125(25):3191–200.

34. Strueber M, Larbalestier R, Jansz P, et al. Results of the post-market Registry to Evaluate the HeartWare Left Ventricular Assist System (ReVOLVE). J Heart Lung Transpl 2014;33(5):486–91.

35. Slaughter MS, Pagani FD, McGee EC, et al. HeartWare ventricular assist system for bridge to transplant: combined results of the bridge to transplant and continued access protocol trial. J Heart Lung Transpl 2013;32(7):675–83.

36. Mehra MR, Naka Y, Uriel N, et al. A fully magnetically levitated circulatory pump for advanced heart failure. N Engl J Med 2017;376(5):440–50.

Surgical Implantation of Intracorporeal Devices
Perspective and Techniques

Colleen Pietras, MD, Pavan Atluri, MD*

KEYWORDS

- Heart failure • Left ventricular assist device (LVAD) • Mechanical circulatory support (MCS)
- Surgical technique • Pump migration

KEY POINTS

- Implantation techniques for HeartMate and HeartWare devices, including open and minimally invasive approaches, are discussed.
- Methods of cannulation for pump implantation, including the option for off-pump as an alternative strategy, are also discussed.
- Pump position and driveline strategy to avoid migration and malfunction are examined.
- The importance of deairing maneuvers and proper weaning from cardiopulmonary bypass is stressed.
- Decision making with concomitant operations is considered.

The history of ventricular assist technology has evolved over the past several decades, creating a natural shift in style design and, therefore, methods and technique used for implantation. Second-generation and third-generation devices are noiseless, continuous-flow, axial, or centrifugal pumps with both improved durability and long-term survival compared with older-generation pulsatile-flow pumps. Surgical maneuvers, although surgeon specific, continue to be an important component to improving patient-reported outcomes and avoiding pump-related complications. No matter which device is implanted, following integral steps and conduct of operation has become the primary standard to care.

STERNAL ENTRY AND EXPOSURE

Among all of the devices described for implantation in the treatment of heart failure today, the 3 most common are the HeartWare HVAD (Medtronic,

Minneapolis, Minnesota) (**Fig. 1**) and the HeartMate (Abbott Laboratories, Abbott Park, Illinois) devices, HeartMate II (**Fig. 2**) and HeartMate 3 (**Fig. 3**). The steps for each implantation are similar with only slight variations. Most commonly, a standard median sternotomy is performed. The pericardium is incised and divided left of midline to several millimeters before reaching the diaphragm, where it is then squared off in either direction. The dissection on the left continues several centimeters above the phrenic nerve to expose the apex of the heart.

Due to the size and structure of the HeartMate II pump, a preperitoneal pocket is created to orient both inflow and outflow cannula in a way that not only optimizes flow but also avoids compression of either ventricle. The incision beyond the diaphragm requires gentle dissection through subcutaneous tissue staying anterior to the posterior rectus sheath. An ideal pump pocket is one in which the incision is extended 7 cm to 10 cm below the xiphoid process and deep so that it

Disclosure Statement: Dr P. Atluri is a consultant for both Abbott and Medtronic.
Division of Cardiovascular Surgery, Hospital of the University of Pennsylvania, 3400 Spruce Street, 6 Silverstein, Philadelphia, PA 19104, USA
* Corresponding author.
E-mail address: Pavan.atluri@uphs.upenn.edu

Cardiol Clin 36 (2018) 465–472
https://doi.org/10.1016/j.ccl.2018.06.012
0733-8651/18/© 2018 Elsevier Inc. All rights reserved.

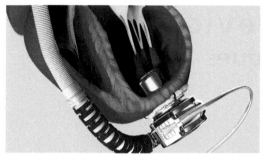

Fig. 1. HVAD. (*Courtesy of* Medtronic Inc, Minneapolis, MN.)

extends laterally under the costal arch.[1] With the lower-profile HeartMate 3 and HVAD, dissection proceeds without entry beyond the xiphoid and

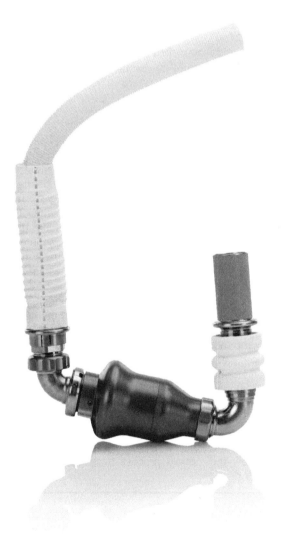

Fig. 2. HeartMate II. (*Courtesy of* Abbott Laboratories, Abbott Park, IL.)

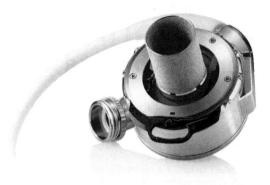

Fig. 3. HeartMate 3. (*Courtesy of* Abbott Laboratories, Abbott Park, IL.)

maintains the integrity of a closed left pleural space. In all cases, this dissection and creation of the driveline tunnel are most often performed prior to the administration of heparin.

THE DRIVELINE

Location of the percutaneous driveline is specific to a patient's anatomy and personal preference. The intention of placement is multifold: to avoid interference with pannus folds and beltlines as well as prevent line fractures and/or ascending infection. The drivelines in all 3 devices are silicone-covered cables with a portion covered in felt. The silicone covering the driveline acts to protect the cable from moisture and, when positioned appropriately, reduces complications associated with line fracture and malfunction. The velour or felt portion of the driveline allows for stability by creating an adherent effect to attach to internal surfaces and is intended to stay within the subcutaneous tissue. The silicone cover, on the other hand, is smooth and resistant to this inflammatory reaction. The recommended driveline placement is, therefore, known as a silicone-to-skin interface (**Fig. 4**). It has been described that maintaining this technique during the implantation of the HeartMate II device allows for a 50% reduction in driveline infections.[2]

Tunneling involves placement of the driveline through the rectus muscle along the anterior axillary line via a tunneling device approximately 2 cm below the costal margin on either side.[3] The driveline is passed through subcutaneous tissue, avoiding entry into the peritoneal space. It then exits through a skin incision at the predetermined location with the felt buried 1 cm to 2 cm from the exit site. An alternative scenario involves tunneling the device through the skin incision, passing through subcutaneous tissue, and entering the pericardial space 2 cm from the costal

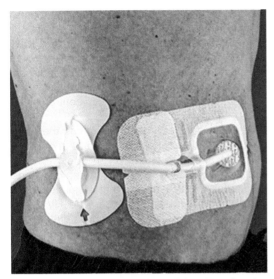

Fig. 4. Silicone-to-skin interface of driveline showing sterile technique, including anchor. (*Courtesy of Centurion Medical Products, Harleysville, PA.*)

margin, connecting the driveline to the end of the tunneling device, and pulling it back out of the incision. Ideally only 1 gentle loop of driveline (**Fig. 5**) within the pericardial space is necessary to accomplish the passage from pump to skin securing the felt out of sight. This obviates the potential for kinking, although further necessitating a more circuitous route away from midline to avoid potential contact with the sternal saw on reentry. Additional techniques have been described and include the rectus-sparing technique[4] and the

double-tunnel technique,[5] both involving a longer passage of driveline in the subcutaneous tissues of the preperitoneal space without a pericardial loop. The idea is to reduce local trauma to the rectus muscle, contain the majority of the felt coating deep within subcutaneous tissue, and reduce the potential for ascending infection to the mediastinum or pump pocket.

The keys for optimal driveline placement include allowing adequate distance between the entry and exit sites with a gentle loop of cord away from the midline. Infection risk is lowered by ensuring the entire felt covering is buried in subcutaneous tissue,[6] and the silicone portion exiting the skin is secured either internally with absorbable suture or externally with polypropylene as a purse-string suture. Whether the driveline is secured with subcuticular sutures, an external bolster, or a small red rubber bumper, the importance in establishing a consistent method of closure that is both atraumatic and tension-free should not be overlooked.

CANNULATION AND CARDIOPULMONARY BYPASS

After the administration of systemic heparin, cannulation sutures are placed in preparation for bypass. Aside from standard arterial access in the aorta, surgeon preference dictates the strategy for either dual-stage or bicaval cannulation for venous drainage. The latter is necessary in the event either mitral or tricuspid valves needs to be addressed or

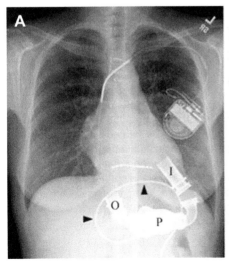
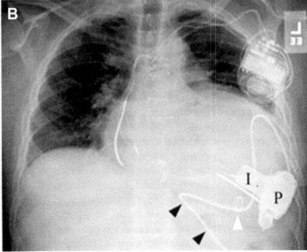

Fig. 5. Chest radiographs demonstrating proper orientation of both pumps (P), HeartMate II (*A*) and HVAD (*B*). Black arrows are the driveline and white arrow is bend relief. I, inflow; O, outflow. (*From* Amin ND, Little BP, Henry TS. Imaging of left ventricular assist devices. Curr Radiol Rep 2015;3:34; with permission; and *Courtesy of* Medtronic Inc, Minneapolis, MN; and Abbott Laboratories, Abbott Park, IL.)

a patent foramen ovale is identified and requires closure. Positioning of the aortic cannula involves leaving room for both the outflow graft and an aortic root vent. In anticipation of future reentry, pledgeted cannulation sutures and unnecessary dissection are avoided when possible.

Once on bypass, the beating heart is gently lifted and the apical dimple can be easily identified lateral to the distal left anterior descending artery. Whether the choice is made to enter here or 1 cm to 2 cm lateral to the apical dimple is guided by transesophageal echocardiogram to ensure the inflow cannula is appropriately aimed in the direction of the mitral valve.[7] Once it is marked, moist laparotomy pads are placed posteriorly and against the diaphragm to keep the apex elevated for continued visualization.

Whether a HeartMate device or HVAD is implanted, the pump is typically assembled on the back table by a trained representative. That said, the surgeon should recheck all connections at the time it is brought to the field for implantation.

INFLOW

The position of the inflow cannula is essential to the long-term success of the pump.[8] The coring device must be inserted and deployed with equal distribution of surrounding muscle to assure proper orientation of the pump once it is seated within the sewing ring. Whether the apex is cored prior to or after the placement of ring sutures is again determined by surgeon preference. In the case of the HeartMate II, however, a VICRYL, 0 suture is often placed in the center of the area marked. This suture is fed through the coring device and held with slight tension while the device is gently twisted into the apex in a perpendicular direction. Individual pledgeted vertical mattress sutures ensure adequate hemostasis around the sewing ring.

With the HeartMate 3 and HVAD, the sewing ring is held against the predetermined location on the distal anterior surface of the left ventricle, as described previously. Individual pledgeted sutures are placed deep into the myocardium, then through the sewing ring in a horizontal mattress fashion. The sutures are tied down and the ring is seated before the apical core is made. The myocardium is incised in the center of the sewing ring and the punch used to remove the core. Careful deployment of the coring device ensures a properly placed pump.[3] In all situations, the core is removed intact and the site carefully inspected so that retained muscle, crossing trabeculae, or thrombus can be removed to avoid future embolic events or pump obstruction.

The number of sutures required depends on the size of the inflow ring. The HeartMate devices typically require 12 Ethibond (Ethicon, Inc, Somerville, NJ) sutures, whereas the HVAD requires 8.[3] All methods entail full-thickness strategically placed sutures directed deep in the myocardium, avoiding unnecessary torque on the needle and misadventure into surrounding coronaries. Each careful step ensures hemostatic control at the end of the bypass run.

After the sutures are tied down and the ring is secure, the inlet cannula is inserted into the left ventricle and, depending on the device, either tied or clipped into place. Each pump has a specific point of attachment that requires appropriate positioning at this time. The HVAD, for example, has a screw that must be directed toward the base of the heart close to and parallel to the left anterior descending artery to make it assessable once the pump is in place.[3] The HeartMate 3, on the other hand, uses a specific locking mechanism, called a slide lock. The slide lock is retracted to be opened prior to inserting the pump in the left ventricle. The pump is then rotated so that the outflow graft is directed toward the right ventricle and the driveline toward midline. Once the pump position is satisfactory, the slide lock is pushed inward to engage and lock it in place. The lock is properly engaged when the yellow zone inside of the lock is no longer visible. The benefit to the slide lock is if the pump requires reorientation, a sterile surgical instrument may be used to unlock the device temporarily.

Research is now emphasizing the importance of proper positioning of the body of the device and its potential benefits in maximizing LVAD flows and reducing adverse events such as right heart failure and pump thrombosis. Studies have shown that ideal placement of the inflow cannula of the HeartMate II is parallel to the apical portion of the interventricular septum at an angle approximately 15° to 30° from the vertical axis.[9] The body of the pump, on the other hand, should be perpendicular to the spine as well as inferior to and parallel with the acute margin of the right ventricle. The elbow of the pump may be fixated with suture around the diaphragm or an adjacent rib to avoid malposition and subsequent obstruction of flow from the left ventricle. Understanding that the pump pocket may contract over time[3] emphasizes the importance of a deep pocket with lateral extension under the costal margin.

OUTFLOW

With each device, the outflow cannula is sized so that it is neither too long to cause kinking nor too short to avoid tension on the outflow anastomosis.

Torsion or twisting of the outflow graft has been described both in the early and late postoperative periods.[10] Aside from varying implantation techniques, possible explanations include abrupt changes in flow characteristics or that over time, cardiac pulsation may be associated with shift or rotation of the cannula. Oversizing the outflow cannula may additionally cause compression on the inferior vena cava. A shorter outflow cannula would shift across the midline not only causing compression of the right ventricle but also creating a potential challenge in anticipation of sternal reentry. Ideally, the cannula is positioned along the right atrial gutter, in the atrioventricular groove, taking a gentle curve around the acute margin. This can be estimated by partial filling of the left ventricle to expand the graft. The outflow graft should be stretched prior to cutting to assess the appropriate length. Once size is determined, the graft is occluded with a vascular clamp and the left ventricle is emptied in anticipation of completing its connection with the aorta.

Using a partial occluding clamp, the aortic anastomosis is sewn with either a 4-0 or a 5-0 polypropylene suture in a running fashion into a beveled graft starting at the heel. The ideal site is distal to the sinotubular junction on the lateral aspect of the greater curvature of the proximal ascending aorta.[11] Once the clamp is in place, an aortotomy is made with a scalpel and extended with the punch device. It is important to first palpate the aorta to avoid entry into a calcified plaque. The incision should be wide enough to accommodate the appropriate cannula (14-mm Vascutek Gelweave graft (VASCUTEK-TERUMO, Inchinnan, Scotland, UK) for HeartMate II/3 and 10-mm Vascutek Gelweave graft for HVAD) to prevent narrowing of the anastomosis and to allow for clear visualization of the back wall for strategically placed sutures. Once the anastomosis is complete, the vascular clamp on the outflow graft is temporarily removed to purge air from the system then reapplied. Depending on which pump is being inserted, the connection to it may already be in place. With the HeartMate II device, the outflow connector is now engaged and tightened while the left ventricle is partially full. This maneuver allows air to escape before completing the circuit. This is also the time to reassess the inflow anastomosis, hemostasis around the ring, and the direction of the inflow cannula. The outflow connector, or bend relief, if not properly brought together, may become partially or fully disconnected. This complication is surprisingly common in older devices and has been identified after symptoms of hemolysis or heart failure.[10] These cases require continued radiologic surveillance and often surgical revision.

DEAIRING AND WEANING FROM CARDIOPULMONARY BYPASS

Other than partial filling of the left ventricle and systematically removing air from the pump and outflow graft prior to its connection, there are several additional strategies that are used to accomplish deairing of the system. An aortic root vent is often used and is placed distal to the inflow anastomosis. A needle may also be inserted in the outflow graft at its highest point proximal to the vascular clamp prior to and during its removal. Flooding the field with saline or carbon dioxide is also used in some circumstances. The purpose of these maneuvers is to avoid catastrophic air embolization. Therefore, deairing and making the transition from cardiopulmonary bypass to ventricular device support becomes one of the most important stages in this operation.[12]

Air removal is a continuous process that involves visual inspection of the right ventricle while observing overall hemodynamics on transesophageal echocardiogram. Typically, there is foresight involved in whether inotropic and vasopressor support as well as pulmonary vasodilator therapy is required. When contemplating weaning from bypass, ideally heart rhythm is regular, core body temperature is over 36°C, pleural spaces are empty, and there is no evidence of surgical bleeding. The patient is placed in the Trendelenburg position and ventilation is resumed. The driveline is now connected to the pump controller. Weaning from bypass should be a slow process starting with minimal support from the implanted pump. Each pump is started at its lowest speed while the clamp from the outflow graft is removed. As bypass is weaned, ventricular assist speed is increased. Adjustments to speed are made accordingly. Transesophageal echocardiography can vitally assist in maintaining optimal volume in the heart while coming off bypass, while monitoring for residual air that may be present. Once this is confirmed by echocardiogram, the aortic root vent may be removed.

In all scenarios encountered, necessary factors to observe when coming off bypass include overall rhythm and hemodynamics, position of the inflow cannula, device flow obtained, septal wall position and potential bowing of the interventricular septum (to the right or left), whether or not the aortic valve is opened or closed, and if there is insufficiency of the mitral or tricuspid valves.[7] Identifying any of these factors in extremis entails reinitiation of cardiopulmonary bypass and either repositioning the pump or having to cross-clamp the aorta to open the heart to repair or replace one or more of the valves.

Intraoperative aortic insufficiency greater than mild is managed with either suture closure of the aortic valve or bioprosthetic aortic valve replacement.[13] An existing mechanical aortic valve is also managed with the latter because both circumstances are considered relative contraindications to VAD implantation. With moderate to severe aortic valve disease that yields chronic progressive enlargement of the left ventricle, it is recommended that the valve either be replaced with a bioprosthesis or the patient's status be upgraded on the transplant list.[14] Percutaneous aortic valve replacement may also be considered as an option.

Even though it is generally agreed on that mitral valve disease is associated with poor left ventricular assist device (LVAD) function, surgical management of the mitral valve at the time of ventricular assist device (VAD) implantation remains controversial. Pulmonary edema may be the result of significant mitral insufficiency, whereas stenosis of the mitral valve leads to right heart failure via elevated left atrial pressures and increased pulmonary vascular resistance.[15] There are few data available regarding the outcomes pertaining to mitral valve repair versus replacement at the time of VAD implantation. Literature supports an increased trend in long-term survival when the mitral valve was addressed in patients receiving their VAD for destination therapy,[15] specifically in the setting of moderate to severe insufficiency.

Surgical approaches vary from mitral valve repair (Alfieri stitch and annuloplasty ring) or replacement with either a bioprosthetic or mechanical valve. Although prior mechanical mitral prosthesis is not an absolute contraindication to LVAD implantation, increased risks include thromboembolism and adverse effects of anticoagulation. One study revealed that mortality after VAD implantation improved when the mitral valve was left alone and that the device alone contributed to improvement in mitral insufficiency.[15] The VAD is responsible for unloading the left ventricle, reducing effective volume, and contributing to leaflet coaptation.

Although there may be no benefit in addressing the mitral valve in regards to mortality, there may be value in abating symptoms and in improving quality of life.[16,17] Even with findings detailing an improvement in postoperative readmission rate after concomitant mitral valve repair,[15] surgical recommendations and technique regarding the management of mitral and tricuspid valve disease continue to be institution specific. Moderate to severe tricuspid regurgitation is most commonly treated with tricuspid valvuloplasty,[18] although replacement has been found to have a comparable long-term outcome.[19]

DECANNULATION

Once a patient has been declared hemodynamically stable with satisfactory flows from the device and surgical bleeding has been ruled out, protamine is given, and the cannulas are removed. Reinforcement of the aortic and venous cannulation sutures often includes pericardial instead of felt pledgets. It is important to remain cognizant of the future possibility of reentry at the time of transplantation.[20] This may involve inserting a GORE-TEX (W.L.Gore & Associates, Inc, Flagstaff, AZ) patch over the pump, the outflow cannula, and/or bend relief. After satisfactory hemostasis, mediastinal and pleural chest tubes are placed paying particular attention to adequate drainage around the pump and, if necessary, the pump pocket. Once the tubes are brought out of the sternum and secured to the skin, the sternum is closed with wires and the sternal incision is closed in layers of Vicryl and monocryl suture.

Dry, sterile dressings are then placed over the mediastinal incision and the chest tube incisions, and the driveline and should be occlusive and include an anchor to prevent strain on the device. Depending on the institution, dressing changes around the driveline may be protocolized but ideally include swabbing with ChloraPrep (2% chlorhexidine gluconate [CHG] and 70% isopropyl alcohol [IPA]) (Becton Dickinson and Company, Franklin Lakes, NJ), addition of a bacteriostatic silver gauze dressing, and an adhesive Foley catheter securement device, such as an anchor.[6]

ALTERNATIVE STRATEGIES

With the evolution of smaller continuous-flow devices and increasing number of high-risk surgical candidates comes the propensity for smaller incisions, less invasive procedures, and shorter operative times. The range of strategy includes ministernotomy, thoracotomy, and beating heart versus off-pump technique. These are specific not only to primary LVAD implantation but also to device exchange. The decision begins with preoperative assessment, that is, pulmonary function test (to assess lung volumes and recovery capacity), transthoracic and/or transesophageal echocardiogram (for knowledge of chamber size, valvular abnormalities, and presence of a patent foramen ovale), noncontrast chest CT (to assess relevant anatomy and the presence of aortic calcifications), angiography (in the presence of coronary disease or assessment of existing graft patency), and vascular ultrasound (to determine extent of peripheral arterial disease).

The preoperative work-up assists in stratifying patients according to their ability to tolerate a minimally invasive approach. In review of one center's experience, recommendations include proceeding with standard median sternotomy if aortic insufficiency is greater than mild, tricuspid regurgitation is greater than moderate, mitral stenosis is significant, or the patient had a previous mechanical aortic valve replacement.[21] With knowledge of a preexisting left ventricular thrombus, a sternotomy with an on-pump technique allows the positioning required to clearly visualize the apex. All clinically significant patent foramen ovales should be closed either surgically or percutaneously with an Amplatzer device (AMPLATZER, St. Jude Medical Inc, St Paul, MN).

On-pump strategies are described as using either a median sternotomy or a left anterior thoracotomy for access to the left ventricle for placement of the sewing ring and an upper hemisternotomy for the outflow anastomosis. This involves preemptively tunneling not only the driveline but also the outflow graft across midline to lie alongside the right ventricle. Cannulation can be performed peripherally or directly through the hemisternotomy.

A preferred off-pump approach that has been described involves a nonfibrillatory technique, inducing periodic bradycardic arrest with rapid ventricular pacing and boluses of intravenous adenosine (30 mg) to core the apex and attach the device.[21] As discussed previously, the outflow graft is tunneled and, depending on the circumstances, the anastomosis performed using a partial cross-clamp on the ascending aorta, descending aorta, innominate,[22] or subclavian artery. The off-pump approaches may be used when aortic access is not possible. It has been speculated that there is a potential protective benefit when the majority of pericardium remains closed, protecting the right ventricle from dilation once the pump is in place.[21]

These strategies are specific to the HVAD and HeartMate 3 given the nature and profile of these pumps. When contemplating a minimally invasive implant or device exchange for the HeartMate II, although the technique may undoubtedly be more difficult, the principles are the same. The pump pocket can be created via a subxiphoid incision. The driveline is tunneled through the same incision beneath the abdominal rectus muscle prior to its closure. Proper positioning in the apex requires a left anterior thoracotomy and transesophageal echocardiography assistance. Attaching the pump, tunneling the outflow graft, and completing the appropriate anastomosis are as described previously. To avoid an unnecessary catastrophic embolic event, the importance of a systematic, complete deairing technique cannot be overemphasized.

SUMMARY

As with the change in VAD technology, there has been a logical adjustment in the methods used for implantation of these devices over time. Poor surgical technique has been associated with worse survival due to infection, pump thrombosis, or systemic embolization.[23] Although often surgeon specific, these implant strategies lead to consistency in the course of each operation. The intent is to eliminate unnecessary complications and improve overall patient survival.

REFERENCES

1. Taghavi S, Ward C, Jayarajan S, et al. Surgical technique influences HeartMate II left ventricular assist device thrombosis. Ann Thorac Surg 2013;96(4): 1259–65.
2. Dean D, Kallel F, Ewald G, et al. Reduction in driveline infection rates: results from the HeartMate II multicenter driveline silicone skin interface (SSI) registry. J Heart Lung Transplant 2015;34(6):781–9.
3. Ranjit J. Implantation of continuous-flow ventricular assist devices: technical considerations. Oper Tech Thorac Cardiovasc Surg 2012;17(2):143–53.
4. Asaki SY, McKenzie ED, Elias B, et al. Rectus-sparing technique for driveline insertion of ventricular assist device. Ann Thorac Surg 2015;100:1920–2.
5. Schibilsky D, Benk C, Haller C, et al. Double tunnel technique for the LVAD driveline: improved management regarding driveline infections. J Artif Organs 2012;15(1):44–8.
6. Cagliostro B, Levin AP, Fried J, et al. Continuous-flow left ventricular assist devices and usefulness of a standardized strategy to reduce drive-line infections. J Heart Lung Transplant 2016;35:108–14.
7. Stulak J, Abou El Ela A, Pagani F. Implantation of a durable left ventricular assist device: how I teach it. Ann Thorac Surg 2017;103:1687–92.
8. Romano M, Haft J, Pagani F. Heartware HVAD: principles and techniques for implantation. Oper Tech Thorac Cardiovasc Surg 2013;18(3):230–8.
9. Adamson RM, Mangi AA, Kormos RL, et al. Principles of HeartMate II implantation to avoid pump malposition and migration. J Card Surg 2015;30(3):296–9.
10. Gruger T, Dupleng F, Dreysse S, et al. Late postpump blood flow obstruction in a novel left ventricular assist device: the unusual case of a twisted outflow graft. J Thorac Cardiovasc Surg 2018;55(1):33–5.
11. Whitson BA. Surgical implant techniques of left ventricular assist devices: an overview of acute and durable devices. J Thorac Dis 2015;7(12):2097–101.

12. Kormos R, Miller L. Mechanical circulatory support. A companion to Braunwald's heart disease. In: Slaughter M, editor. Surgical methods for mechanical circulatory support, 11, 1st edition. Philadelphia: Elsevier Saunders; 2012. p. 141–61.

13. Smith LA, Yarboro LT, Kennedy JL. Left ventricular assist device implantation strategies and outcomes. J Thorac Dis 2015;7(12):2088–96.

14. Stepanenko A, Potapov EV, Weng Y, et al. Concomitant surgery during ventricular assist device implantation. Ann Cardiothorac Surg 2014;3(6):630–1.

15. Robertson J, Naftel D, Myers S, et al. Concomitant mitral valve procedures in patients undergoing implantation of continuous flow left ventricular assist devices: an INTERMACS database analysis. J Heart Lung Transplant 2018;37:79–88.

16. Stulak J, Tchantchaleishvili V, Haglund N, et al. Uncorrected preoperative mitral valve regurgitation is not associated with adverse outcomes after continuous-flow left ventricular assist device implantation. J Heart Lung Transplant 2015;34:718–23.

17. Kassis H, Cherukuri K, Agarwal R, et al. Significance of residual mitral regurgitation after continuous flow left ventricular assist device implantation. JACC Heart Fail 2017;5:81–8.

18. Rojas SV, Hanke JS, Haverich A, et al. Chronic ventricular assist device support: surgical innovation. Curr Opin Cardiol 2016;31(3):308–12.

19. Deo S, Hasin T, Altarabsheh S, et al. Concomitant tricuspid valve repair or replacement during left ventricular assist device implant demonstrates comparable outcomes in the long term. J Card Surg 2012;27:760–6.

20. Gallo M, Trivedi J, Sobieski M, et al. Surgical technique for ventricular device exchange: from HeartMate II to HVAD. ASAIO J 2017;63:364–6.

21. Maltais S, Davis ME, Haglund N. Minimally invasive and alternative approached for long-term LVAD placement: the Vanderbilt strategy. Ann Cardiothorac Surg 2014;3(6):563–9.

22. Hanke J, Rojas S, Martens A, et al. Minimally invasive left ventricular assist device implantation with outflow graft anastomosis to the innominate artery. J Thorac Cardiovasc Surg 2015;149: 69–70.

23. Kilic A, Acker MA, Atluri P. Dealing with surgical left ventricular assist device complications. J Thorac Dis 2015;7(12):2158–64.

Temporary Circulatory Support and Extracorporeal Membrane Oxygenation

Kimber Eleuteri, MSN, ACNP[a],*,
Michael Mathias Koerner, MD, PhD[b],
Douglas Horstmanshof, MD[c], Aly El Banayosy, MD[c]

KEYWORDS

- Cardiogenic shock • Temporary mechanical circulatory support • ECMO • V-A ECMO
- Decompensated heart failure • Acute on chronic heart failure

KEY POINTS

- The treatment of cardiogenic shock continues to plague providers, with high mortality rates and complex clinical presentations, making it challenging to successfully intervene.
- Temporary mechanical circulatory support should be considered early in the progression of cardiogenic shock and deployed quickly to improve patient outcomes and mortality.
- Veno-arterial extracorporeal membrane oxygenation is a viable form of temporary mechanical circulatory support and can provide systemic support and improved end-organ function.

INTRODUCTION

Despite significant advances in medical care, the prognosis for patients with refractory cardiogenic shock (CS) remains grim. High mortality rates, especially in those with an underlying diagnosis of acute on chronic heart failure, continue to plague providers when attempting to intervene and treat this acutely ill cohort of patients. CS is the most severe form of acute heart failure, causing a low cardiac output state and launching a cascade of symptoms, including systemic hypoperfusion, end-organ failure, systemic inflammatory response, and eventually death if left untreated.[1-3] Derangements within the circulatory system as the body attempts to compensate for low blood pressure (BP) by vasoconstricting are ultimately counteracted by pathologic vasodilation, triggering systemic inflammation and circulatory dysfunction. Myocardial oxygen demand increases in the setting of drastically reduced contractile function, creating an environment of intensified wall stress and diminished coronary blood flow. Diagnostic criteria have been established for CS, and those include (1) systolic BP less than 90 mm Hg for more than 30 minutes or vasopressors required to achieve a BP greater than or equal to 90 mm Hg, (2) pulmonary congestion or elevated left ventricular (LV) filling pressures, and (3) signs of impaired end-organ perfusion, which include cold and clammy skin, oliguria, increased serum lactate, and altered mental status.[4,5] Despite earlier intervention with rapid reperfusion, revascularization,

Disclosures: K. Eleuteri is currently an employee at Medtronic with no financial conflicts of interest. The other authors have nothing to disclose.
[a] Mechanical Circulatory Support, Medtronic, 500 Old Connecticut Path, Framingham, MA 01701, USA; [b] Cardiovascular Intensive Care, Integris Baptist Medical Center, 3300 Northwest Expressway, Oklahoma City, OK 73112, USA; [c] Department of Heart Failure Cardiology, Integris Baptist Medical Center, 3300 Northwest Expressway, Oklahoma City, OK 73112, USA
* Corresponding author. 245 Simpson Road, Marlborough, MA 01752.
E-mail address: keleuteri@gmail.com

Cardiol Clin 36 (2018) 473–485
https://doi.org/10.1016/j.ccl.2018.06.002
0733-8651/18/© 2018 Elsevier Inc. All rights reserved.

inotrope and vasopressor therapy, and mechanical circulatory support, 1-year mortality rates remain high at almost 50%.[3–5] Acute myocardial infarction with associated ventricular dysfunction accounts for 50% to 80% of all CS cases, with other causes, such as myocarditis, valvular disease, drug overdose, aortic dissection, and exacerbation of chronic heart failure, contributing to this high morbidity rate.[4,6]

Noninvasive treatment strategies to help mitigate the deterioration of decompensated heart failure and the progression of CS include diuretic therapy in escalating doses, inotropes, and vasodilators. Inotropic agents are beneficial in that they have minimal vasodilatory effect and provide afterload reduction, thus improving overall cardiac output.[3] Clinically, the objective of therapy is to maintain end-organ perfusion without creating worsening ischemia or myocardial oxygen demand. Once these conventional measures have been maximized and CS continues to progress, temporary mechanical circulatory support (tMCS) therapy should be considered and initiated as early as possible.

MULTIDISCIPLINARY TEAM

Because of the wide range of therapies that a patient may require, a team-based approach tends to be optimal when managing the CS patient because each member is able to offer individual expertise for the combined effort of comprehensive care. The team may include an interventional cardiologist, a heart failure cardiologist, a cardiothoracic surgeon, an intensivist, an anesthesiologist, advanced practice clinicians including nurse practitioners and physician assistants, ICU nurses, and other clinical support staff.[3,6] This multidisciplinary team is crucial in determining timing of intervention and appropriate patient and device selection when required. Goals for the multidisciplinary team should focus on rapid identification of CS and the underlying etiology. Team-based patient management requires a primary leader, who should be a qualified cardiovascular intensivist with training in heart failure, CT surgery, or critical care. This individual's key roles include deciphering appropriateness of patient referral, triaging of the patient based on acuity, rapidly assessing end-organ function based on laboratory and diagnostic testing, and determining proper device strategy for the clinical scenario of the patient.[2,3]

MORTALITY AND PREDICTION SCORES

As the general population continues to age and the number of heart failure cases continues to rise,

more patients will require acute intervention for decompensated heart failure and refractory CS. Scoring systems may be helpful at predicting mortality rates and outcomes as well as stratifying patient level of shock to determine the level of therapy required. Much like other risk-predicting scores for disease severity and organ dysfunction in critically ill patients, such as acute physiology and chronic health evaluation (APACHE), simplified acute physiology score (SAPS), multiple organ dysfunction score (MODS) and sequential organ failure assessment (SOFA) scores, studies, such as the CardShock and survival after veno-arterial ECMO registry, attempt to classify patient levels of shock using a scoring system to predict outcomes and mortality risk.[7–10]

TEMPORARY MECHANICAL CIRCULATORY SUPPORT

The application of a tMCS device provides time to determine whether the patient has the potential for improvement and recovery from the inciting event, or whether they will require additional support in the form of durable MCS or cardiac transplantation.[8–11] Much like the rapidly evolving field of durable MCS, tMCS technology has allowed for expanded application in more critical situations warranting short-term hemodynamic support and end-organ perfusion. The ease of application and cannulation, as well as the ability to place percutaneously at the patient bedside, has helped usher in the use of these devices in the acute care setting.[5,9–11] More contemporaneous percutaneous MCS devices have greatly reduced the time between decision for use and actual application compared with earlier, pulsatile predecessors. The Clinical Expert Consensus Statement on the Use of Percutaneous Mechanical Circulatory Support Devices Study in 2015[12] confirmed that the use of percutaneous MCS devices was superior to medical management alone and should be considered when managing patients with refractory CS. National trends on the use of tMCS from 2007 to 2011 have shown an overwhelming growth rate of 1511%.[10,11,13,14]

The decision to use a tMCS device must be made quickly and thoroughly in the setting of acute CS, ultimately avoiding the sequala of circulatory collapse, inflammatory activation, and end-organ failure. Recognizing the severity and degree of CS and proactively determining short-term and long-term goals of tMCS will help establish what type of device is most suitable for the specific patient scenario, because there are multiple devices that offer a wide range of hemodynamic support. Devices range from limited cardiac output augmentation with the intra-aortic balloon pump

(IABP), to full systemic support with extracorporeal membrane oxygenation (ECMO), with each type of device having distinct benefits and disadvantages.[3,11,15] Factors to consider for safe and effective device selection include (1) the ability and expertise of the practitioner, (2) the availability of a tMCS device at an institution, (3) the presence of an experienced team to manage the tMCS patient, (4) the resources available to maintain the tMCS patient in the ICU, (5) a positive risk/benefit ratio for the use of the device, and (6) a device that must be economical and cost effective. Despite the ease of applicability and the cost effectiveness of tMCS devices, there are some contraindications that are ubiquitous and should be considered when treatment decisions are established (**Table 1**).

Over the past decade as continuous-flow MCS devices evolved, it became clear that postoperative adverse event rates and complications were too high to justify the routine implantation of costly durable devices in the sickest patients, specifically Interagency Registry for Mechanically Assisted Circulatory Support (INTERMACS) Profile 1 patients. More recently, a shift has occurred that places greater emphasis on the use of tMCS devices for sicker, INTERMACS 1 patients and favors the implantation of durable VADs in less acutely ill patients.[16] All commercially available devices help to restore cardiac output and BP to some extent, so it is important to determine the degree of hemodynamic *support* required.[9] Percutaneous MCS devices, discussed later, allow for rapid deployment, immediate hemodynamic stability, and improvement in end-organ circulation. Early and prompt use of tMCS has been shown to yield drastically better survival outcomes as opposed to delaying MCS treatment in lieu of other less-invasive maneuvers.[16–19]

SHORT-TERM PERCUTANEOUS MECHANICAL CARDIOGENIC SHOCK DEVICES
Intra-aortic Balloon Pump

The IABP is the most widely used form of temporary, percutaneous MCS, and accounts for more than 50,000 implants annually.[5,8,17,19,20] The goal of this therapy is to assist with coronary artery perfusion by means of counterpulsation during diastole. The balloon is rapidly inflated during diastole and rapidly deflated immediately prior to systole, reducing LV afterload. The IABP console provides helium, which inflates the polyethylene balloon that is at the end of a peripherally inserted, 7.5F to 8.0F catheter. Helium, due to its low viscosity, can be shuttled back and forth quickly, and, in the case of balloon rupture, can be absorbed rapidly into the bloodstream. It can be easily inserted via the femoral artery and initiated quickly. Although, because of the need to keep the lower extremity immobile during use, some practitioners opt to insert the IABP via the axillary or subclavian arteries, allowing the patient to ambulate when supported for longer periods of time.[14,15,19–22]

Timing of the inflation and deflation is synchronized with the cardiac cycle. It can be triggered by ECG or arterial pressure waveform. Because the IABP only offers modest cardiac output support (0.5–1 L/min), and demonstrated no substantial improvement in survival outcomes at 30 days in the Intra-Aortic Balloon Couterpulsation in Acute Myocardial Infarction Complicated by Cardiogenic Shock II trial, the recommendations for its use in CS patients was downgraded from a class I to a class III device by the European Society of Cardiology, and a class IIa by the American Heart Association and American College of Cardiology.[6,11,13,23,24] Despite that IABP therapy has little impact on mortality in the CS cohort of patients after acute myocardial infarction, it may be beneficial as a bridge to more advanced therapies.

Impella Device Platform

The Impella devices (Abiomed, Danvers, Massachusetts) are small, axial flow pumps that can be inserted peripherally, and deployed across the aortic valve into the LV. LV support by Impella

Table 1
Contraindications of temporary mechanical circulatory support

Relative Contraindications	Absolute Contraindications
1. Advanced age	1. Nonrecoverable neurologic disease or injury
2. Peripheral vascular disease	2. Systemic malignancy with life expectancy <2 y
3. Inability to take or receive anticoagulation	3. Nonrecoverable CS patients who are not candidates for durable MCS or cardiac transplantation
4. Mechanical heart valves	4. Noncardiac disease with a known high mortality rate
5. Severe aortic insufficiency	5. Aortic dissection

Data from Gilotra NA, Stevens GR. Temporary mechanical circulatory support: a review of the options, indications, and outcomes. Clin Med Insights Cardiol 2015;8(Suppl 1):75–85.

devices include the Impella 2.5, the Impella Cardiac Power (Impella CP or Impella 3.5), and the Impella 5.0. These nonpulsatile micropumps propel blood from the LV into the ascending aorta using the Archimedes screw principle, which is the rotation of a small, rotating screw-shaped surface inside a small, hollow tube that crosses the aortic valve.[11,20,22,24,25] The tip of the Impella is a pigtail that provides stabilization of the device in the LV and is placed via the femoral artery so that the inlet resides in the LV and the outlet rests in the ascending aorta. The pump, which is connected to the console, allows for pressure monitoring and can be adjusted based on the desired degree of hemodynamic support. All devices are preload dependent and are able to provide optimal LV unloading. One benefit of the use of the 5.0 is that it can be inserted via the axillary artery, which allows the patient to be mobile and ambulate while on therapy.[1,20–22,25] None of these peripheral devices can be placed or initiated at the patient bedside and must be inserted in a cardiac catheterization laboratory or hybrid suite under fluoroscopic guidance (**Table 2**). Echocardiographic visualization is also helpful for confirming the position of the catheter which is important to help decrease the risk of malposition or migration. Some of the more apparent advantages of the Impella devices are peripheral insertion, direct ventricular decompression, duration of support up to 21 days, and ability to support mobile patients with an axillary or central cannulation scenario. Disadvantages of this therapy are immobilization of patient with femoral cannulation, costly therapy, hemolysis concerns, catheter migration with frequent need for reimaging and repositioning, and no pulmonary support.[23–25] Seeking confirmation of the benefit of the Impella 2.5 for the treatment of post-MI patients with CS, the Impella-EUROSHOCK registry was established. Results showed an improvement in overall end-organ perfusion; however, it failed to show any benefit or impact on survival rates, with a 30-day mortality of 64.2%.[23,25]

The newest Impella device, the Impella RP (Abiomed) offers right ventricular (RV) support in the setting of RV dysfunction and failure. It is the first percutaneous pump designed for right heart support and can provide up to 14 days of support in both adult and pediatric patients with a body surface area of greater than or equal to 1.5 m^2 per manufacturer guidelines. The Impella RP is designed to provide up to 4 L/min of right heart support, with the inlet resting in the right atrium and the outlet sitting in the main pulmonary artery. It is beneficial at providing right heart support in the setting of acute right heart failure and can be applied immediately after durable LV assist device (LVAD) implant, post-MI, heart transplant, or cardiac surgery.[19,23,26]

There are currently no peer-reviewed studies that address Impella weaning. A brief description for a weaning procedure can be found in the manufacturer guidelines.

Tandem Heart

The TandemHeart (Cardiac Assist, Pittsburgh, Pennsylvania) is an extracorporeal, centrifugal, continuous-flow pump, which pulls blood from the left atrium (LA) and returns it to the femoral artery. The 21F inflow cannula is inserted via the femoral vein and advanced into the LA via a transseptal puncture and contains 14 side holes and a large end hole that helps to facilitate the aspiration of blood from the LA back to the pump. The outflow cannula is typically 15F to 19F and is placed in the femoral artery. The circuit is then connected to an extracorporeal pump.[6,9,14,19,22] The pump has a hydrodynamic bearing that allows for the levitation of the spinning impeller, which spins at speeds of 3000 rpm to 7500 rpm. It requires a continuous heparin infusion to provide cooling and lubrication, which helps to stave off thrombus formation.[6,11,14] An external console or driver controls the pump. Both the native heart and pump work together providing a combined blood flow to the aorta. The procedure must be performed in the cardiac catheterization laboratory by a skilled and experienced practitioner. The TandemHeart helps improve cardiac output and BP by decreasing afterload and preload, effectively reducing LV end-diastolic pressure (LVEDP) and providing optimal LV unloading.[1,10,11] One of the unique benefits of the TandemHeart is that it bypasses the LV, so there is no concern for mechanical aortic valve or LV thrombus. It also has the advantage of providing biventricular or isolated RV support with newer technology.

Careful attention and monitoring must be performed to assure that the catheter does not migrate, because dislodgement can cause severe systemic deterioration, acute tamponade, and device malfunction, thus necessitating complete immobility to avoid such devastating events.[11]

Similar to the Impella device, there are currently no peer-reviewed studies that address weaning specifics for the TandemHeart. Some references for the procedure can be found in manufacturer guidelines.

Table 2
Comparison of contemporaneous percutaneous mechanical circulatory support devices

	Intra-aortic Balloon Pump	Impella 2.5	Impella CP	Impella 5.0	TandemHeart	Veno-arterial Extracorporeal Membrane Oxygenation
Flow rates (L/min)	Max 0.5–1	Max 2.5	Intermediate support: 3.7–4.0	Max 5.0	Max 4.0–5.0	Max 7.0 or full systemic support
Physiologic and hemodynamic impact	Augmentation of cardiac output and coronary artery perfusion, improvement in LV stroke volume and BP, reduction of LVEDP	LV unloading/reduction of LVEDP, improved cardiac output, improved blood BP. Can help with LV unloading when used with V-A ECMO	Reduction of LVEDP, LV unloading, improvement of CO and BP	Reduction of LVEDP, improvement in end-organ function, improvement of CO and BP	LV unloading/reduction of LVEDP, improvement of CO and BP, improved tissue and end-organ perfusion	Biventricular support, rapid restoration of circulation, gas exchange improvement
Degree of hemodynamic support	Low	Moderate	Moderate	High	High	High
Pump speed (rpm)	Balloon inflation: intrinsic heart rate	Max 51,000	Max 51,000	Max 33,000	Max 7500	Max 5000
Pump design	Pneumatic	Axial flow	Axial flow	Axial flow	Centrifugal	Centrifugal

(continued on next page)

Table 2
(continued)

	Intra-aortic Balloon Pump	Impella 2.5	Impella CP	Impella 5.0	TandemHeart	Veno-arterial Extracorporeal Membrane Oxygenation
Cannula size	7F–8F	12–13F	14F	21F	15F–19F (arterial) 21F (venous)	15F–21F (arterial) 17F–25F (venous)
Insertion/placement	Percutaneous (femoral artery). Can also be inserted via axillary or subclavian	Percutaneous (femoral artery)	Percutaneous (femoral artery)	Peripheral surgical cutdown (femoral or axillary artery)	Percutaneous (femoral artery + femoral vein for LA cannula)	Percutaneous (femoral artery and vein) or central cannulation
Time to initiation	Very low	Low	Low	High, with axillary cut down and graft	High	Moderate
Ability to cannulate at bedside?	Yes	No	No	No	No	Yes
Ability to be mobile?	Yes, for axillary and subclavian approaches	No	No	Yes, if axillary approach	No	Yes, if centrally cannulated. Some anecdotal reports of mobilization with peripheral inserted ECMO
Cost	Low	Medium	Medium	High	High	Low

Abbreviations: CO, cardiac output; Max, maximum.
Data from Refs.[4,12,14,21]

Extracorporeal Membrane Oxygenation

The management of patients with severe CS has been revolutionized by the introduction of ECMO, which provides short-term support to patients with end-organ dysfunction secondary to acute systemic hypoperfusion. ECMO is an extracorporeal device that is comprised of a continuous-flow, centrifugal pump and membrane oxygenator to assist with carbon dioxide extraction and oxygenation. This is achieved by removing deoxygenated, venous blood from the patient, pumping it through a membrane oxygenator and returning it via the arterial circulation system, essentially providing full cardiopulmonary support.[1,11,15,22,23] Because of the pioneering efforts of both Bartlett with pediatric respiratory failure patients and Hill,[27] using ECMO to support an adult acute respiratory distress syndrome patient almost 5 decades ago, ECMO therapy has become a mainstay for the treatment of both respiratory and cardiac failure patients.

Over the past decade, veno-arterial (V-A) ECMO has been shown a viable and effective treatment of patients suffering from refractory CS. Due to technologic improvements, such as biocoated tubing for improved hemocompatibility, magnetically levitated pumps, and low-pressure drop oxygenators, this therapy has experienced tremendous growth, with a 433% increase of use between 2006 and 2011.[28,29] Data from the Extracorporeal Life Support Organization (ELSO) 2013 registry report showed that ECMO use was increasing, and adults that had received ECMO support from 1989 to 2015 showed an all-comer survival rate of 42% to hospital discharge. Some single-center observations have reported up to 80% survival rates after 30 days. The American Heart Association Guidelines for Cardiopulmonary Resuscitation concur that the application of ECMO for cardiac arrest or shock is appropriate, and the benefit of its use outweighs the risks associated with the therapy itself.[20,29–33] In those patients who present with refractory CS due to acute etiologies, ECMO offers the possibility of recovery, whereas in patients with a chronic HF etiology, ECMO is considered a bridge to bridge (to another durable device) or a bridge to transplant. Current clinical guidelines from the European Society of Cardiology recommend consideration of ECMO use in patients with CS as a bridge to stabilization until hemodynamic parameters are normalized. The concept of bridge to decision, as well as the ability to rapidly deploy the therapy, has helped ECMO to become a mainstay of CS support.[29] Other positive features of ECMO therapy include the ability to cannulate peripherally, ease of insertion at the bedside, and its portability.

Choosing to place a critically ill patient on V-A ECMO for CS is a multifactorial decision that must be made thoroughly and promptly, while considering any relative or absolute contraindications (see **Table 1**). Among many of the known mortality predictors for critically ill patients, SOFA score has been used successfully to predict mortality of CS patients supported on V-A ECMO, with lower scores demonstrating better survival rates.[34] The lack of data evaluating survival scores necessitates more prospective studies to confirm the success of their utility in predicting outcomes of this critically ill patient population. Most recently, the ExtraCorporeal Membrane Oxygenation in the Therapy of Cardiogenic Shock trial was initiated to study the timing impact of the application of V-A ECMO and whether independent application of ECMO versus adjunct therapy was superior when treating CS patients. This is a multicenter, randomized, prospective trial that started enrolling patients in 2014 with expected final patient follow-up in 2019.[29]

The Extracorporeal Membrane Oxygenation Circuit and Application

The size of the arterial cannula in V-A ECMO dictates the degree of circulatory support delivered to the patient, allowing for more flow with a larger cannula. The 2015 ELSO guidelines recommend the use of precannulation echocardiogram to evaluate both the left and the right ventricles and exclude other reasons for shock, such as severe aortic regurgitation and massive pulmonary embolism. A precannulation ultrasound of the vessels helps determine vessel diameter as well as confirm the common femoral artery above the bifurcation to avoid cannulating the profunda.[35,36] Real-time ultrasound also helps confirm proper placement of the distal perfusion catheter, assuring that it is in the superficial femoral artery and not in the deep femoral artery, where leg ischemia would most likely ensue.

The ECMO system includes a centrifugal pump, a circuit of arterial and venous tubing, a membrane oxygenator, and an oxygen air blender. Use of newer ECMO technology allows for a shorter and simplified circuit, without any connectors or bridges, minimizing the amount of interface between artificial material and blood.[33,35] Coated circuit tubing helps to improve biocompatibility, thus lowering the risk of platelet and fibrin deposition. Membrane oxygenators are used to promote O_2 and CO_2 exchange and have a blood and gas phase separated by a membrane. There are 3 types of oxygenators: (1) silicone membrane, (2) microporous hollow fiber (typically used in cardiopulmonary bypass), and (3) polymethylpentene hollow-fiber membranes. Polymethylpentene oxygenators are highly efficient, tend to last longer, are low-pressure drop, and have lower rates of thrombus formation, leakage, and hemolysis. All are designed for prolonged use, have a low priming volume (200–300 mL) and a large surface area for gas exchange (1.5–2 m^2). Oxygenators contain inflow and outflow connections for the circuit blood, the sweep gas, and water from the heating unit.[33,36–38]

The ECMO system used in the ICU is one that can be managed by ICU nursing staff and midlevel providers after extensive training and does not require perfusionist oversight. This helps with overall cost savings as well as resource management. A newer, miniaturized system, the Cardio-Help System (Maquet Getinge Group, Wayne, New Jersey) allows for ease in portability as well as providing other features, such as the ability to monitor pressure, oxygen saturation, hemoglobin, and bubble detection. Integrated sensors provide a continuous monitoring of pressures and flow rate, with the ability to individually set alarm limits to assure a high degree of safety during use. In the case of a pump failure, there is an emergency hand crank to allow for ongoing support while pump replacement is being performed. The ease of applying this system is also advantageous, because the entire circuit comes packaged in one piece and allows for easy and rapid priming.[33,34]

Established Extracorporeal Membrane Oxygenation Programs

Developing a hub-and-spoke system allows for 1 main, experienced, and staffed hospital (hub) to assist with and manage patients residing in smaller, community-based hospitals (spoke). Remote hospitals are able to initiate conventional critical care support and maintain the patient until a mobile unit can arrive, stabilize the patient with ECMO, and return them to the tertiary care center. This care delivery system allows for a larger number of critically ill patients to access management and oversight by an experienced ECMO team. As the hub provider, a 24/7, 365-day-per-year program is required, with the support of hospital administration, because it warrants a dedicated ICU bed,

specially trained staff, and available physicians to manage incoming patients for the entire process of ECMO application and transport. Successful ECMO programs should have (1) knowledgeable practitioners, (2) a multidisciplinary team, (3) specialized facilities with dedicated staff, (4) accessible equipment, (5) practice guidelines and standards of care, and (6) easily transportable equipment.[39,40]

Extracorporeal Membrane Oxygenation Patient Management

Application of V-A ECMO involves different cannulation strategies, depending on the acuity of shock and the expectation of patient recovery. Peripheral cannulation uses a femoral approach to access the right atrium via the femoral vein. For the purpose of this review, percutaneous application of V-A ECMO is discussed, with which the authors have extensive experience.

Frequent and ongoing evaluation of a patient's cardiac and respiratory status are monitored while on V-A ECMO support. Hemodynamic parameters are monitored via the Swan-Ganz catheter and arterial line and should reflect an adequate mean arterial BP greater than 60 mm Hg, a pulmonary artery wedge pressure (PCWP) of less than 22 mm Hg to 24 mm Hg, and an mixed venous oxygen saturation (Svo_2) greater than 60%.[33,35] An arterial line should be placed in the right radial artery, because this assures an acceptable level of cerebral oxygenation.[9,33,35] Ongoing laboratory work should include arterial blood gas, Svo_2, lactic acid, complete blood cell count, plasma-free hemoglobin (hemolysis marker), lactate dehydrogenase (hemolysis marker), comprehensive metabolic profile, and activated partial thromboplastin time (aPTT).[37] Anticoagulation is achieved with a continuous infusion of heparin, and aPTT levels should be evaluated every 4 hours to 6 hours, with a goal of aPTT range between 50 seconds and 60 seconds in closed ECMO circuits without bridges or connectors.[33,35] If there are ongoing bleeding issues or suspected thrombus formation, an anti-Xa level should be assessed, because this provides a direct measure of heparin activity. Some centers use Xa or TEG for monitoring anticoagulation in the ECMO patient. In cases of severe bleeding in patients supported with a simple, closed circuit without connections, it is safe to stop heparin completely.

Patients should be sedated for the initial application of ECMO support; however, sedation should be weaned as soon as possible, to allow for ongoing neurologic assessment and ability to wean from mechanical ventilation. Daily chest radiographs and echocardiography help assure that volume status is optimal, and LV unloading is adequate.[33,35] Balancing fluid administration and inotrope and vasopressor use can be challenging. Maintaining the patient in an euvolemic state, as well as maintaining adequate MAP and flows, is paramount, and requires constant vigilance for titrating and weaning. The lowest dose of vasopressor/inotropes that support an adequate MAP should be considered, because high-dose vasopressors can create diminished circulation and perfusion complications in the extremities.

Once a patient has been stabilized, and there is some indication that there is improvement in clinical status, next-step discussions should ensue and should include weaning to recovery, transitioning the patient from ECMO to a durable MCS device, or transplant. The authors describe the use of a specific protocol that screens patients that may be optimal candidates to transition to durable MCS and, in their experience, have achieved 100% survival (>6 months) in this patient cohort.

Weaning

The weaning trial should be performed when there is some indication that the patient is stabilized and has clinically acceptable return of cardiac and end-organ function. Daily transthoracic echocardiograms (TTEs) or transesophageal echocardiogram (TEE) should be performed to monitor the LV function trend and RV contractility in conjunction with hemodynamic readings.

Criteria for patient weaning from full ECMO support (ramp-down)

- Inotropes at the lowest level
- Euvolemia
- Acceptable return of cardiac function (ejection fraction >25%)
- Svo_2 greater than 60%
- Signs of end-organ recovery (liver and kidney function trending to baseline)
- PCWP $\leq$20 mm Hg
- Normal lactate levels
- Fraction of inspired oxygen $\leq$50% in intubated patients
- Optimal heart rate and rhythm

ECMO weaning protocol[33]

1. TTE or TEE as well as full hemodynamic measurements should be performed with full ECMO support (100%)
2. Drop ECMO support/flow to 75% from baseline
3. Again, obtain TEE or TTE and hemodynamic measurements after 3 minutes
4. If the patient remains hemodynamically stable as evidenced by
   a. MAP greater than 60 mm Hg
   b. PCWP less than 20 mm Hg
   c. Svo_2 greater than 55%
   d. Central venous pressure less than 15 mm Hg
   e. Heart rate remains below 120 bpm
5. Then, drop ECMO support to 50% from baseline
6. Repeat TTE/TEE and hemodynamic measurements after 3 minutes
7. If the patient remains stable as described above, drop ECMO to 25% from baseline
8. Repeat TTE/TEE and hemodynamic measurements after 3 minutes
9. If the patient remains stable, administer 2500 U to 5000 U heparin, and completely clamp the ECMO circuit for 3 minutes
10. Repeat TTE/TEE and hemodynamic measurements including thermodilution and Fick cardiac output
11. Patients are deemed weanable if they meet the following criteria:
    a. No sign of volume overload
    b. Minimal inotropic support
    c. LVEF greater than 25%
    d. CI $\geq$2.4 L/min/m2
    e. MAP $\geq$65 mm Hg
    f. PCWP less than 18 mm Hg
    g. Central venous pressure less than 15 mm Hg

COMPLICATIONS

Complications remain common in the V-A ECMO–supported patient. Both patient illness and duration of ECMO support place an already critically ill patient at risk for developing subsequent serious complications.[40,41] It can be difficult to attribute whether the overall complication rates are related to the severity of the disease state inherent in patients requiring ECMO or whether it is related to the ECMO therapy itself. It can be assumed that complications that are more mechanical in nature, such as lower extremity ischemia or compartment syndrome requiring fasciotomy or amputation, are related to the actual application of ECMO, where other, more general clinical features of CS, such as acute renal failure and neurologic complications, can be attributed to the underlying CS.[42]

One of the biggest concerns with V-A ECMO therapy is the effect of retrograde flow in the aorta toward the LV. In some patients, this phenomenon causes increased LV afterload and ultimately, worsening LV function. Eventually, the LV dilates, LA pressures rise, and pulmonary edema ensues. Once the LV is unable to contract appropriately, the aortic valve may not open, creating blood stagnation and placing the patient at risk for developing thrombus, and, ultimately, stroke. Monitoring and achieving clinically acceptable LV unloading in V-A ECMO patients is essential.[22,43,44] Implanting an LV venting catheter may be helpful with LV unloading and may be achieved surgically, peripherally, or percutaneously. Techniques include atrial septostomy, transaortic catheter venting, venting via pulmonary artery drainage, and indirect LV venting via IABP, TandemHeart, or Impella.[44]

Another concerning potential complication with the use of percutaneous V-A ECMO is distal limb ischemia. Using a large-bore catheter and impeding blood circulation to the extremity below the femoral artery can cause lower limb ischemia and compartment syndrome and, if left untreated, can ultimately lead to amputation. Patients with smaller femoral vessels as well as those who require high-dose vasopressors are at risk for compromised circulation. Limb ischemia typically presents as pain, paresthesia, and/or paralysis; however, these clinical manifestations are difficult to confirm if the patient is sedated or comatose.[28,38] Frequent extremity assessments of the cannulated limb are crucial, and include pulse checks, capillary refill checks, and temperature checks, especially if the patient has no or very weak pulses due to low BP, or low to no pulsatility. The authors have reported experience with the effective use of a noninvasive somatic oximeter (INVOS Cerebral/Somatic Oximetry Adult Sensors, Medtronic, Minneapolis, MN) to monitor the amount of oxygenated blood circulating to the lower extremities.[33,38] This technology can help to identify changes in peripheral circulation and allow for immediate intervention. Another measure to help to limit limb ischemia is the use of an antegrade perfusion catheter when percutaneously cannulating for V-A ECMO. The occurrence of limb ischemia with femoral cannulation has been reported in up to 20% of patients; however, the authors report less than a 5% incidence with the use of an antegrade perfusion catheter.[38] Some centers initiate V-A ECMO via cannulation of the subclavian or axillary artery to reduce the risk of lower limb ischemia. This is controversial, however, because this technique can create its own set of complications, including upper extremity edema (**Table 3**).

There is a wide variation in antithrombotic treatment of ECMO patients. Unfractionated heparin is most frequently used for ECMO patients if not contraindicated, whereas direct thrombin inhibitors are used in less than 10% of patients.[41,45] Antiplatelet agents are not consistently used for ECMO patients, and, in the authors' experience, these agents are used only in recently stented patients and not given routinely. Some patients develop heparin-induced thrombocytopenia and require direct thrombin inhibitors, such as bivalirudin or argatroban, despite the limited amount of data on safety and efficacy of these agents.[41,45] One of the biggest concerns of under anticoagulating is clot formation within the ECMO circuit, with the most common site the oxygenator. As discussed previously, if a provider chooses to use a simple, closed circuit without connectors, lower levels of anticoagulation can be maintained without thrombus issues.

FUTURE DIRECTIONS OF TEMPORARY MECHANICAL CIRCULATORY SUPPORT

The field of MCS is growing rapidly, with the development of newer technologies for both durable and short-term support devices. The development of smaller devices with lower adverse event profiles (see **Table 2**) and the ability to be easily and rapidly applied at the patient bedside or outside of the hospital, is necessary. There needs to be a paradigm shift in the way that CS patients are managed, in that conventional therapy should be applied quickly, and the consideration for tMCS should be made much earlier in the process, to avoid patient deterioration beyond medical assistance and support. Priority needs to be focused on device selection and appropriate patient selection and identification. Recognizing that not all patients are the same has a direct impact on what type of device is chosen for a specific patient scenario. Current work is being done by the European Mechanical Circulatory Support Summit Cardiogenic Shock Working Group, who are developing algorithms to help stratify a heterogeneous group of patients based on their level of acuity to identify the best

Table 3
Short-term mechanical circulatory support complications

Intra-aortic Balloon Pump	Impella	Tandemheart	Veno-arterial Extracorporeal Membrane Oxygenation
• Limb ischemia[1,9,11,17] • Bleeding[9,17,20] • Infection • Hematoma[17] • Vascular complications[1,11,20] • Thrombocytopenia[11,20] • Coagulopathies[11] • Acute kidney injury[11] • Aortic dissection[21] • Bowel ischemia[11] • Embolism[11]	• Bleeding[1,9,11,22] • Tamponade[22] • Infection • Stroke[22] • Aortic valve injury[14,20] • Hematoma at insertion site[11,14,17] • Limb ischemia[9,11,22] • Thrombocytopenia[1] • Aortic dissection • Hemolysis[1,9,11,14,17,20,22] • Coagulopathies[1] • Pseudoaneurysm[1,11] • AV fistula[1,11] • LV perforation[14] • Thrombosis[22]	• Perforation of the posterior wall, aortic root, or the coronary sinus[1] • Limb ischemia[9,17,20–22] • Vascular injury[17] • Hemolysis[11] • Tamponade[11,14,17,20] • Hematoma at insertion site[14,17] • Bleeding[1,9,14,17] • Infection[1,22] • Arrhythmias[17,22] • Thrombo or air embolism[11,14,17,20] • Stroke[22] • Coagulopathy[11,22]	• Lower extremity ischemia[1,9,20,22,35,44] • Upper extremity hypoxia[1,20] • Compartment syndrome[9,35,36,43] • Hemolysis[9,11,21] • LL Amputation[9] • Stroke[11,21,30,35] • Pseudoaneurysm[40] • Bleeding[9,11,22,35,36] • Neurologic complications[20,21,30,35,36] • Acute kidney injury[21] • Tamponade in postcardiotomy patients[22] • Significant infection[9,22] • Hematoma[40] • Arterial thrombus[22] • Venous thrombus[11,20,22] • LV distention[14,17,22,43] • Thrombosis of circuit[11,20,35,36]

type of tMCS therapy to be used. Anecdotal reports support the application of tMCS for acute CS patients; however, there continues to be a lack of consensus about patient and device selection as well as patient management, necessitating well-designed, prospective clinical trials to determine the safety, effectiveness, and impact of tMCS on patient survival and to confirm the utility and viability of this advanced and technical therapy.

REFERENCES

1. Ergle K, Parto P, Krim SR. Percutaneous ventricular assist devices: a novel approach in the management of patients with acute cardiogenic shock. Ochsner J 2016;16:243–9.
2. Mebazaa A, Tolppanen H, Mueller C, et al. Acute heart failure and cardiogenic shock: a multidisciplinary practical guidance. Intensive Care Med 2016;42:147–63.
3. Doll JA, Ohman EM, Patel MR, et al. A team-based approach to patients in cardiogenic shock. Catheter Cardiovasc Interv 2016;88:424–33.
4. Thiele H, Ohman EM, Desch S, et al. Management of cardiogenic shock. Eur Heart J 2015;36:1223–30.
5. Takayama H, Takeda K, Doshi D, et al. Short-term continuous – flow ventricular assist devices. Curr Opin Cardiol 2014;29(3):265–74.
6. Csepe TA, Kilic A. Advancements in mechanical circulatory support for patients in acute and chronic heart failure. J Thorac Dis 2017;9(10):4070–83.
7. Harjola VP, Lassus J, Sionis A, et al, on behalf of the CardShock study investigators, GREAT network. Clinical picture and risk prediction of short-term mortality in cardiogenic shock. Eur J Heart Fail 2015;17:501–9.
8. den Uil CA, Akin S, Jewbali LS, et al. Short – term mechanical circulatory support as a bridge to durable left ventricular assist device implantation in refractory cardiogenic shock: a systematic review and meta – analysis. Eur J Cardiothorac Surg 2017;52:14–25.
9. Lawson WE, Koo M. Percutaneous ventricular assist devices and ECMO in the management of acute decompensated heart failure. Clin Med Insights Cardiol 2015;9(S1):41–8.
10. Shah P, Smith S, Harft JQ, et al. Clinical outcomes of advances hart failure patients with cardiogenic shock treated with Temporary circulatory support before durable LVAD implant. ASAIO J 2016. https://doi.org/10.1097/MAT. 0000000000000309.
11. Rihal CS, Naidu S, Givertz MM, et al, on behalf of the Society for Cardiovascular Angiography and Interventions, Heart Failure Society of America, Society for Thoracic Surgeons, American Heart Association, and American College of Cardiology. 2015 SCAI/ ACC/HFSA/STS clinical expert consensus statement on the use of percutaneous mechanical circulatory support devices in cardiovascular care (Endorsed by the American Heart Association, the Cardiological Society of India, and Sociedad Latino Americana de Cardiologia Intervencion; Affirmation of Value by the Canadian Association of Interventional Cardiology-Association Canadienne de Cardiologie d'intervention). J Card Fail 2015;21(6):499–518.
12. Rihal CS, Naidu S, Givertz MM, et al. Consensus statement. J Card Fail 2015;21(6):499–518.
13. Thiele H, Zeymer U, Neumann FJ, et al. Intra-aortic balloon counterpulsation in acute myocardial infarction complicated by cardiogenic shock (IABP-SHOCK II); Final 12-month results of a randomized, open-label trial. Lancet 2013;382:1638–45.
14. Saffarzadeh A, Bonde P. Options for temporary mechanical circulatory support. J Thorac Dis 2015;7(12):2102–11.
15. Stretch R, Sauer CM, Yuh DD, et al. National trend in the utilization of short – term mechanical circulatory support. J Am Coll Cardiol 2014;64(14):1407–15.
16. Khera R, Cram P, Lu X, et al. Trends in the use of percutaneous ventricular assist devices: analysis of national inpatient sample data, 2007-2012. JAMA Intern Med 2015;175:941–50.
17. Nagpal AD, Singal RK, Arora RC, et al. Temporary mechanical circulatory support in cardiac critical care: a state of the art review and algorithm for device selection. Can J Cardiol 2017;33:110–8.
18. Shah P, Pagani FD, Desai SS, et al, on behalf of the Mechanical Circulatory Support Research Network. Outcomes of patients receiving temporary circulatory support before durable ventricular assist device. Ann Thorac Surg 2017;103:106–13.
19. Basir MB, SchreiberTL Grines CL, Dixon SR, et al. Effect of early initiation of mechanical circulatory support on survival in cardiogenic shock. Am J Cardiol 2017;119:845–51.
20. Gilotra NA, Stevens GR. Temporary mechanical circulatory support: a review of the options, indications, and outcomes. Clin Med Insights Cardiol 2015;8(Suppl 1):75–85.
21. Touchan J, Guglin M. Temporary mechanical circulatory support for cardiogenic shock. Curr Treat Options Cardiovasc Med 2017;19:77, 16.
22. Mandawat A, Rao SV. Percutaneous mechanical circulatory support devices in cardiogenic shock. Circ Cardiovasc Interv 2017. https://doi.org/10.1161/CIRCINTERNVETIONS.116.004337.
23. Miller PE, Solomon MA, McAreavery D. Advanced percutaneous mechanical circulatory support devices for cardiogenic shock. Crit Care Med 2017;45(11):1922–9.
24. Hall SA, Uriel N, Carey SA, et al. Use of a percutaneous temporary circulatory support device as a bridge to decision during acute decompensation

of advanced heart failure. J Heart Lung Transplant 2017. https://doi.org/10.1016/j.healun.2017.09.020.

25. Lima B, Kale P, Ganzalez-Stawinski GV, et al. Effectiveness and safety of the impella 5.0 as a bridge to cardiac transplantation or durable left ventricular assist device. Am J Cardiol 2016;117:1622–8.

26. Anderson MB, Goldstein J, Milano C, et al. Benefits of a novel percutaneous ventricular assist device for right heart failure: the prospective RECOVER RIGHT study of the Impella RP device. J Heart Lung Transplant 2015;34(12):1549–60.

27. Walfson PJ. The development and use of extracorporeal membrane oxygenation in neonates. Ann Thorac Surg 2003;76:S2224–9.

28. Mohite PN, Fatullayev J, Maunz O, et al. Distal limb perfusion: achilles' heel in peripheral venoarterial extracorporeal membrane oxygenation. Artif Organs 2014;38:940–4.

29. Ostadal P, Rokyta R, Kruger A, et al. Extra corporeal membrane oxygenation in the therapy of cardiogenic shock (ECMO-CS): rationale and design of the multicenter randomized trial. Eur J Heart Fail 2017;19(Suppl. 2):124–7.

30. Lorusso R, Gelsomino S, Parise O, et al. Venoarterial extracorporeal membrane oxygenation for refractory cardiogenic shock in elderly patients: trends in application and outcome from the extracorporeal life support organization (ELSO) registry. Ann Thorac Surg 2017;104:62–9.

31. Lorusso R, Barili F, DiMauro M, et al. In-hospital neurologic complications in acute patients undergoing venoarterial extracorporeal membrane oxygenation: results from the extracorporeal life support organization registry. Crit Care Med 2016;44(10):e964–72.

32. Terri S, Andrew G, Amandeep S, et al. Veno-arterial extracorporeal membrane oxygenation (VA-ECMO) for emergency cardiac support. J Crit Care 2018;44:31–8.

33. Ghodsizad A, Koerner MM, El-Banayosy A, et al. Extracorporeal membrane oxygenation (ECMO): an option for cardiac recovery from advanced cardiogenic shock. Heart Surg Forum 2017;20(6):E274–7.

34. Czobor P, Venturini JM, Parikh KS, et al. Sequential organ failure assessment score and presentation predicts survival in patients treated with percutaneous veno-arterial extracorporeal membrane oxygenation. J Invasive Cardiol 2016;28(4):133–8.

35. Ghodsizad A, Koerner MM, Brehm CE, et al. The role of extracorporeal membrane oxygenation circulatory support in the 'crash and burn' patient: from implantation to weaning. Curr Opin Cardiol 2014;29:275–80.

36. Sidebotham D, Allen SJ, McGeorge A, et al. Venovenous extracorporeal membrane oxygenation in adults: practical aspects of circuits, cannulae, and procedures. J Cardiothorac Vasc Anesth 2012;26:893–909.

37. Aoyama N, Imai H, Kurosawa T, et al. Therapeutic strategy using extracorporeal life support, including appropriate indication, management, limitation and timing or switch to ventricular assist device in patients with acute myocardial infarction. J Artif Organs 2014;17:33–41.

38. Banfi C, Pozzi M, Brunner ME, et al. Veno – arterial extracorporeal membrane oxygenation; an overview of different cannulation techniques. J Thorac Dis 2016;8(9):E875–85.

39. Moll V, Teo EYL, Grenda DS, et al. Rapid development and implementation of an ECMO program. ASAIO J 2016;62:354–8.

40. Zangrillo A, Landoni G, Biondi-Zoccai G, et al. A meta-analysis of complications and mortality of extracorporeal membrane oxygenation. Crit Care Resusc 2013;15(3):172–8.

41. Kreuziger LB, Massicotte MP. Mechanical circulatory support: balancing bleeding and clotting in high-risk patients. Hematology 2015;2015:61–8.

42. Wong JK, Melvin AL, Joshi DJ, et al. Cannulation-related complications on veno-arterial extracorporeal membrane oxygenation: prevalence and effect on mortality. Artif Organs 2017;41(9):827–34.

43. Soleimani B, Pae WE. Management of left ventricular distension during peripheral extracorporeal membrane oxygenation for cardiogenic shock. Perfusion 2012;27:326–31.

44. Meani P, Gelsomino S, Natour E, et al. Modalities and effects of left ventricle unloading on extracorporeal life support: a review of the current literature. Eur J Heart Fail 2017;19(Suppl. 2):84–91.

45. Petricevic M, Milicic D, Boban M, et al. Bleeding and thrombotic events in patients undergoing mechanical circulatory support: a review of literature. Thorac Cardiovasc Surg 2015;63:636–46.

Candidate Selection for Durable Mechanical Circulatory Support

Jennifer A. Cowger, MD, MS*, Gillian Grafton, DO

KEYWORDS

- Left ventricular assist device support • Heart failure • Mortality • Risk stratification

KEY POINTS

- Heart failure (HF) risk stratification is important for guiding the timing of durable mechanical circulatory support (MCS), and it is integral to the shared decision-making process with HF patients and families.
- HF risk stratification includes estimating patient morbidity and mortality with ongoing medical management alone versus that of MCS.
- Although several HF risk models have been devised, accuracy of the tools for predicting outcome in the advanced HF population remains poor.
- Patients with recurrent HF admissions, hemodynamic instability, progressive end-organ dysfunction, or frequent ventricular arrhythmias may benefit from MCS evaluation.
- The operative period is the highest risk for mortality in MCS patients. Although many risk scores exist, advanced age, medical comorbidities, preoperative right ventricular dysfunction, renal dysfunction, and measures of hemodynamic instability are common covariates of mortality after MCS.

INTRODUCTION

The evolution of mechanical circulatory support (MCS) for management of end-stage heart failure (HF) has been rapid, imparting an exponential impact on patient survival and quality of life. Compared with a survival rate of 54% in patients supported with the first-generation pulsatile-flow HeartMate (Abbott, Abbott Park, Illinois) XVE left ventricular assist device (LVAD), survivals averaged 76% and 83% at 2 years for patents supported with the second-generation axial-flow HeartMate II (HMII) LVAD and third-generation centrifugal-flow HeartMate 3 LVAD, respectively.[1,2] In addition to marked improvements in device technology, surgical technique, and patient management, gains in patient survival after LVAD implant have been achieved through refinement of patient selection. This article focuses on the critical interplay of preexisting patient comorbidities and instantaneous hemodynamic status in determining the risk versus benefit of MCS. This article expands on predictors of operative risk and correlates of long-term success on MCS.

IMPORTANCE OF RISK PREDICTION

HF encompasses a wide spectrum of patient phenotypes. Some patients with HF have no or minimal limitations to their functional capacity (New York Heart Association [NYHA] classes I–II), whereas others have severe shortness of breath

Disclosures: Henry Ford receives institutional research funds from Abbott and Medtronic. Dr J.A. Cowger is a paid speaker and consultant for Medtronic (Minnesota); she is a paid speaker for Abbott and research related travel support from Abbott (Illinois); and she is on the Scientific Advisory Board for Procyrion (Texas). Dr G. Grafton has no disclosures otherwise.
Department of Cardiology, Henry Ford Hospital, 2799 West Grand Boulevard, Detroit, MI 48202, USA
* Corresponding author. Henry Ford Hospital, 2799 West Grand Boulevard, K 14, Detroit, MI 48202.
E-mail address: Jennifercowger@gmail.com

with minimal exertion (NYHA classes III–IV). Patient clinical status can vary from long-term stability with excellent 5-year prognosis to rapid decompensation with impending mortality. Forecasting patient risk for death from HF is often challenging but is nevertheless critical for timing of the implementation of advanced HF therapies (including transplant and MCS) to ensure the best outcomes for these complex patients.

Information gleaned for prognostication is integral to shared decision making with patients and their families, especially during the complex process of education about MCS and as part of informed consent. Although there are models used to estimate average HF patient risk as a starting point for shared decision making, patient-specific details are crucial for a more precise estimation of patient morbidity and mortality. In the evaluation for durable MCS, practitioners must present the risk of ongoing medical management of HF compared with the risks of surgical implantation of the LVAD and the sizable morbidity and mortality associated with long-term MCS. Although this article focuses on mortality risk prediction, the impact of morbidities encountered during LVAD support as well as the impact on quality of life and functional capacity are summarized in the articles, Saima Aslam's article, "Ventricular Assist Device Infections," and Tonya Elliott and Lori G. Edwards's article, "Ambulatory Ventricular Assist Device Patient Management," and Ju H. Kim and colleagues article, "Continuous-Flow Left Ventricular Assist Device–Related Gastrointestinal Bleeding," and Ajay Kadakkal and Samer S. Najjar's article, "Neurologic Events in Continuous-Flow Left Ventricular Assist Devices," in this issue. It is important that all these factors are taken into consideration and are discussed and well outlined in the shared decision-making process between advanced HF patients and the practitioner.[3–6]

Assessing Patient Morbidity and Mortality from Medical Management of Heart Failure

The first step in assessing candidacy for durable MCS is assessing patient risk of death from ongoing medical management of HF. For those with advanced HF (encompassing late stage C and stage D HF), survival is uniformly poor but also highly variable. A meta-analysis of 20 studies encompassing 2877 patients requiring extracorporeal membrane oxygenation for management of postcardiotomy shock demonstrated survivals of 34% at discharge.[7] In the population of patients who are less critically ill but are dependent on inotropes at home, survival averages were marginally better, at 25% to 60% at

12 months.[2,8,9] The more complex patients to prognosticate are those who are less ill with severe systolic dysfunction—the ambulatory patient with systolic HF.

Several clinical trials, cohort studies, and registries have identified markers of mortality in ambulatory patients with HF.[10–16] Commonly identified risks include advanced patient age, renal dysfunction, hyponatremia, major comorbidities (eg, chronic obstructive pulmonary disease and diabetes), recurrent HF admissions, recurrent ventricular dysrhythmias, lower systolic blood pressures, poor functional capacity (reduced peak oxygen consumption or 6-minute walk test distance), and/or advanced NYHA class. The utility of an individual parameter to prognostic risk, however, is often poor due to the presence of many coexistent positive or negative risk factors. To allow for a more individualized estimation of patient risk using a set of patient-specific characteristics, various risk prediction models have been devised (**Table 1**).[11,13,15,17–19] Two of the most commonly used tools include the Meta-Analysis Global Group in Chronic Heart Failure (MAGGIC) risk score and the Seattle Heart Failure Model (SHFM).[11,13] The MAGGIC model was devised using data from 39,372 patients with HF enrolled into 30 different cohort studies.[13] Patients in the MAGGIC cohort included both reduced left ventricular ejection and preserved left ventricular ejection fractions (LVEF), but average mortality was high at 40% over a median follow-up of 2.5 years. Using 13 predictors of mortality (see **Table 1**), MAGGIC can be used to estimate an individual's probability of dying within 1 and 3 years.[13] The SHFM was derived from patients enrolled into the Prospective Randomized Amlodipine Survival Evaluation (PRAISE) study, which included 1125 patients with an LVEF less than or equal to 30% and NYHA class IIIb to class IV symptoms.[11,20] The SHFM was then validated in 9902 patients enrolled into 5 other trials, including those with preserved systolic function and NYHA class II to class IV.[11] Mortality variables are shown in **Table 1**, and when entered into the online model, practitioners are given 1-year, 2-year, and 5-year mortality estimates.[21] Both MAGGIC and the SHFM tools have been independently validated to assess risk, but the accuracy in the subset of patients with advanced HF remains suboptimal.[10,22–24] For example, when the SHFM was examined in 445 patients referred for cardiac transplant, the SHFM showed acceptable discrimination (which captures the ability of a model to correctly identify patients with vs without event-free survival) but poor calibration (which measures how close the mortality values predicted by the

Table 1
Risk models and their associated predictors of heart failure mortality with ongoing medical management

	NYHA Class in Derivation Cohort	LVEF Evaluated	Predictors of Death:			Tested in LVAD candidates?
			Demographic	Clinical	Lab	
Seattle HF Model[11,21]	II-IV	<30%	Age, gender, weight, systolic BP	NYHA class, LVEF, HF medications, QRS >120	Hemoglobin, Lymphocyte%, uric acid, total cholesterol, sodium	Yes, under-estimates actual mortality %
MAGGIC[13]	I-IV (85% were II-III)	Any LVEF, Mean 37%	Age, NYHA class, gender, body mass index	smoker, diabetic, COPD, HF meds, HF diagnoses last 18 months	Creatinine	No
Lee Score[19]	Not Reported	53% had LVEF <40%	Age, systolic BP, respiratory rate	cardiovascular disease, dementia, cirrhosis, cancer, COPD	BUN, Creatinine, Hemoglobin, sodium	No
HF Survival Score[15]	Mean 2.8	LVEF <40%	Heart rate, mean BP	Ischemic cardiomyopathy, LVEF, IVCD, pVO$_2$	sodium	Yes with first generation pumps, devised originally for transplant risk
ADHERE[18]	Not Reported	66% had LVEF <40%	Systolic BP	None	BUN, Creatinine	No
Shocked[17]	I-IV (72% were III)	LVEF <40%	Age	NYHA, LVEF, Atrial fibrillation, COPD, Diabetes, chronic kidney disease	None	No

Common variables across models are highlighted by color.
Abbreviations: ADHERE, Acute Decompensated Heart Failure National Registry; BP, blood pressure; BUN, blood urea nitrogen; COPD, chronic obstructive pulmonary disease; CRT, cardiac resynchronization therapy; IVCD, intraventricular conduction delay on ECG.

model matched those observed), underestimating patient mortality.[22] The SHFM model was applied to patients enrolled into the Risk Assessment and Comparative Effectiveness of Left Ventricular Assist Device and Medical Management in Ambulatory Heart Failure Patients (ROADMAP) study, which was a nonrandomized, observational study comparing optimal medical management versus LVAD in non–inotrope-dependent patients with advanced systolic HF with NYHA class IIIb/IV symptoms.[23,25] The model was predictive of overall survival (C statistic 0.71) but again underestimated clinical deterioration necessitating LVAD.[23,25]

The overall poor performance of HF models in those with advanced HF is likely multifactorial. Models derived from clinical trials tend to self-select patients who are healthier than most patients considered for MCS. Patients in the derivation cohort of the SHFM, for example, were excluded if they received inotropes within 72 hours of enrollment and patients had not received intravenous (IV) vasodilators or diuretics within 24 hours of enrollment.[11,20] In addition, HF mortality rates have

changed greatly in the past 10 years to 15 years with the introduction of new HF therapies (eg, biventricular pacing and angiotensin-neprilysin inhibitors). The Heart Failure Survival Score (a model developed in ambulatory HF patients for the purpose of cardiac transplant risk stratification) and the PRAISE cohort (from which the SHFM was derived) were derived prior to the widespread introduction of β-blockers or use of biventricular pacing.[15,20] Thus, models derived from early cohorts may not perform well in HF patients due to improvements in guideline-directed therapies.

In patients with non–inotrope-dependent, ambulatory systolic HF, the patient's preoperative Interagency Registry for Mechanically Assisted Circulatory Support (INTERMACS) Profile has some potential utility for risk stratification (**Table 2**).[26,27] INTERMACS Profiles characterize patients' global clinical status, ranging from critical cardiogenic shock (INTERMACS Profile 1) to advanced NYHA III (Profile 7).[26] Ambulatory patients encompass Profiles 4 to 7. Using this simple classification, Stewart and colleagues[27] demonstrated an event-survival free of 52% in

Table 2
INTERMACS Profiles

Interagency Registry for Mechanically Assisted Circulatory Support Profile	Descriptor	New York Heart Association Class Assumed	Modifier Options
1	Crash and burn: critical cardiogenic shock. Includes life-threatening hypotension, organ hypoperfusion, or elevated lactate	IV	TCS, A
2	Sliding fast on inotropes: declining organ function or inability to restore volume on inotropes	IV	TCS, A
3	Inotrope dependent, stable: at home or in hospital. Stable blood pressure and organ function on inotropes but unable to wean due to recurrent HF.	IV	A, TCS if hospitalized, FF if home
4	Resting symptoms at home on oral therapy: stable but diuretic doses fluctuate often.	IV	FF, A
5	Housebound: exercise intolerant. Comfortable at rest but symptoms occur with minimal activity. Often have evidence of volume overload and/or renal dysfunction.	Ambulatory IV	FF, A
6	Walking wounded: exertion limited. Meaningful activity limited. No evidence of volume overload.	IIIb	FF, A
7	Advanced class III	III	A only

The INTERMACS Profiles and the associated short-hand patient description and New York Heart Association class are shown. Modifiers are optional descriptors used to label those with recurrent admissions.

Abbreviations: A, arrhythmias; FF, frequent flyer; TCS, temporary circulatory support.

Data from Stevenson LW, Pagani FD, Young JB, et al. INTERMACS profiles of advanced heart failure: the current picture. J Heart Lung Transplant 2009;28:535–41; and Stewart GC, Kittleson MM, Patel PC, et al. INTERMACS (Interagency Registry for Mechanically Assisted Circulatory Support) profiling identifies ambulatory patients at high risk on medical therapy after hospitalizations for heart failure. Circ Heart Fail 2016;9:e003032.

patients categorized as Profile 4 versus 78% and 86% in patients in Profiles 5 and 6 to 7, respectively. In the ROADMAP study, patients in Profile 4 (LVAD = 67% vs medical = 28%) and the combined Profile 5 to 7 (LVAD = 76% vs medical = 49%) who underwent LVAD had better event-free survival at 2 years then patients in the same Profile(s) who chose medical management.[28]

Finally, the utility of 6-minute walk test distance and/or cardiopulmonary stress testing cannot be ignored in the ambulatory HF patient.[16] Patients often underestimate the severity of their physical limitations. Impaired ventilatory efficiency (Ve/Vco$_2$ [expired volume per unit time/carbon dioxide production] slope >34) or reduced peak oxygen uptake (peak oxygen consumption on cardiopulmonary stress test [pVo$_2$] ≤50% predicted) on cardiopulmonary stress testing identifies a high-risk HF patient[15,29,30] independent of NYHA class. In addition, the test can identify other contributors to

HF exercise intolerance, including pulmonary limitations and chronotropic incompetence. Although providing less overall information, the 6-minute walk test is an easy, quick, and validated measure for assessing HF mortality risk. Six-minute walk test distances has been shown to correlate with pVo$_2$ measures on cardiopulmonary testing and a value less than 300 m is generally considered to confer increased mortality in patients with HF.[31]

Left Ventricular Assist Device Operative Mortality Assessment

Predicting an MCS candidate's operative mortality with LVAD can be even more challenging. A patient's ability to undergo anesthesia needs to be predicted: the response of the right ventricle to the increased preload and global wall stress applied during LVAD support; the ability of the congested, fibrotic, and/or ischemic liver to produce hemostatic factors during surgery; and the hemocompatibility

Table 3
Risk models and their associated predictors of mortality after left ventricular assist device implant

	LVAD type	Predictors of Death:		
		Demographic	Clinical	Lab
Lietz-Miller Score[38]	HeartMate XVE	None	Vasodilator therapy, mean pulmonary pressure, no inotrope	Albumin, BUN, INR, Platelet, hematocrit, AST
HMII Risk Score[32-26]	HMII and HVAD separately	Age	Center volume	Albumin, Creatinine, INR
MELD[47,48]	- XVE - HMII	None	None	Sodium, Creatinine, Bilirubin, INR
MELDx[49,50]	HMII HVAD	None	None	Sodium, Creatinine, Bilirubin
Bayesian model*[42,51]	HMII and HVAD	None	Previous cardiac surgery, IV Inotrope, Destination therapy, INTERMACS profile, ECMO, dialysis, Intubation cardiac arrest	Hemoglobin, Creatinine, prealbumin, INR
INTERMACS 7th report[37]	HMII HVAD	Age, female, BMI	History of stroke, preop ventilator, NYHA IV, Destination Therapy, History of cardiac surgery, INTERMAC 1 or 2, dialysis, high right atrial pressure	Creatinine, Albumin, BUN, Bilirubin

Common variables across models are highlighted by color. INTERMACS multivariable predictors are also shown but are not part of a risk scoring model.

Abbreviations: AST, aspartate aminotransferase; BMI, body mass index; BUN, blood urea nitrogen; ECMO, extracorporeal membrane oxygenation.

a Bayesian models included many risk factors entered for each patient. The variables listed are those common to most models studied for mortality after LVAD at various time points.

between the device and patient. Despite all these unknowns, several risk correlates have been identified for assessing an MCS candidates operative LVAD mortality risk (**Table 3**).[23,32-38]

One of the most important prognostic factors is the patient's preoperative INTERMACS Profile. Although heterogeneity exists between practitioners in patient Profile categorization and mortality overlap can be seen between contiguous categories (such as INTERMACS Profile 1 vs Profile 2), patients in Profile 1 to Profile 2 (spectrum of cardiogenic shock) have been shown to have higher mortality than those individuals in Profile 3 (inotrope dependent) and combined Profiles 4 to 7 (ambulatory, non–inotrope-dependent HF).[37,39–41] Other patient characteristics that have been correlated with increased LVAD operative mortality include preoperative need for temporary circulatory support, vasopressors, and/or ventilatory support—interventions common to many patients grouped into INTERMACS Profiles 1 to 2.[37,42] In addition, advanced patient age, body mass index, transplant

intent, female gender, renal dysfunction, intrinsic coagulopathy, malnutrition/sarcopenia, frailty, prior sternotomy/cardiac surgery, and right ventricular dysfunction are important markers of LVAD operative risk.[35,37,42] The role of right ventricular failure in imparting morbidity and mortality after LVAD cannot be ignored. This topic is outlined in detail by Brent C. Lampert's article, "Perioperative Management of the Right and Left Ventricle," and Diyar Saeed's article, "Right Ventricular Failure and Biventricular Support Strategies," in this issue. Finally, center volume and surgical experience have an impact on patient outcomes,[43–45] which are critical for referring providers to be aware of.

From many these univariable predictors, multivariable risks scores for predicting an LVAD candidate's operative survival have been devised. The individual components of popular risk scores are outlined in **Table 3**.[23,32–37] The HMII Risk Score was derived from 583 patients enrolled into the combined bridge to transplant and destination therapy HMII trial cohorts.[34] The score was then internally validated in 539 HMII patients.[34] The markers of risk included older age, higher creatinine, lower serum albumin, and higher international normalized ratio (INR). The HMII risk score has been externally validated in HMII patients and studied in the HeartWare ventricular assist device HVAD (Medtronic, Minneapolis, Minnesota) population omitting INR, which can be influenced by anticoagulation use in the preoperative setting.[23,32,33,35] Three studies demonstrated moderate model discrimination (C statistic 0.6–0.7),[23,32,33] whereas others have demonstrated poorer performance.[36,46] The Model for End-Stage Liver Disease ([MELD], composed of serum creatinine, bilirubin, sodium, and INR) and the MELDx (omitting INR) have also been applied other models highlighting the importance of multi-system dysfunction (liver and/or right ventricle and renal) and coagulopathy on the impact of MCS outcomes.[47–50] Finally, Loghmanpour and colleagues[42,51] have used bayesian network modeling and machine learning algorithms to predict patient risk for MCS mortality using several patient preoperative variables. Although potentially time consuming for patient data entry, these models potentially have the ability to provide more accurate estimates of patient level mortality than traditional, simplified risk scores.

Correlates of Long-Term Survival on Mechanical Circulatory Support

Few studies have examined correlates of long-term survival after MCS implant.[42,52] Because operative survival is obligatory for long-term survival, the risk factors having an impact on operative risk, discussed previously, remain important. In the derivation of the HMII Risk Score, center experience was the only preoperative variable independently associated with increased long-term mortality when the risk analysis was restricted to those who survived the operative (90 day) period.[34] The Penn-Columbia Risk Score combines patient age, body mass index and laboratory parameters (bilirubin and creatinine) with preoperative echocardiography measures of aortic insufficiency and right ventricular function to generate a tiered risk of 1-year mortality. The model was not restricted to operative survivors and independent validation and comparison of discrimination and calibration is pending.[52] Finally, preoperative comorbidities (including pulmonary disease, diabetes, orthopedic limitations, and cognition) likely have additional impact on long-term patient survival. To date, models have not included a detailed evaluation of comorbidities and further study is warranted because patients live longer and longer on device support.

SUMMARY

Assessing HF patient mortality risks is integral to the process of shared decision making with patients and their families. Patient assessment and informed consent discussion must include the risks of ongoing HF medical therapy and the alternative risks of the MCS operation, including the complications encountered during long-term device support. Advanced patient age, renal dysfunction, poor functional status, concomitant medical comorbidities, and unstable hemodynamics are common mortality risks for HF and LVAD mortality. Although several models exist for estimating patient-specific HF or LVAD mortality, reduced accuracy limits clinical utility to a generalized attribution of risk. In addition to mortality, quality of life and morbidity must be considered in the shared decision-making process for managing patients with advanced HF.

REFERENCES

1. Mehra MR, Goldstein DJ, Uriel N, et al. Two-year outcomes with a magnetically levitated cardiac pump in heart failure. N Engl J Med 2018;378:1386–95.
2. Rose EA, Gelijns AC, Moskowitz AJ, et al. Long-term use of a left ventricular assist device for end-stage heart failure. N Engl J Med 2001;345:1435–43.
3. Cowger JA, Naka Y, Aaronson KD, et al. Quality of life and functional capacity outcomes in the MOMENTUM 3 trial at 6 months: a call for new metrics for left ventricular assist device patients. J Heart Lung Transplant 2018;37:15–24.
4. Grady KL, Meyer PM, Dressler D, et al. Longitudinal change in quality of life and impact on survival after left ventricular assist device implantation. Ann Thorac Surg 2004;77:1321–7.
5. Grady KL, Naftel DC, Myers S, et al. Change in health-related quality of life from before to after destination therapy mechanical circulatory support is similar for older and younger patients: analyses from INTERMACS. J Heart Lung Transplant 2015;34:213–21.
6. Arnold SV, Jones PG, Allen LA, et al. Frequency of poor outcome (Death or Poor Quality of Life) after left ventricular assist device for destination therapy: results from the INTERMACS registry. Circ Heart Fail 2016;9 [pii:e002800].
7. Wang L, Wang H, Hou X. Clinical outcomes of adult patients who receive extracorporeal membrane oxygenation for postcardiotomy cardiogenic shock: a systematic review and meta-analysis. J Cardiothorac Vasc Anesth 2018. [Epub ahead of print].
8. Stevenson LW. Clinical use of inotropic therapy for heart failure: looking backward or forward? Part II: chronic inotropic therapy. Circulation 2003;108:492–7.

9. Stevenson LW. Clinical use of inotropic therapy for heart failure: looking backward or forward? Part I: inotropic infusions during hospitalization. Circulation 2003;108:367–72.

10. Alba AC, Agoritsas T, Jankowski M, et al. Risk prediction models for mortality in ambulatory patients with heart failure: a systematic review. Circ Heart Fail 2013;6:881–9.

11. Levy WC, Mozaffarian D, Linker DT, et al. The Seattle heart failure model: prediction of survival in heart failure. Circulation 2006;113:1424–33.

12. Ouwerkerk W, Voors AA, Zwinderman AH. Factors influencing the predictive power of models for predicting mortality and/or heart failure hospitalization in patients with heart failure. JACC Heart Fail 2014; 2:429–36.

13. Pocock SJ, Ariti CA, McMurray JJ, et al. Predicting survival in heart failure: a risk score based on 39 372 patients from 30 studies. Eur Heart J 2013;34: 1404–13.

14. Aaronson KD, Cowger J. Heart failure prognostic models: why bother? Circ Heart Fail 2012;5:6–9.

15. Aaronson KD, Schwartz JS, Chen TM, et al. Development and prospective validation of a clinical index to predict survival in ambulatory patients referred for cardiac transplant evaluation. Circulation 1997;95: 2660–7.

16. Matthews JC, Dardas TF, Aaronson KD. Heart transplantation: assessment of heart failure mortality risk. Curr Heart Fail Rep 2007;4:103–9.

17. Bilchick KC, Stukenborg GJ, Kamath S, et al. Prediction of mortality in clinical practice for medicare patients undergoing defibrillator implantation for primary prevention of sudden cardiac death. J Am Coll Cardiol 2012;60:1647–55.

18. Fonarow GC, Adams KF Jr, Abraham WT, et al. Risk stratification for in-hospital mortality in acutely decompensated heart failure: classification and regression tree analysis. JAMA 2005; 293:572–80.

19. Lee DS, Austin PC, Rouleau JL, et al. Predicting mortality among patients hospitalized for heart failure: derivation and validation of a clinical model. JAMA 2003;290:2581–7.

20. Packer M, O'Connor CM, Ghali JK, et al. Effect of amlodipine on morbidity and mortality in severe chronic heart failure. Prospective randomized amlodipine survival evaluation study group. N Engl J Med 1996;335:1107–14.

21. Levy W. Seattle heart failure model. 2006. Available at: https://depts.washington.edu/shfm/?width=1280&height=720. Accessed May 24, 2018.

22. Kalogeropoulos AP, Kelkar A, Weinberger JF, et al. Validation of clinical scores for right ventricular failure prediction after implantation of continuous-flow left ventricular assist devices. J Heart Lung Transplant 2015;34:1595–603.

23. Lanfear DE, Levy WC, Stehlik J, et al. Accuracy of seattle heart failure model and heartmate II risk score in non-inotrope-dependent advanced heart failure patients: insights from the ROADMAP study (Risk Assessment and Comparative Effectiveness of Left Ventricular Assist Device and Medical Management in Ambulatory Heart Failure Patients). Circ Heart Fail 2017;10 [pii:e003745].

24. Rahimi K, Bennett D, Conrad N, et al. Risk prediction in patients with heart failure: a systematic review and analysis. JACC Heart Fail 2014;2:440–6.

25. Estep JD, Starling RC, Horstmanshof DA, et al. Risk assessment and comparative effectiveness of left ventricular assist device and medical management in ambulatory heart failure patients: results from the ROADMAP study. J Am Coll Cardiol 2015;66:1747–61.

26. Stevenson LW, Pagani FD, Young JB, et al. INTERMACS profiles of advanced heart failure: the current picture. J Heart Lung Transplant 2009;28:535–41.

27. Stewart GC, Kittleson MM, Patel PC, et al. INTERMACS (Interagency Registry for Mechanically Assisted Circulatory Support) profiling identifies ambulatory patients at high risk on medical therapy after hospitalizations for heart failure. Circ Heart Fail 2016;9 [pii:e003032].

28. Shah KB, Starling RC, Rogers JG, et al. Left ventricular assist devices versus medical management in ambulatory heart failure patients: an analysis of INTERMACS Profiles 4 and 5 to 7 from the ROADMAP study. J Heart Lung Transplant 2018;37(6):706–14.

29. Malhotra R, Bakken K, D'Elia E, et al. Cardiopulmonary exercise testing in heart failure. JACC Heart Fail 2016;4:607–16.

30. Mancini D, LeJemtel T, Aaronson K. Peak VO(2): a simple yet enduring standard. Circulation 2000; 101:1080–2.

31. Du H, Wonggom P, Tongpeth J, et al. Six-minute walk test for assessing physical functional capacity in chronic heart failure. Curr Heart Fail Rep 2017; 14:158–66.

32. Adamo L, Nassif M, Tibrewala A, et al. The Heartmate Risk Score predicts morbidity and mortality in unselected left ventricular assist device recipients and risk stratifies INTERMACS class 1 patients. JACC Heart Fail 2015;3:283–90.

33. Adamo L, Tang Y, Nassif ME, et al. The heartmate risk score identifies patients with similar mortality risk across all INTERMACS profiles in a large multicenter analysis. JACC Heart Fail 2016;4:950–8.

34. Cowger J, Sundareswaran K, Rogers JG, et al. Predicting survival in patients receiving continuous flow left ventricular assist devices: the HeartMate II risk score. J Am Coll Cardiol 2013;61:313–21.

35. Cowger JA, Castle L, Aaronson KD, et al. The heartmate II risk score: an adjusted score for evaluation of all continuous-flow left ventricular assist devices. ASAIO J 2016;62:281–5.

36. Kanwar MK, Lohmueller LC, Kormos RL, et al. Low accuracy of the heartmate risk score for predicting mortality using the INTERMACS registry data. ASAIO J 2017;63:251–6.

37. Kirklin JK, Naftel DC, Pagani FD, et al. Seventh INTERMACS annual report: 15,000 patients and counting. J Heart Lung Transplant 2015;34:1495–504.

38. Lietz K, Long JW, Kfoury AG, et al. Outcomes of left ventricular assist device implantation as destination therapy in the post-REMATCH era: implications for patient selection. Circulation 2007;116:497–505.

39. Cowger J, Shah P, Stulak J, et al. INTERMACS profiles and modifiers: heterogeneity of patient classification and the impact of modifiers on predicting patient outcome. J Heart Lung Transplant 2016;35:440–8.

40. Boyle AJ, Ascheim DD, Russo MJ, et al. Clinical outcomes for continuous-flow left ventricular assist device patients stratified by pre-operative INTERMACS classification. J Heart Lung Transplant 2011;30:402–7.

41. Kirklin JK, Pagani FD, Kormos RL, et al. Eighth annual INTERMACS report: special focus on framing the impact of adverse events. J Heart Lung Transplant 2017;36:1080–6.

42. Loghmanpour NA, Kanwar MK, Druzdzel MJ, et al. A new Bayesian network-based risk stratification model for prediction of short-term and long-term LVAD mortality. ASAIO J 2015;61:313–23.

43. Cowger JASJ, Shah P, Dardas TF, et al. Impact of center LVAD volume on outcomes after implant. JACC Heart Fail 2017;5:691–9.

44. Shah N, Chothani A, Agarwal V, et al. Impact of annual hospital volume on outcomes after left ventricular assist device (LVAD) implantation in the contemporary era. J Card Fail 2016;22:232–7.

45. Davis KF, Hohmann SF, Doukky R, et al. The impact of hospital and surgeon volume on in-hospital mortality of ventricular assist device recipients. J Card Fail 2016;22:226–31.

46. Thomas SS, Nahumi N, Han J, et al. Pre-operative mortality risk assessment in patients with continuous-flow left ventricular assist devices: application of the HeartMate II risk score. J Heart Lung Transplant 2014;33:675–81.

47. Deo SV, Daly RC, Altarabsheh SE, et al. Predictive value of the model for end-stage liver disease score in patients undergoing left ventricular assist device implantation. ASAIO J 2013;59:57–62.

48. Matthews JC, Pagani FD, Haft JW, et al. Model for end-stage liver disease score predicts left ventricular assist device operative transfusion requirements, morbidity, and mortality. Circulation 2010;121:214–20.

49. Yang JA, Kato TS, Shulman BP, et al. Liver dysfunction as a predictor of outcomes in patients with advanced heart failure requiring ventricular assist device support: use of the Model of End-stage Liver Disease (MELD) and MELD eXcluding INR (MELD-XI) scoring system. J Heart Lung Transpl 2012;31:601–10.

50. Critsinelis A, Kurihara C, Volkovicher N, et al. MELD-XI scoring system to predict outcomes in patients who undergo LVAD implantation. Ann Thorac Surg 2018. [Epub ahead of print].

51. Loghmanpour NA, Druzdzel MJ, Antaki JF. Cardiac Health Risk Stratification System (CHRiSS): a Bayesian-based decision support system for left ventricular assist device (LVAD) therapy. PLoS One 2014;9:e111264.

52. Birati EY, Hanff TC, Maldonado D, et al. Predicting long term outcome in patients treated with continuous flow left ventricular assist device: the penn-columbia risk score. J Am Heart Assoc 2018;7:e006408.

Perioperative Management of the Right and Left Ventricles

Brent C. Lampert, DO

KEYWORDS

- Left ventricular assist device (LVAD) • Heart failure • Preoperative care • Intraoperative care
- Right ventricular failure • Extracorporeal membrane oxygenation (ECMO)

KEY POINTS

- The greatest risk of death after left ventricular assist device is within the early postoperative period, with in-hospital deaths accounting for two-thirds of all deaths in the first year.
- Preoperative strategies to reduce mortality emphasize medical and mechanical support of the left and right ventricles to improve volume status and organ perfusion; improving nutrition, hematologic abnormalities, and renal function; and reducing infection risks.
- Intraoperative approaches highlight anesthesia related issues, management of concomitant valve disease, right ventricular failure, and weaning from cardiopulmonary bypass.
- Early postoperative efforts concentrate on augmenting right ventricular function, addressing pulmonary hypertension, supporting other end-organ recovery, and quickly identify potential complications.

INTRODUCTION

A majority of patients with heart failure with reduced ejection fraction respond to guideline-directed medical therapy and device therapy. Despite optimal treatment, however, approximately 10% of patients progress to advanced heart failure characterized by progressive symptoms, poor quality of life, poor prognosis, and high risk of recurrent hospitalizations.[1] For appropriately selected patients with advanced heart failure, left ventricular assist devices (LVADs) can provide significant improvements in survival and quality of life.[2,3] As a consequence, rates of LVAD implantation have grown tremendously over the past decade.[4]

Even with improvements in device technology, risk stratification, and patient management,

LVAD support remains associated with high morbidity and mortality.[4] There has been a modest improvement in intermediate and long-term survival in recent years, but short-term mortality after LVAD implant remains high and is essentially unchanged over eras (Fig. 1).[4] The greatest risk of death after LVAD remains during the implant hospitalization with in-hospital deaths accounting for two-thirds of all deaths in the first year.[5]

Numerous preoperative risk factors correlate with adverse outcomes after LVAD implantation. These include older age, presence of cardiogenic shock Interagency Registry for Mechanically Assisted Circulatory Support (INTERMACS) Profiles 1 to 2 (Table 1), need for concurrent right ventricular (RV) support, preimplant dialysis, and increased surgical complexity.[4] Other laboratory findings predictive of in-hospital death after

Disclosure Statement: Dr B.C. Lampert is a consultant for Abbott and has received travel grants from Abiomed and Medtronic.
Division of Cardiovascular Medicine, The Ohio State University Wexner Medical Center, 473 West 12th Avenue, Suite 200, Columbus, OH 43210, USA
E-mail address: Brent.Lampert@osumc.edu

Cardiol Clin 36 (2018) 495–506
https://doi.org/10.1016/j.ccl.2018.06.004
0733-8651/18/© 2018 Elsevier Inc. All rights reserved.

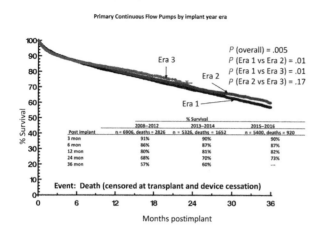

INTERMACS Continuous Flow LVAD/BiVAD Implants: 2008–2016, n = 17633

Fig. 1. Kaplan-Meier survival after continuous flow ventricular assist device implant, stratified by era at the time of implant. BiVAD, biventricular assist device. (*From* Kirklin JK, Pagani FD, Kormos RL, et al. Eighth annual INTERMACS report: special focus on framing the impact of adverse events. J Heart Lung Transplant 2017;36(10):1081; with permission.)

LVAD implant include decreased platelets, elevated international normalized ratio (INR), elevated creatinine, leukocytosis, hypoalbuminemia, and elevated transaminases.[5] These variables are often used to assist in LVAD patient selection and have been combined into numerous risk scores to predict which patients will be successful with LVAD support.[5,6] Numerous perioperative strategies to modify these known risk factors have evolved in an effort to improve LVAD outcomes.

OPTIMIZATION OF THE LEFT VENTRICLE

Previously reserved for short-term support of patients in cardiogenic shock, LVADs have improved sufficiently to allow for intermediate and long-term support in patients waiting for cardiac transplant or as destination therapy in the transplant ineligible. Yet, patients in progressive cardiogenic shock have worse survival (**Fig. 2**) and longer lengths of stay than "less sick" inotrope dependent patients.[4,7] Accordingly, the percentage of LVAD implants in stable, inotrope dependent patients (INTERMACS Profile 3) has steadily increased since 2008.[4] Despite this, delays in the recognition of advanced heart failure or delayed referral to a tertiary center have kept the proportion of patients implanted in cardiogenic shock (INTERMACS Profile 1) stable at 14% to 16%.[4] With limited medical options to optimize left ventricular (LV) function in cardiogenic shock, there is a definitive role for temporary mechanical circulatory support in these situations. Temporary

Table 1
Interagency Registry for Mechanically Assisted Circulatory Support Profiles

Profile	Description	Details
1	Critical cardiogenic shock: crashing and burning	Life-threatening hypotension despite rapidly escalating inotropic support, with critical organ hypoperfusion
2	Progressive decline: sliding on inotropes	Declining function despite intravenous inotrope support
3	Stable but inotrope dependent: dependent stability	Stable on continuous intravenous inotrope support
4	Resting symptoms: frequent flyer	Patient experiences daily symptoms of congestion at rest or with activities of daily living
5	Exertion intolerant: housebound	Patient comfortable at rest and with activities of daily living but unable to engage in any other activity
6	Exertion limited: walking wounded	Patient has fatigue after the first few minutes of any meaningful activity
7	Advanced NYHA class III: NYHA IIIb	Patients living comfortably with meaningful activity limited to mild physical exertion

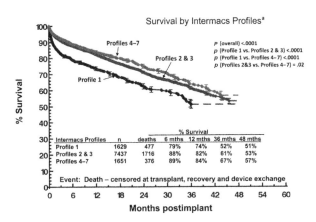

INTERMACS **Continuous Flow LVAD/BiVAD Implants: 2013–2016, n = 10,726**

Fig. 2. Kaplan-Meier survival curves, stratified by INTERMACS Profile at the time of implant. BiVAD, biventricular assist device. [a] 9 patients with unspecified Patient Profile at time of implant. (*From* Kirklin JK, Pagani FD, Kormos RL, et al. Eighth annual INTERMACS report: special focus on framing the impact of adverse events. J Heart Lung Transplant 2017;36(10):1082; with permission.)

mechanical support allows time to decide on a more definitive therapy (bridge to decision) or to optimize patients prior to durable LVAD placement. The ideal timing, duration, and particular temporary support device type, however, remain unknown. Devices commonly used include intra-aortic balloon pumps (IABPs), extracorporeal membrane oxygenation (ECMO), surgically implanted temporary mechanical circulatory support, and percutaneous circulatory devices.

Intra-aortic Balloon Pump

The IABP is the most commonly used mechanical support device. It is widely available, easily and quickly placed, relatively inexpensive, and does not require continuous monitoring by technical support personnel. The IABP, however, provides only a small amount of hemodynamic support. In cardiogenic shock complicating myocardial infarction, where IABP has been the most frequently used, it has shown limited clinical benefit. For instance, in the 600 patient IABP-SHOCK (Intraaortic balloon support for myocardial infarction with cardiogenic shock) trial, the use of IABP did not significantly reduce 30-day mortality in patients with cardiogenic shock complicating myocardial infarction.[8] The need for IABP prior to LVAD implantation is also known to correlate with worse outcomes.[4] Despite this, IABP remains a commonly used strategy to bridge patients or optimize them before LVAD implantation. One small series of 54 patients demonstrated that in patients developing cardiogenic shock more than half were stabilized with IABP support as a bridge to LVAD.[9] Other small series have shown some benefit for the use of prophylactic IABP in INTER-MACS Profile 2 patients[10] and the safety of long-term IABP support as a bridge to LVAD implant.[11]

Extracorporeal Membrane Oxygenation

ECMO is a cardiopulmonary support system that drives blood through an externalized artificial membrane where it removes carbon dioxide and adds oxygen to blood. The pulmonary circulation is bypassed and oxygenated blood can return to the patient via an arterial (venoarterial [VA]) or venous (venovenous [VV]) route (**Fig. 3**). In addition to supporting gas exchange, VA ECMO can support cardiac output and unload both the RV and LV. Peripheral ECMO cannulas can also be placed bedside in an emergency using a cut-down technique and some high-volume centers will place them within catheterization laboratory.

With preoperative cardiogenic shock a significant risk factor for post-LVAD mortality, uncertainty over the likelihood of a durable LVAD reversing the end-organ dysfunction due to cardiogenic shock, and the high cost of durable LVADs, VA-ECMO as emergency temporary circulatory support can successfully bridge patients to a durable LVAD.[12–16] In particular, the use of ECMO prior to LVAD implantation can successfully improve patients from INTERMACS Profile 1 to characteristics more akin to that of the INTERMACS Profile 3.[17] Despite improved hemodynamics and end-organ function, however, post-LVAD morbidity and mortality in patients bridged with ECMO seems similar to INTERMACS Profile 1.[18]

Despite success with this strategy, observational studies have reported overall survival rates of only 20% to 50% in patients receiving ECMO for cardiogenic shock.[19–21] Risk factors for these patients are not fully understood and appropriate patient selection for using ECMO as a bridge to LVAD implantation remains a significant challenge. Additional considerable questions include the

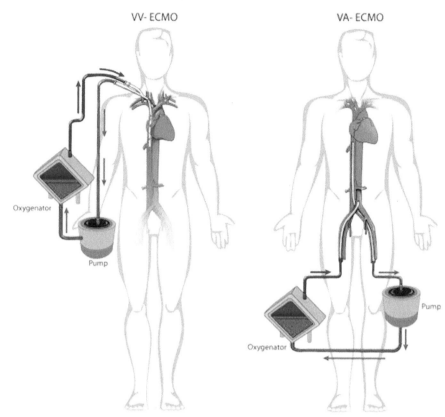

Fig. 3. Commonly implemented VV (*left*) and VA (*right*) ECMO circuit cannulation schemes. (*Adapted from* Squiers JJ, Lima B, DiMaio JM. Contemporary extracorporeal membrane oxygenation therapy in adults: fundamental principles and systematic review of the evidence. J Thorac Cardiovasc Surg 2016;152:23; with permission.)

ethics of and approach to weaning ECMO support from otherwise alert patients who end up not being a candidate for durable LVAD support.

Percutaneous Circulatory Devices

Impella system

The Impella system (Abiomed, Danvers, Massachusetts) is placed retrograde across the aortic valve into the LV. This axial flow pump has a miniature impeller pump that draws blood out of the LV ejecting it into the ascending aorta. The Impella CP provides up to 4 L/min of flow and is placed via a cardiac catheterization procedure. The Impella 5.0 provides 5 L/min of flow but is larger and requires surgical cut down of the femoral or axillary artery for placement. There are few data on the use of the Impella system to optimize patients prior to durable LVAD implantation, but 1 small single-center study demonstrated a 75% survival using the Impella 5.0 to bridge patients to cardiac transplant or durable LVAD implantation.[22] Another retrospective evaluation of 58 patients across 3 centers using Impella 5.0 in patients with

cardiogenic shock demonstrated 67% survival to the next therapy. In this analysis, 20 patients received a durable LVAD with a 65% 1-year survival postimplant.[23]

Tandem heart

The TandemHeart System (CardiacAssist, Pittsburgh, Pennsylvania) is a percutaneously implanted left atrial to aorta bypass system (**Fig. 4**). One limitation of the TandemHeart is difficulty of implant; the left atrium is accessed by transeptal puncture, requiring a skilled operator. Blood is then pumped through an external centrifugal pump into the ileofemoral system. The TandemHeart unloads the heart providing up to 4 L/min of cardiac output support and has been shown to have greater effects on hemodynamics than IABP.[24,25] Small series have demonstrated success using TandemHeart to bridge patients to durable LVAD or transplantation.[26]

Surgical Temporary Mechanical Support

The CentriMag (Abbott, St. Paul, Minnesota) is the most commonly used ventricular assist system as

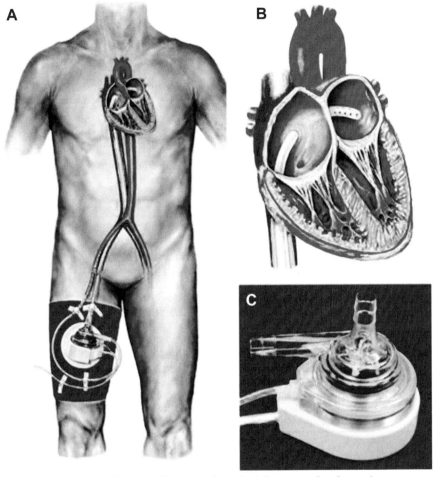

Fig. 4. TandemHeart (*A*) consists of a 21-Fr inflow cannula in the left atrium after femoral venous access and transeptal puncture (*B*) and a 15-Fr to 17-Fr arterial cannula in the iliac artery. The externalized centrifugal motor (*C*) rotates at maximal speed of 7500 rotations per minute delivering 4 liters/min of continuous flow. (*Courtesy of* CardiacAssist, Inc, Pittsburgh, PA.)

a bridge to decision device for patients with refractory cardiogenic shock. This magnetically levitated centrifugal flow pump can be used to support both the RV and LV. Generally, placement of a Centri-Mag requires a median sternotomy but has the advantage of not having stringent anticoagulation requirements if higher flows are able to be maintained. Bridge to decision therapy using a Centri-Mag has been shown to be feasible in a variety of refractory cardiogenic shock settings.[27]

OPTIMIZATION OF THE RIGHT VENTRICLE

Most patients with advanced LV dysfunction have some degree of RV dysfunction and RV failure complicates up to 40% of LVAD implants.[28–30] Acute RV failure after LVAD implant is defined by the INTERMACS as documented elevations of central venous pressure (CVP) and its manifestations, such as edema, ascites, or worsening hepatic or renal dysfunction (**Table 2**).[31] There is also increasing recognition of chronic RV failure occurring weeks to months after LVAD implantation.[32] RV failure after LVAD is associated with increased mortality and can contribute to multiple complications, including coagulopathy, altered drug metabolism, malnutrition, diuretic resistance, and worsened quality of life. Multiple risk scores using clinical, echocardiographic, and hemodynamic factors exist to predict RV failure, but no single variable has been effective to entirely guide patient selection.[32]

Numerous strategies have arisen to optimize RV function prior to LVAD implantation.[33] These largely focus on modifying the laboratory and hemodynamic abnormalities related to RV failure. Elevated CVP has commonly been associated with RV failure post-LVAD implantation and

Table 2
Interagency Registry for Mechanically Assisted Circulatory Support definition of right ventricular failure

RVF definition	Symptoms or findings of persistent RVF characterized by both of the following
	• Elevated CVP documented by
	   ○ Right atrial pressure >16 mm Hg on right heart catheterization
	   ○ Significantly dilated inferior vena cava with no inspiratory variation on echocardiography
	   ○ Elevated JVP
	• Manifestations of elevated CVP characterized by
	   ○ Peripheral edema (≥2+)
	   ○ Ascites or hepatomegaly on examination or diagnostic imaging
	   ○ Laboratory evidence of worsening hepatic (total bilirubin >2.0) or renal dysfunction (creatinine >2.0)

Severity scale	
Mild	Patient meets both criteria for RVF plus • Postimplant inotropes, inhaled nitric oxide or intravenous vasodilators not continued beyond postoperative day 7 after VAD implant and • No inotropes continued beyond postoperative day 7 after VAD implant
Moderate	Patient meets both criteria for RVF plus • Postimplant inotropes, inhaled nitric oxide or intravenous vasodilators continued beyond postoperative day 7 and up postoperative day 14 after VAD implant
Severe	Patient meets both criteria for RVF plus • CVP or right atrial pressure >16 mm Hg and • Prolonged postimplant inotropes, inhaled nitric oxide or intravenous vasodilators continued beyond postoperative day 14 after VAD implant
Severe–acute	Patient meets both criteria for RVF plus • CVP or right atrial pressure >16 mm Hg and • Need for RVAD at any time after VAD implant or • Death during VAD implants hospitalization with RVF as primary cause

Abbreviations: JVP, jugular venous pressure; RVF, right ventricular failure; VAD, ventricular assist device.

hemodynamic guided heart failure management to lower CVP is strongly recommended for at risk patients. The optimal preoperative CVP has not been described, but a CVP greater than 15 mm Hg is associated with RV failure.[30] Aggressive diuresis, or ultrafiltration if diuresis is infective, can be used to lower CVP. Strategies to optimize RV afterload may also improve hemodynamics. Pulmonary vasodilators, such as inhaled nitrous oxide and phosphodiesterase-5 inhibitors, have been shown to improve pre-LVAD implantation hemodynamics, but their effect on reducing postimplant RV failure remains uncertain.[34,35] Perioperative inotrope support and the avoidance of β-blockers may also decrease the risk of RV failure.

Despite rigorous patient selection and preoperative optimization, RV failure necessitating mechanical support with a RV assist device (RVAD) still occurs and is associated with worse outcomes.[4] Elective RVAD implantation, however, correlates with better long-term survival and survival to transplant than emergent implant and should be considered in high risk patients.[36,37] Multiple technologies originally designed for LV support have been modified for temporary RV support. IABP can improve RV hemodynamics and echocardiographic indices prior to LVAD implantation.[38] Preoperative use of IABP has been shown to stabilize patients with RV failure and improve post-VAD outcomes.[9,10] As well as the tradition femoral access for IABP, an alternative approach of axillary or subclavian insertion to allow for patient ambulation and avoidance of deconditioning before LVAD implantation has been successfully described.[39] The Impella 5.0 is another mechanical support option used to effectively bridge patients with borderline RV function to LVAD.[22] The Impella RP is a percutaneously inserted axial flow pump designed specifically for short-term RV support that can be used to optimize or bridge patients to durable LVAD.[40] For refractory shock requiring intensified mechanical support, the CentriMag and TandemHeart have both been used for temporary RV support.[40,41] Bridge-to-transplant patients with refractory biventricular failure should be considered for planned biventricular support or total artificial heart. The total artificial heart can improve survival, but its use is not approved for patients who are ineligible for transplant.[42]

OTHER PREOPERATIVE OPTIMIZATION
Nutrition

Malnutrition can increase the risk of postoperative infection and delayed wound healing and has been associated with increased mortality after cardiac surgery.[43] Specially, serum albumin less than 3.3 mg/dL is associated with a 6.6-fold increase in mortality after LVAD implantation, making it a considerable risk factor.[5] Screening for malnutrition in patients prior to LVAD implantation should include at least measures of serum albumin and prealbumin.[33] When a malnourished patient is identified, a nutritional evaluation and appropriate nutritional interventions should be considered. If clinical status allows, LVAD implantation should be delayed to maximize nutritional status.[33] Significant malnutrition, however, is often a consequence of advanced heart failure. It rarely occurs in isolation, frequently associated with abnormal liver function and other known significant risk factors. There is no evidence that aggressive nutritional support for days to weeks before LVAD implantation improves outcomes, and potential improvements in nutritional status should be weighed against the risks of the time needed to make meaningful improvement, delaying surgery.

Coagulation and Hematologic Disorders

Bleeding is a common complication with LVAD implantation owing to RV failure causing hepatic dysfunction, frequent use of antiplatelets, and anticoagulant medications, and previous sternotomies in these patients. Elevated INR not due to pharmacologic therapy should be evaluated prior to implant to determine etiology. Hypercoagulable assessment and hematology assessment should also be completed in appropriate patients. If the clinical scenario allows, correction of elevated INR or low platelet count should be done prior to surgery. Unless there is a strong indication for their use, thienopyridine antiplatelet agents should also be stopped at least 5 days prior to surgery.[33] Testing for heparin-induced thrombocytopenia should be considered for patients with a platelet count less than,150,000 or those who have had a 20% decrease in their baseline platelet count.[33]

Infection

Infection remains a leading cause of morbidity and mortality in LVAD patients.[4] Numerous preoperative factors common in advanced heart failure contribute to an increased risk of infection. These include malnutrition, renal failure, prolonged hospitalizations, and the need for indwelling catheters and intravenous lines. Patients considered for LVAD implantation should be assessed for signs of infection and any infection should be eradicated prior to implantation. Dental assessment and nasal swab to screen for methicillin-resistant *Staphylococcus aureus* with treatment as indicated should be a part of this evaluation.[33,44] All unnecessary lines and catheters should also be removed prior to LVAD implantation.[33,44] Finally, preoperative antibiotic prophylaxis with broad spectrum gram-negative and gram-positive coverage should be given.[33,44]

Renal Function

Renal dysfunction is common at the time of LVAD implantation. It results from a combination of intrinsic renal disease, elevated right atrial pressure, renal hypoperfusion, and heart failure related neurohormonal activation. Advanced renal dysfunction requiring chronic dialysis after LVAD implant presents technical challenges, because few dialysis centers are willing to accept LVAD patients. Moreover, it is associated with high levels of morbidity and mortality making improving renal function particularly important to preoperative optimization.[45,46] Complicating the preoperative assessment is that renal function may improve with the improved hemodynamics after LVAD implantation. For example, in the HeartMate II bridge to transplant trial, renal function improved over 6 months after LVAD implantation. The baseline renal function was only moderately impaired, however, in this cohort with a mean creatinine of 1.4 mg/dL $\pm$ 0.5 mg/dL and the impact of LVAD implantation on patients with more advanced renal disease is unknown.[47] Moreover, the improvement in renal function may be temporary. A large review of INTERMACS data demonstrated that despite substantial early improvement in renal function, by 1 year the estimated glomerular filtration rate was only 6.7% above the preimplant value.[48]

Patients with low urine output or worsening creatinine should have hemodynamic-guided optimization prior to LVAD implantation.[33] Aggressive diuresis and inotropic support should be initiated if clinically indicated. Once patients are optimized, assessment of serum creatinine, serum urea nitrogen, and 24-hour urine collection for creatinine clearance and proteinuria should be obtained. If aggressive medical therapy does not result in acceptable renal function, temporary mechanical support can be considered. Permanent dialysis, however, is generally considered a contraindication for LVAD placement.[33] Exceptions may be made at some centers to implant an LVAD in select dialysis patients being considered for combination heart kidney transplantation.

INTRAOPERATIVE OPTIMIZATION

There are many technical considerations during LVAD implantation that influence surgical and long-term outcomes. Key matters include anesthesia-related issues, management of concomitant valve disease, RV failure, and weaning from cardiopulmonary bypass.

Anesthesia Management

Management of anesthesia for patients undergoing LVAD implantation requires a thorough understanding of the pathophysiology of cardiogenic shock and the unique challenges associated with mechanical support. Due to a combination of autonomic dysfunction, advanced biventricular dysfunction, and frequent use of long-acting angiotensin-converting enzyme inhibitors, patients with heart failure are susceptible to significant hypotension with anesthesia induction. Further contributing to hypotension is that intubation and positive pressure ventilation may increase RV afterload and decrease venous return. In addition to standard monitoring, an arterial catheter and pulmonary artery catheter should be used to allow for continuous monitoring during induction and throughout the surgery. Prior to anesthesia induction, defibrillators should be turned off. Before patient is placed on cardiopulmonary bypass, a comprehensive transesophageal echocardiogram (TEE) should be performed. In addition ato assessing valvular function, TEE can evaluate for the presence of patent foramen ovale (PFO), intracardiac thrombi, or severe aortic atherosclerosis. The TEE also provides baseline assessment of RV size and function. During the surgery, TEE can provide intracardiac air surveillance and evaluate proper position of the LVAD inflow cannula and septal position. Additionally, TEE can monitor the degree of LV unloading throughout the procedure and during the immediate postbypass period.

Concomitant Valve Disease

Valve pathology commonly exists in patients undergoing LVAD implantation and the intraoperative approach to treating it remains a subject of debate. Tricuspid regurgitation (TR) is common in advanced heart failure. It results from pulmonary hypertension with chronic right heart pressure and volume overload, atrial fibrillation, presence of transvalvular leads, and advancing age. Correction of TR may improve RV function

and is frequently performed at the time of LVAD implantation. No consensus exits, however, on which patient should have tricuspid valve repair. Generally, patients with moderate to severe TR have repair done at the time of LVAD implant.[33,49,50] TV annulus greater than 40 mm[51] and the presence of atrial fibrillation,[52] however, have also been suggested as criteria to guide TV repair.

Conversely, a large review of more than 2000 patients in The Society of Thoracic Surgeons National Database found that TV procedures in LVAD patients with moderate to severe TR did not reduce early mortality or the need for an RVAD but were associated with more postoperative renal failure and prolonged intensive care unit and hospital lengths of stay.[53] INTERMACS has also reported that concomitant cardiac surgery at the time of LVAD implant is associated with increased early mortality.[54] Further investigation is needed to guide TV repair at the time of LVAD implantation.

Functional mitral valve regurgitation is a common consequence of advanced heart failure.[55] LV unloading from the LVAD regularly decreases LV size and improves mitral regurgitation, and concurrent mitral valve surgery is infrequently done. Concomitant mitral valve procedures have not been associated with increased survival but may provide some benefit of improved quality of life in highly selected patients.[56] Mitral valve stenosis is rarely encountered in advanced heart failure patients, but if present should be corrected at the time of implant so it does not limit LVAD filling or maintain pulmonary hypertension.

Significant aortic regurgitation can create a circuitous flow of blood from the LVAD outflow cannula back through the incompetent valve into the LV, causing systemic hypoperfusion. Prolonged LVAD support can worsen preexisting aortic regurgitation or contribute to de novo regurgitation from reduced systolic excursion and resulting valve deterioration.[57,58] Patients expected to be on LVAD support for an extended period of time with more than mild aortic regurgitation should have it corrected at the time of LVAD implantation.[33] Options for surgical management of aortic regurgitation include repair by sewing the leading edges together or replacing the valve with a biological prosthesis.[33]

Unloading of the LV with an LVAD can create a pressure gradient from the right to left atrium exaggerating right to left shunting through a PFO resulting in systemic hypoxemia. In addition to echo evaluation, careful direct inspection for a PFO should be done at the time of surgery. If present, the PFO should be closed at the time of LVAD implantation.[33]

Right Ventricular Dysfunction

In addition to the preoperative RV optimization strategies (discussed previously), several intraoperative approaches can minimize the risk of RV failure. Intraoperative RV hypoperfusion can contribute to worsening RV failure. Hypoperfusion can be the result of air emboli or systemic hypotension. Deairing maneuvers and TEE surveillance for air emboli should be used. Preserving adequate systemic blood pressure with a combination of epinephrine, norepinephrine, and vasopressin can also protect the RV. Treatment of obstructive coronary artery disease of the right coronary artery or grafts supplying the RV distribution should also be considered.

Perioperative bleeding should be minimized as excessive transfusions can result in pulmonary edema or transfusion-related lung injury, increasing RV afterload.[59] Reduced cardiopulmonary bypass times and aggressive inotrope support when weaning from bypass to LVAD support may also reduce the incidence of RV failure.[51] Finally, some centers administer inhaled nitric oxide or prostacyclin as a pharmaceutical bridge for those with preexisting pulmonary hypertension and struggling RV function.

Weaning from Cardiopulmonary Bypass

When the LVAD implant is completed, pharmacologic cardiac support is initiated and weaning from bypass commences allowing the LV to be adequately filled. The LVAD is started when the patient is off bypass or at minimal flows.[33] The device speed is then gradually increased with diligent attention to optimize LV decompression without excessive leftward shift of the interventricular septum. TEE is used to monitor the position of the interventricular septum, degree of LV decompression, mitral regurgitation, aortic insufficiency, and RV function. According to the TEE findings, LVAD speed settings, fluid requirements, and inotrope needs can be adjusted. To avoid increased pulmonary vasoconstriction and stress on the RV, optimal oxygenation and acid base balance should be achieved prior to separation from bypass. Pulmonary vasodilators such as inhaled nitric oxide or prostaglandin can also be used to reduce RV afterload. CVP should be closely monitored with care to avoid over distention of the RV. In general, a CVP of less than or equal to 14 mm Hg is preferred.

EARLY POSTOPERATIVE OPTIMIZATION

The primary goals of early postoperative optimization are to augment RV function, support other end-organ recovery, and quickly identify potential complications. Most patients have at least 1 adverse event in the first 60 days after LVAD implant with the most common events being bleeding and infection.[60] Several strategies can be used to minimize these risks.

Invasive arterial and pulmonary artery catheter monitoring should be maintained in the early postoperative period to allow for optimization of diuresis, pharmacologic cardiac support, and pump speed. Therapies should be adjusted to balance maintenance of appropriate intravascular volume while avoiding anemia, hypovolemia, and RV overload. Cardiac index greater than 2.2 L/min/m^2 and mean arterial pressure 70 mm Hg to 90 mm Hg should be targeted.[33] Low pump output and significant CVP elevations greater than 20 mm Hg necessitate urgent echocardiographic evaluation to rule out tamponade or other technical complications. Triggers of pulmonary hypertension (acidosis and hypoxia) that may compromise RV function should be remediated. Bleeding should be controlled by correcting any coagulopathies as needed. Bleeding that is not controlled despite correcting coagulopathies should be surgically evaluated. Blood transfusions for anemia should be individualized based on the clinical scenario.[33] Extubation should be attempted within 24 hours after LVAD implantation in otherwise stable patients but close monitoring of oxygenation and ventilation is imperative to avoid provocation of RV failure. Invasive lines and drains should also be removed as soon as the patient's condition allows to minimize infectious complications. If the clinical situation allows, patients should also be fed and out of bed to a chair on postoperative day 1.

SUMMARY

LVADs provide substantial improvements in survival and quality of life in select advanced heart failure patients. With improved technology, patient selection, and management strategies, the rate of LVAD implantation continues to grow. LVAD support, however, remains associated with significant morbidity and mortality with the greatest risk of death occurring during the implant hospitalization. Numerous strategies are used throughout the perioperative period minimize this risk. Medical and mechanical support options are used for both RV and LV optimization, but absolute criteria for their use remain uncertain. Other preoperative strategies emphasize improving nutrition, hematologic abnormalities, infection risk, and renal function. Intraoperative approaches highlight anesthesia related issues, management of concomitant valve disease, RV failure, and weaning from cardiopulmonary bypass. Finally, early postoperative efforts concentrate on augmenting RV function, supporting other end-organ recovery, and quickly identify potential complications.

REFERENCES

1. Metra M, Ponikowski P, Dickstein K, et al. Advanced chronic heart failure: a position statement from the study group on advanced heart failure of the heart failure association of the european society of cardiology. Eur J Heart Fail 2007;9(6–7):684–94.

2. Rose EA, Gelijns AC, Moskowitz AJ, et al. Long-term use of a left ventricular assist device for end-stage heart failure. N Engl J Med 2001;345(20):1435–43.

3. Rogers JG, Aaronson KD, Boyle AJ, et al. Continuous flow left ventricular assist device improves functional capacity and quality of life of advanced heart failure patients. J Am Coll Cardiol 2010; 55(17):1826–34.

4. Kirklin JK, Pagani FD, Kormos RL, et al. Eighth annual INTERMACS report: special focus on framing the impact of adverse events. J Heart Lung Transplant 2017;36(10):1080–6.

5. Lietz K, Long JW, Kfoury AG, et al. Outcomes of left ventricular assist device implantation as destination therapy in the post-REMATCH era: implications for patient selection. Circulation 2007;116(5): 497–505.

6. Cowger J, Sundareswaran K, Rogers JG, et al. Predicting survival in patients receiving continuous flow left ventricular assist devices: the HeartMate II risk score. J Am Coll Cardiol 2013;61(3):313–21.

7. Cowger J, Shah P, Stulak J, et al. INTERMACS profiles and modifiers: heterogeneity of patient classification and the impact of modifiers on predicting patient outcome. J Heart Lung Transplant 2016; 35(4):440–8.

8. Thiele H, Zeymer U, Neumann FJ, et al. Intraaortic balloon support for myocardial infarction with cardiogenic shock. N Engl J Med 2012;367(14): 1287–96.

9. Sintek MA, Gdowski M, Lindman BR, et al. Intra-aortic balloon counterpulsation in patients with chronic heart failure and cardiogenic shock: clinical response and predictors of stabilization. J Card Fail 2015;21(11):868–76.

10. Imamura T, Kinugawa K, Nitta D, et al. Prophylactic intra-aortic balloon pump before ventricular assist device implantation reduces perioperative medical expenses and improves postoperative clinical course in INTERMACS profile 2 patients. Circ J 2015;79(9):1963–9.

11. Koudoumas D, Malliaras K, Theodoropoulos S, et al. Long-term intra-aortic balloon pump support as bridge to left ventricular assist device implantation. J Card Surg 2016;31(7):467–71.

12. Pagani FD, Lynch W, Swaniker F, et al. Extracorporeal life support to left ventricular assist device bridge to heart transplant: a strategy to optimize survival and resource utilization. Circulation 1999; 100(19 Suppl):II206–10.

13. Pagani FD, Aaronson KD, Dyke DB, et al. Assessment of an extracorporeal life support to LVAD bridge to heart transplant strategy. Ann Thorac Surg 2000;70(6):1977–84 [discussion: 1984–5].

14. Hoefer D, Ruttmann E, Poelzl G, et al. Outcome evaluation of the bridge-to-bridge concept in patients with cardiogenic shock. Ann Thorac Surg 2006; 82(1):28–33.

15. Toda K, Fujita T, Kobayashi J, et al. Impact of preoperative percutaneous cardiopulmonary support on outcome following left ventricular assist device implantation. Circ J 2012;76(1):88–95.

16. Russo CF, Cannata A, Lanfranconi M, et al. Veno-arterial extracorporeal membrane oxygenation using levitronix centrifugal pump as bridge to decision for refractory cardiogenic shock. J Thorac Cardiovasc Surg 2010;140(6):1416–21.

17. Schibilsky D, Haller C, Lange B, et al. Extracorporeal life support prior to left ventricular assist device implantation leads to improvement of the patients INTERMACS levels and outcome. PLoS One 2017; 12(3):e0174262.

18. Shah P, Pagani FD, Desai SS, et al. Outcomes of patients receiving temporary circulatory support before durable ventricular assist device. Ann Thorac Surg 2017;103(1):106–12.

19. Combes A, Leprince P, Luyt CE, et al. Outcomes and long-term quality-of-life of patients supported by extracorporeal membrane oxygenation for refractory cardiogenic shock. Crit Care Med 2008;36(5): 1404–11.

20. Chang CH, Chen HC, Caffrey JL, et al. Survival analysis after extracorporeal membrane oxygenation in critically ill adults: a nationwide cohort study. Circulation 2016;133(24):2423–33.

21. Pontailler M, Demondion P, Lebreton G, et al. Experience with extracorporeal life support for cardiogenic shock in the older population more than 70 years of age. ASAIO J 2017;63(3):279–84.

22. Lima B, Kale P, Gonzalez-Stawinski GV, et al. Effectiveness and safety of the impella 5.0 as a bridge to cardiac transplantation or durable left ventricular assist device. Am J Cardiol 2016; 117(10):1622–8.

23. Hall SA, Uriel N, Carey SA, et al. Use of a percutaneous temporary circulatory support device as a

bridge to decision during acute decompensation of advanced heart failure. J Heart Lung Transplant 2018;37(1):100–6.

24. Thiele H, Sick P, Boudriot E, et al. Randomized comparison of intra-aortic balloon support with a percutaneous left ventricular assist device in patients with revascularized acute myocardial infarction complicated by cardiogenic shock. Eur Heart J 2005; 26(13):1276–83.

25. Burkhoff D, Cohen H, Brunckhorst C, et al, TandemHeart Investigators Group. A randomized multicenter clinical study to evaluate the safety and efficacy of the TandemHeart percutaneous ventricular assist device versus conventional therapy with intraaortic balloon pumping for treatment of cardiogenic shock. Am Heart J 2006;152(3):469. e1-8.

26. Kar B, Gregoric ID, Basra SS, et al. The percutaneous ventricular assist device in severe refractory cardiogenic shock. J Am Coll Cardiol 2011;57(6): 688–96.

27. Takayama H, Soni L, Kalesan B, et al. Bridge-to-decision therapy with a continuous-flow external ventricular assist device in refractory cardiogenic shock of various causes. Circ Heart Fail 2014;7(5): 799–806.

28. Dang NC, Topkara VK, Mercando M, et al. Right heart failure after left ventricular assist device implantation in patients with chronic congestive heart failure. J Heart Lung Transplant 2006; 25(1):1–6.

29. Patel ND, Weiss ES, Schaffer J, et al. Right heart dysfunction after left ventricular assist device implantation: a comparison of the pulsatile HeartMate I and axial-flow HeartMate II devices. Ann Thorac Surg 2008;86(3):832–40 [discussion: 832–40].

30. Kormos RL, Teuteberg JJ, Pagani FD, et al. Right ventricular failure in patients with the HeartMate II continuous-flow left ventricular assist device: incidence, risk factors, and effect on outcomes. J Thorac Cardiovasc Surg 2010;139(5):1316–24.

31. Interagency registry for mechanically assisted circulatory support (INTERMACS). Appendix A: Adverse event definitions: Adult and pediatric patients (2013). Available at: http://www.uab.edu/medicine/intermacs/intermacs-documents. Accessed January 16, 2018.

32. Lampert BC, Teuteberg JJ. Right ventricular failure after left ventricular assist devices. J Heart Lung Transplant 2015;34(9):1123–30.

33. Feldman D, Pamboukian SV, Teuteberg JJ, et al. The 2013 international society for heart and lung transplantation guidelines for mechanical circulatory support: executive summary. J Heart Lung Transplant 2013;32(2):157–87.

34. Argenziano M, Choudhri AF, Moazami N, et al. Randomized, double-blind trial of inhaled nitric oxide in LVAD recipients with pulmonary hypertension. Ann Thorac Surg 1998;65(2):340–5.

35. Tedford RJ, Hemnes AR, Russell SD, et al. PDE5A inhibitor treatment of persistent pulmonary hypertension after mechanical circulatory support. Circ Heart Fail 2008;1(4):213–9.

36. Fitzpatrick JR 3rd, Frederick JR, Hiesinger W, et al. Early planned institution of biventricular mechanical circulatory support results in improved outcomes compared with delayed conversion of a left ventricular assist device to a biventricular assist device. J Thorac Cardiovasc Surg 2009; 137(4):971–7.

37. Morgan JA, John R, Lee BJ, et al. Is severe right ventricular failure in left ventricular assist device recipients a risk factor for unsuccessful bridging to transplant and post-transplant mortality. Ann Thorac Surg 2004;77(3):859–63.

38. Ntalianis A, Kapelios CJ, Kanakakis J, et al. Prolonged intra-aortic balloon pump support in biventricular heart failure induces right ventricular reverse remodeling. Int J Cardiol 2015;192:3–8.

39. Tanaka A, Tuladhar SM, Onsager D, et al. The subclavian intraaortic balloon pump: a compelling bridge device for advanced heart failure. Ann Thorac Surg 2015;100(6):2151–7 [discussion: 2157–8].

40. Kapur NK, Paruchuri V, Korabathina R, et al. Effects of a percutaneous mechanical circulatory support device for medically refractory right ventricular failure. J Heart Lung Transplant 2011; 30(12):1360–7.

41. Bhama JK, Kormos RL, Toyoda Y, et al. Clinical experience using the levitronix CentriMag system for temporary right ventricular mechanical circulatory support. J Heart Lung Transplant 2009;28(9): 971–6.

42. Copeland JG, Smith RG, Arabia FA, et al. Cardiac replacement with a total artificial heart as a bridge to transplantation. N Engl J Med 2004;351(9): 859–67.

43. Engelman DT, Adams DH, Byrne JG, et al. Impact of body mass index and albumin on morbidity and mortality after cardiac surgery. J Thorac Cardiovasc Surg 1999;118(5):866–73.

44. Kusne S, Mooney M, Danziger-Isakov L, et al. An ISHLT consensus document for prevention and management strategies for mechanical circulatory support infection. J Heart Lung Transplant 2017; 36(10):1137–53.

45. Sandner SE, Zimpfer D, Zrunek P, et al. Renal function and outcome after continuous flow left ventricular assist device implantation. Ann Thorac Surg 2009;87(4):1072–8.

46. Topkara VK, Dang NC, Barili F, et al. Predictors and outcomes of continuous veno-venous hemodialysis use after implantation of a left ventricular

assist device. J Heart Lung Transplant 2006;25(4): 404–8.

47. Russell SD, Rogers JG, Milano CA, et al. Renal and hepatic function improve in advanced heart failure patients during continuous-flow support with the HeartMate II left ventricular assist device. Circulation 2009;120(23):2352–7.

48. Brisco MA, Kimmel SE, Coca SG, et al. Prevalence and prognostic importance of changes in renal function after mechanical circulatory support. Circ Heart Fail 2014;7(1):68–75.

49. Piacentino V 3rd, Troupes CD, Ganapathi AM, et al. Clinical impact of concomitant tricuspid valve procedures during left ventricular assist device implantation. Ann Thorac Surg 2011;92(4):1414–8 [discussion: 1418–9].

50. Maltais S, Topilsky Y, Tchantchaleishvili V, et al. Surgical treatment of tricuspid valve insufficiency promotes early reverse remodeling in patients with axial-flow left ventricular assist devices. J Thorac Cardiovasc Surg 2012;143(6):1370–6.

51. Krishan K, Nair A, Pinney S, et al. Liberal use of tricuspid-valve annuloplasty during left-ventricular assist device implantation. Eur J Cardiothorac Surg 2012;41(1):213–7.

52. Anwer LA, Tchantchaleishvili V, Poddi S, et al. Atrial fibrillation should guide prophylactic tricuspid procedures during left ventricular assist device implantation. ASAIO J 2017. [Epub ahead of print].

53. Robertson JO, Grau-Sepulveda MV, Okada S, et al. Concomitant tricuspid valve surgery during implantation of continuous-flow left ventricular assist devices: a society of thoracic surgeons database analysis. J Heart Lung Transplant 2014;33(6): 609–17.

54. Kirklin JK, Naftel DC, Pagani FD, et al. Seventh INTERMACS annual report: 15,000 patients and counting. J Heart Lung Transplant 2015;34(12): 1495–504.

55. Patel JB, Borgeson DD, Barnes ME, et al. Mitral regurgitation in patients with advanced systolic heart failure. J Card Fail 2004;10(4):285–91.

56. Robertson JO, Naftel DC, Myers SL, et al. Concomitant mitral valve procedures in patients undergoing implantation of continuous-flow left ventricular assist devices: an INTERMACS database analysis. J Heart Lung Transplant 2018;37(1):79–88.

57. Pak SW, Uriel N, Takayama H, et al. Prevalence of de novo aortic insufficiency during long-term support with left ventricular assist devices. J Heart Lung Transplant 2010;29(10):1172–6.

58. Mudd JO, Cuda JD, Halushka M, et al. Fusion of aortic valve commissures in patients supported by a continuous axial flow left ventricular assist device. J Heart Lung Transplant 2008;27(12):1269–74.

59. Goldstein DJ, Beauford RB. Left ventricular assist devices and bleeding: adding insult to injury. Ann Thorac Surg 2003;75(6 Suppl):S42–7.

60. Genovese EA, Dew MA, Teuteberg JJ, et al. Incidence and patterns of adverse event onset during the first 60 days after ventricular assist device implantation. Ann Thorac Surg 2009;88(4):1162–70.

Ventricular Assist Device Infections

Saima Aslam, MD, MS

KEYWORDS

• VAD infection • Driveline infection • Ventricular assist device

KEY POINTS

- Ventricular assist device (VAD) infections are common and associated with increased morbidity and mortality.
- The International Society for Heart and Lung Transplantation's criteria should be used to diagnose a VAD-specific and VAD-related infection.
- VAD infections are biofilm based and difficult to eradicate.
- Treatment strategies for VAD infection include intravenous antibiotics followed by oral suppression in tandem with surgical debridement.
- Prevention strategies center on patient selection, surgical strategies, and driveline management.

INTRODUCTION

Ventricular assist devices (VADs) are well established as a therapy for heart failure and are increasingly used on a global scale both for destination therapy and as a bridge to transplant. The International Society for Heart and Lung Transplantation Registry for Mechanically Assisted Circulatory Support's (IMACS) first report published outcomes of almost 6000 VAD recipients who received an implant between 2013 and 2014 in 31 countries.[1] A recent report from the Interagency Registry for Mechanically Assisted Circulatory Support (INTERMACS) (which publishes data on VADs placed in the United States) published outcomes of more than 15,000 VAD recipients over a 9-year period.[2]

As VADs have evolved over the past 2 decades, so has the epidemiology of infection. Previous first-generation pulsatile-flow devices were associated with high rates of bacterial and fungal infection, the latter being associated with up to a 90% mortality rate.[3] However, changes in device type and size as well as improvement in surgical techniques have led to a decreased incidence of infection. **Fig. 1** demonstrates the significant difference in freedom from bacteremia between the current continuous-flow devices when compared with the older pulsatile VADs.[4] Within the category of continuous-flow devices, there has been a significant decline in the rate of sepsis in the recent era as well: from 8.22 per 100 patient months in the era 2008 to 2011 to 7.28 per 100 patient months in the era 2012 to 2014.[2] Despite the decline in event rate, infection remains an important cause of morbidity and mortality in these patients. The incidence of infection-related death is highest in the early postoperative period and then subsides; but with a longer support period, the incidence increases again, as noted in **Fig. 2**.[2] In fact, infection is the third most common cause of death 1 year following device placement after neurologic complications and multisystem organ failure; the rate of infection steadily increases up to 4 years of follow-up.[2]

In addition to the morbidity associated with the infection itself, VAD infections are also implicated in complications, such as device thrombosis, stroke, intracerebral hemorrhage, and gastrointestinal bleeding. It is difficult to state this conclusively

Disclosure Statement: None relevant.

Division of Infectious Diseases and Global Public Health, University of California, San Diego, 4510 Executive Drive, Suite P-725, MC 7745, San Diego, CA 92121, USA

E-mail address: saslam@ucsd.edu

Cardiol Clin 36 (2018) 507–517
https://doi.org/10.1016/j.ccl.2018.06.005

cardiology.theclinics.com

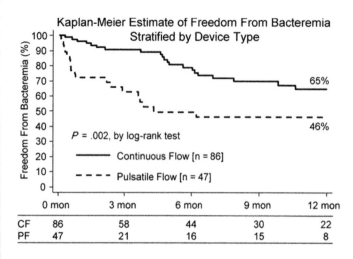

Fig. 1. Significant difference in freedom from bacteremia between pulsatile and continuous-flow VADs. CF, continuous flow; PF, pulsatile flow. (*Adapted from* Schaffer, Allen JG, Weiss ES, et al. Infectious complications after pulsatile-flow and continuous-flow left ventricular assist device implantation. J Heart Lung Transplant 2011;30(2):168; with permission.)

based on current evidence, as some of these complications may also predispose to infection.[5,6]

VENTRICULAR ASSIST DEVICE INFECTIONS AND DIAGNOSTIC CRITERIA

The International Society of Heart and Lung Transplantation (ISHLT) published a consensus paper in 2011 that clearly defined infections in VAD recipients and put forth diagnostic criteria in order to standardize such definitions with the goal of making comparison of infection rates simpler across different studies and clinically relevant.[7]

Infection is divided in 3 main categories: VAD-specific, VAD-related, and non-VAD infections.

- VAD-specific infections are those that are related directly to the device hardware and are specific to VAD recipients. This category includes infections of the driveline, surgical pocket, pump, and cannula and may present as a continuum.

- VAD-related infections are those that can occur in patients without VADs but warrant special considerations in a VAD recipient because of the presence of hardware. This category includes infections such as bacteremia, mediastinitis, and endocarditis.
- Non-VAD infections are those that are unrelated to the indwelling device and consist of infections such as pneumonia, urinary tract infection, and *Clostridium difficile* infection.

Detailed diagnostic criteria and definitions for VAD-specific and VAD-related infections were published by the ISHLT in 2011.[7] In brief, driveline infection (DLI) can be considered to be superficial if the infection is superficial to the fascial/muscle layers or deep if it is present within these tissue planes. Pump and/or cannula infections are diagnosed based on direct microbiological cultures from the device and/or blood cultures along with appropriate clinical presentation and imaging

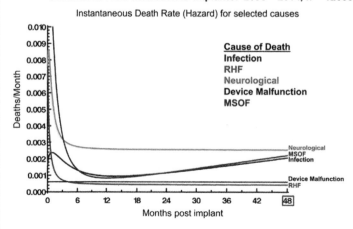

Fig. 2. Hazard function curves indicating the instantaneous risk of death overtime showing the bimodal pattern related to infection following VAD placement. BiVAD, biventricular assist device; LVAD, left VAD; MSOF, multisystem organ failure; RHF, right heart failure. (*From* Kirklin JK, Naftel DC, Pagani FD, et al. Seventh INTERMACS annual report: 15,000 patients and counting. J Heart Lung Transplant 2015;34(12):1498; with permission.)

criteria (such as fluid collection within the pump pocket).

Infection in VAD recipients occurs from a variety of different sources as illustrated earlier based on the timing of infection. In general, infection within the first 3 months following implant is commonly related to sources such as central venous and urinary catheters, postoperative pneumonia, and *C difficile* infection and may be from the device itself as well.[8] Later-onset infections tend to be associated with the device, most commonly driveline infections.[4,8,9]

In clinical practice, however, one type of infection may coexist or lead to another type of infection. The difficulty is particularly acute with the occurrence of bloodstream infection in a VAD recipient. It is important to parse out if the bloodstream infection arose from an infected VAD versus a different source, as the treatment duration may be different in each case. Additionally, there is concern that once a bloodstream infection arises, it has the potential to seed the device and set up a series of events that may lead to device infection as well as thrombosis.

The most common VAD-specific infections are driveline infections with an overall event rate of 14% to 48% between various studies, and these tend to increase as a function of support duration.[2,9–12] Bacteremia is less common; a recent study of approximately 10,000 VAD recipients from the IMACS' database noted an incidence of 12%.[8] Patients who survived an episode of bacteremia within the first 3 months after device implant still had a significantly higher mortality rate at 2 years.[8] Hemorrhagic stroke is now recognized as a complication of bacteremia in left VAD patients. Several studies have noted that bacteremia and/or pump infection were independent risk factors for hemorrhagic stroke and death from neurologic complications.[5,6,13,14]

MICROBIOLOGY

The 2 key pathogens associated with VAD-specific and -related infections are *Staphylococcus aureus* and *Pseudomonas aeruginosa*. Other organisms noted in various studies include *Staphylococcus epidermidis*, *Enterococcus* species, other gram-negative bacilli such as *Klebsiella* species, *Escherichia coli*, as well as *Candida* species. Candida infections are associated with very high mortality, up to 90%.[3] **Table 1** shows the relative distribution of organisms across recent studies. A common clinical problem is the issue of superinfection, that is, the development of a new infection while patients are on suppressive antibiotics therapy for a primary VAD infection.[15,16]

Table 1
Microbiological distribution of pathogenic organisms causing ventricular assist device infections

Organism	Device Infection
Staphylococci	31%–42%
Enterococci	14.5%
Pseudomonas aeruginosa	23.5%–31.0%
Other gram-negative bacilli	5.0%–27.5%
Candida species	4.3%–10.0%

Data from Refs.[4,9,15,48]

PATHOGENESIS

VAD-specific infections, including deep driveline infections and pump/cannula infections, arise from biofilms, which comprise microorganisms embedded within an extracellular polysaccharide matrix on the device surface. Certain organisms, such as *S aureus*, exhibit microbial surface components recognizing adhesive matrix molecules on their surface that facilitate adhesion to tissues and neointimal surfaces, which may explain the proclivity of such organisms to cause device infections. Biofilm-based infections are often refractory to treatment with antibiotics alone; at times, device removal is the only way to ensure a cure. However, device removal is not always feasible or practical and considerably inflates expense. Systemic antibiotics are able to clear planktonic organisms that have been released from the biofilm but often are unable to effectively treat biofilm-embedded organisms. This inability may be related to the degree of penetration of various antibiotics into the biofilm, changes in bacterial metabolism, antimicrobial resistance, impaired host defenses, and local alterations in the microenvironment of the biofilm that impair the activity of the antimicrobial agent. The minimal inhibitory concentrations for biofilm-embedded bacteria can be up to 1000-fold higher than those pertaining to the same organisms when grown in broth medium.[17,18] **Fig. 3** shows a scanning electron micrograph of a *S aureus* biofilm on a VAD.

RISK FACTORS FOR INFECTION

A variety of different risk factors have been identified, some of which are amenable to infection-prevention strategies and others may be used for risk adjustment. Patient characteristics associated with an increased risk of device infection include older age, obesity or high body mass index (BMI), presence of diabetes mellitus, renal

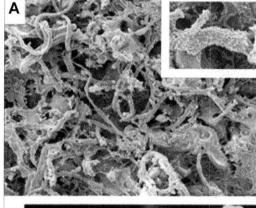

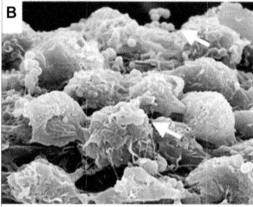

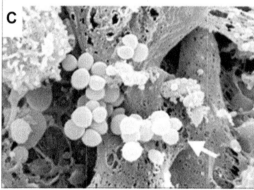

Fig. 3. Scanning electron microscopy of the pseudo-neointimal surface lining an explanted VAD polyurethane membrane (HeartMate, Abbott Laboratories, Abbott Park, IL). (*A*) Low-power view of the VAD's textured polyurethane membrane lined with extracellular matrix and cellular components. Inset: higher-power view of polyurethane fibers and adherent cells. (*B*) Cellular components of the pseudoneointimal surface (high power). Disks (9 mm) from the device were incubated with *S aureus* for 1 hour. White arrows indicate *S aureus* adhering to cells. (*C*) *S aureus* attached to cells or matrix material (high power). Disks from the device (9 mm) were incubated with *S aureus* for 1 hour. (*From* Gordon R, Quagliarello V, Lowy FD, et al. Ventricular assist device-related infections. Lancet Infect Dis 2006;6:431; with permission.)

insufficiency, severity of heart failure at the time of VAD placement (highest risk with INTERMACS profile 1), low serum albumin, presence of frailty, hypogammaglobulinemia, indwelling central lines (especially in the femoral location), and trauma to the driveline exit site.[2,4,8,11,19–21] T-cell dysfunction, especially associated with first-generation devices, were noted to have an association with device infection, especially candidiasis.[22–24] Surgical factors, such as concomitant surgery at the time of VAD placement, the velour-skin interface of the driveline, and location of the driveline exit site, are associated with DLI as is the duration of device support (higher risk of infection with longer durations).[2,8,25,26]

PREVENTION STRATEGIES

Given the dire outcomes of established VAD infection, there has been considerable effort made at prevention strategies. These strategies are reviewed in distinct categories: (1) preoperative risk factor modification, (2) antibiotic prophylaxis at time of surgery, (3) surgical techniques, and (4) long-term driveline management strategies.

Preoperative risk factor modification: A variety of risk factors, detailed earlier, are associated with an increased risk of developing a VAD infection. Some of these may be amenable to modification before VAD placement, such as losing weight in obese patients (in whom VAD placement is not emergent), optimizing nutritional status (perhaps with the use of enteral nutrition via a feeding tube for those with a low BMI), optimizing blood sugar control in diabetics, treatment of open wounds or ulcers, minimizing the use of urinary and vascular catheters, choosing nonfemoral locations for vascular catheters when needed, and using tunneled rather than nontunneled catheters when an anticipated need for vascular catheters is greater than 14 days. Screening and treatment of methicillin-resistant *S aureus* has been shown to reduce the risk of infection in patients undergoing cardiothoracic surgery, though not specifically VAD surgery, and can be considered in this setting as well.[27] Screening for active infections, by means of chest radiograph, urinalysis, as well as blood culture in patients with indwelling catheters, is helpful so that such patients can be treated before the insertion of the VAD. Dental evaluation is also recommended, especially if patients have a history of poor dentition.

Antibiotic prophylaxis at time of surgery: Wide variation in the use of antibiotic and antifungals as perioperative prophylaxis exists. There are no randomized trials to guide the choice and duration of antibiotic prophylaxis at the time of VAD implant

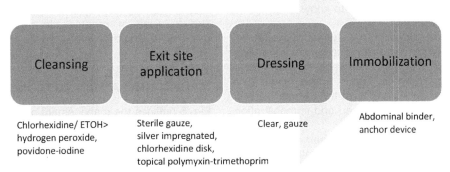

Fig. 4. Available strategies in the management of the driveline exit site. ETOH, ethyl alcohol.

surgery. A recent consensus document from the ISHLT recommends antibiotics that have staphylococcal activity, such as vancomycin or cefazolin, for prophylaxis for a maximum period of 48 hours following surgery.[28] Routine coverage for fungi or gram-negative bacteria is not recommended, unless warranted by local institutional infection epidemiology patterns.

Surgical techniques: Along with evolution in the type of VADs, surgical implantation techniques have evolved as well. Reduction in DLI rates are noted when the velour portion of the driveline is tunneled into the subcutaneous fascia and the silicone portion is at the skin interface.[25,26] A longer C-shaped loop as well as an exit side on the left side of the abdomen has been associated with a reduced risk of DLI as well.[25] Retroauricular and chest wall approaches for the driveline exit site have been developed, though single-center studies did not note a difference in the DLI rate

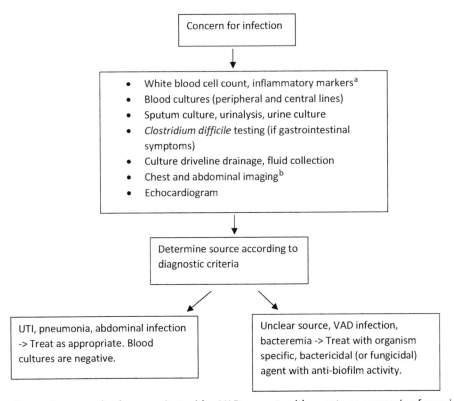

Fig. 5. The diagnostic approach when a patient with a VAD presents with symptoms concerning for an infection. [a] Sedimentation rate (erythrocyte sedimentation rate), C-reactive protein. [b] Generally computed tomography scans recommended. UTI, urinary tract infection.

when compared with the traditional abdominal exit site.[29,30] With the advent of third-generation VADs, a mini-thoracotomy approach has been developed, though it is too early to know its effect on infection rate.[31,32]

Long-term driveline management strategies: Many different driveline management strategies have been used with success in the clinical setting. As shown in **Fig. 4**, these range from agents used for cleansing of the exit site as well as the type of dressing used and immobilization device.

Some institutions package their own kits for ease of patient use as an outpatient, though commercial kits are available as well. Recent kits include chlorhexidine/alcohol as a cleaning agent, silver impregnated gauze/pads, absorptive and antiinfective dressings around the DLI, which is usually covered by a clear see-through dressing (to assess for drainage and so forth). Foley-type small anchors are recommended rather than an abdominal binder. These kits are noted to be comfortable and easy to

use and demonstrated to reduce the rate of DLI compared with previous management practices at local institutions.[33–35] Frequency of dressing changes ranges from daily to weekly, and the use of prophylactic oral antibiotics has not been shown to reduce the risk of DLI.[36,37]

MANAGEMENT APPROACH TO INFECTION

Fig. 5 outlines the management approach to the workup of suspected infection in a VAD recipient. Recommended testing at the time of presentation includes basic laboratory testing, microbiological cultures, and imaging. Computed tomography (CT) scans of the chest and abdomen are preferred to look for induration around the driveline or an abscess either associated with the driveline or pump. Additional imaging modalities have been noted to be useful in diagnosing VAD-specific infections as well; these include 18F-fluoro-2-deoxy-D-glucose PET visually correlated with CT, gallium single-photon

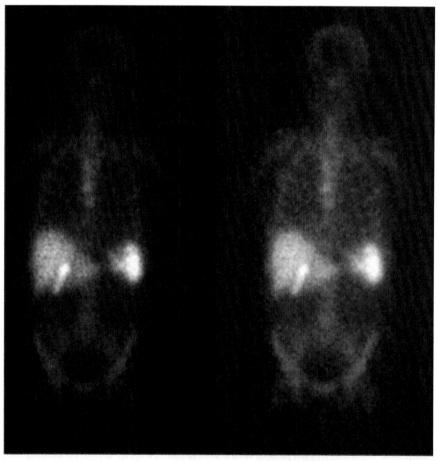

Fig. 6. Indium-labelled white blood cell scan image showing increased uptake along the driveline in a patient with *Pseudomonas aeruginosa* DLI. (*Courtesy of* Saima Aslam, MD, San Diego, CA.)

Table 2
Management of bacterial ventricular assist device–specific and –related infections

Infection Types	Medical Management	Surgical Management
Superficial DLI	Treat with IV or oral antibiotics for a minimum of 2 wk or until infection has resolved (drainage, redness, tenderness, and so forth). Reinforce patient and caretaker education about DL immobilization techniques.	Not applicable
Deep DLI (or unclear depth)/ pocket infection	Treat with IV antibiotics until clinical stabilization and improvement of infection (usually 6–8 wk), followed by long-term oral suppression therapy.	Surgical debridement with or without wound VAC may be needed. Recommend abscess drainage. New DL exit site away from previous infection may be required.
VAD pump and/or cannula	Treat with IV antibiotics for at least 6–8 wk. If bacteremia resolves, recommend oral suppression (if possible) until transplantation in BTT patients. If intraoperative cultures are positive, recommend 4–6 wk of IV antibiotics following transplantation; if they are negative, recommend 2 wk of oral antibiotics following transplant. In DT, IV antibiotic treatment is followed by long-term oral antibiotic suppression.	Surgical drainage and debridement may be required to control infection. Source control is as follows: in BTT, explant of the device for HT; in DT, explant/exchange of the device for control of infection.
Persistent bacteremia/ relapsing infection, despite adequate antimicrobial and surgical therapy	In BTT, IV antibiotics should continue until after HT, with continuation of antibiotics following HT as previously mentioned based on intraoperative cultures. In DT, IV antibiotic treatment is followed by long-term oral antibiotic suppression, though at times oral options are not available and IV therapy is continued beyond 8 wk. Duration of antibiotics treatment after device exchange depends on the clinical course and pathogen. Longer course (4–6 wk) may be offered in positive intraoperative cultures or recent preoperative bacteremia, and a shorter course (14 d) may be offered in the absence of such conditions.	Strong consideration should be made for device explant/ exchange. One could consider bridging patients with a percutaneous device so that infection control is achieved before new VAD placement.
VAD-related bacteremia	Duration of antibiotics depends on the source, organism, and clearing of bacteremia. CRBSI secondary to *Staphylococcus aureus* is treated for 4–6 wk, and the catheter is removed. If not *S aureus*, blood cultures become negative within 24–48 h and there are no signs of metastatic infection; 2 wk from the first negative blood culture may be adequate (eg, urinary tract source). If no source is identified, treatment may be considered as with VAD pump and cannula infection.	
Bacterial mediastinitis	Duration of antibacterial therapy is at least 6–8 wk after last surgical debridement.	Surgical debridement is often indicated. Open chest and VAC wound closure may be needed.
Infective endocarditis	Duration of antibacterial therapy is the same as for VAD pump and cannula infection.	Surgical intervention may be required.

Abbreviations: BTT, bridge to transplant; CRBSI, catheter-related bloodstream infection; DL, driveline; DT, destination therapy; HT, heart transplant; IV, intravenous; VAC, vacuum-assisted closure.

Adapted from Kusne S, Mooney M, Danziger-Isakov L, et al. An ISHLT consensus document for prevention and management strategies for mechanical circulatory support infection. J Heart Lung Transplant 2017;36(10):1147–8; with permission.

Table 3
Management of fungal ventricular assist device–specific and –related infections

Infection Type	Medical Management	Surgical Management
Candida sp superficial DLI	Routine blood cultures should be performed to diagnose/rule out concomitant fungemia. Superficial infection in clinically stable patients with negative blood cultures should be treated with an azole for a minimum of 2 wk.	Not applicable
Candida sp deep (or unclear depth) DLI/pocket infection	Routine blood cultures should be performed to diagnose/rule out concomitant fungemia. It should be treated with an echinocandin or L-AmB for 6–8 wk, followed by long-term oral suppressive therapy thereafter. If device is replaced surgically or after HT, antifungal agents should be continued for a minimum of 6 wk and possibly longer if surgical cultures are positive.	Surgical drainage may be required for control of extensive infection with or without a wound VAC. Routine device replacement in the setting of an FI is not recommended. If the device requires replacement, then the new driveline needs to be placed in a different site.
Candida sp pump/cannula infection	Recommend treatment with an echinocandin or L-AmB for 8–12 wk from the first negative blood culture, followed by long-term suppression with an oral agent. Flucytosine can be added to L-AmB in select patients. If device exchange or HT occurs, then antifungal agents should be continued for a minimum of 6 wk and possibly longer if surgical cultures are positive following surgery.	Routine device replacement in the setting of an FI is not recommended. Device exchange or placement on the cardiac transplant list is recommended if patients have a relapse despite appropriate treatment (antifungal agent, dose, and duration).
Candidemia	Investigations are recommended to determine the precise source, including microbiologic cultures (driveline, pocket, and CVC) and imaging. Empirical therapy with an echinocandin or L-AmB is recommended. Once identification and sensitivity testing has occurred, patients are clinically stable, and blood cultures are negative, antifungal agents should be de-escalated to the narrowest spectrum agent possible. If the source of the candidemia is a CVC, it has been removed, blood cultures become negative within 24–48 h, and there is no obvious metastatic infection, then 2–4 wk of antifungal therapy is recommended from the date of first negative blood culture. A complete ophthalmologic examination for endophthalmitis before discontinuation of therapy is recommended.	Not applicable
Candida sp mediastinitis/infective endocarditis	The type and duration of antifungal therapy for mediastinitis and infective endocarditis is the same as for a VAD pump/cannula infection.	Thorough surgical debridement of mediastinitis with an open chest ± a VAC wound closure is recommended.

Abbreviations: CVC, central venous catheter; FI, fungal infection; L-AmB, liposomal amphotericin B; VAC, vacuum-assisted closure.

Adapted from Husain S, Sole A, Alexander BD, et al. The 2015 International Society for Heart and Lung Transplantation guidelines for the management of fungal infections in mechanical circulatory support and cardiothoracic organ transplant recipients: executive summary. J Heart Lung Transplant 2016;35(3):276–7; with permission.

emission CT/CT and indium-labelled white blood cell scintigraphy (**Fig. 6**).[38,39]

Empirical antimicrobial therapy should be active against *S aureus* and *P aeruginosa* and also informed by institutional epidemiologic patterns. Therapeutic drug monitoring is recommended for certain antimicrobial agents, such as vancomycin (steady-state trough of 15–20 mg/L is recommended), aminoglycosides (trough varies based on dosing frequency and specific drug used), voriconazole (goal steady-state trough 1–5 mg/L), and posaconazole (goal steady-state trough >1.25 mg/L).[40,41] Drug interactions with anticoagulation may be pertinent as well. This point is particularly true for warfarin, which has known drug interactions with quinolones, trimethoprim-sulfamethoxazole, clarithromycin, and metronidazole.[42]

The ISHLT's recent consensus document provides details on the treatment duration for various VAD-specific and VAD-related infections.[28] General concepts to keep in mind when selecting an antimicrobial agent are as follows:

- Organism-specific antimicrobial agent
- Bactericidal/fungicidal drugs rather than bacteriostatic/fungistatic agents
- Biofilm penetration (even if not an actual VAD infection but for, eg, catheter-related bacteremia; an antimicrobial with known biofilm activity may affect chances of the organism seeding the device)
- Dose: high doses of drugs recommended, especially when treating a biofilm-based infection to maximize antibiotic penetration
- Duration: As cure of VAD-specific infection is not expected, long-term suppression is recommended with oral antibiotics once the acute phase of the infection has been treated for 6 to 8 weeks of intravenous antibiotics (or longer in the case of fungal infection).

Detailed recommendations for the management of bacterial infections based on severity and location are presented in **Table 2**. For patients with a VAD-specific or VAD-related fungal infection, the ideal clinical management is outlined in **Table 3**.

VAD infection is a potential criterion to increase the listing urgency for patients on the heart transplant waitlist. Outcomes of patients with VAD infection following heart transplant are comparable with those without pretransplant VAD infection in most studies, though a few have noted inferior outcomes.[16,43–47]

SUMMARY

VAD support is critical in the care of end-stage heart failure and as a bridge to heart transplantation. Ongoing evolution in device type in particular as well as surgical and medical management of such patients has led to an overall improvement in infection rates. Despite this, device infection is an important cause of morbidity and mortality; ongoing innovation in the prevention and management of such infections remains crucial in reducing the burden of disease.

REFERENCES

1. Kirklin JK, Cantor R, Mohacsi P, et al. First annual IM-ACS report: a global International Society for Heart and Lung Transplantation Registry for Mechanical Circulatory Support. J Heart Lung Transplant 2016; 35(4):407–12.
2. Kirklin JK, Naftel DC, Pagani FD, et al. Seventh INTERMACS annual report: 15,000 patients and counting. J Heart Lung Transplant 2015;34(12): 1495–504.
3. Aslam S, Hernandez M, Thornby J, et al. Risk factors and outcomes of fungal ventricular-assist device infections. Clin Infect Dis 2010;50(5):664–71.
4. Schaffer JM, Allen JG, Weiss ES, et al. Infectious complications after pulsatile-flow and continuous-flow left ventricular assist device implantation. J Heart Lung Transplant 2011;30(2):164–74.
5. Aggarwal A, Gupta A, Kumar S, et al. Are blood stream infections associated with an increased risk of hemorrhagic stroke in patients with a left ventricular assist device? ASAIO J 2012;58(5):509–13.
6. Trachtenberg BH, Cordero-Reyes AM, Aldeiri M, et al. Persistent blood stream infection in patients supported with a continuous-flow left ventricular assist device is associated with an increased risk of cerebrovascular accidents. J Card Fail 2015; 21(2):119–25.
7. Hannan MM, Husain S, Mattner F, et al. Working formulation for the standardization of definitions of infections in patients using ventricular assist devices. J Heart Lung Transplant 2011;30(4): 375–84.
8. Aslam S, Xie R, Cowger J, et al. Bloodstream infections in mechanical circulatory support device recipients in the International Society of Heart and Lung Transplantation Mechanically Assisted Circulation Support Registry: Epidemiology, risk factors, and mortality. J Heart Lung Transplant 2018;37(8): 1013–20.
9. Nienaber JJ, Kusne S, Riaz T, et al. Clinical manifestations and management of left ventricular assist device-associated infections. Clin Infect Dis 2013; 57(10):1438–48.

10. Pereda D, Conte JV. Left ventricular assist device driveline infections. Cardiol Clin 2011;29(4):515–27.
11. Zierer A, Melby SJ, Voeller RK, et al. Late-onset driveline infections: the Achilles' heel of prolonged left ventricular assist device support. Ann Thorac Surg 2007;84(2):515–20.
12. Raymond AL, Kfoury AG, Bishop CJ, et al. Obesity and left ventricular assist device driveline exit site infection. ASAIO J 2010;56(1):57–60.
13. Yoshioka D, Sakaniwa R, Toda K, et al. Relationship between bacteremia and hemorrhagic stroke in patients with continuous-flow left ventricular assist device. Circ J 2018;82(2):448–56.
14. Frontera JA, Starling R, Cho SM, et al. Risk factors, mortality, and timing of ischemic and hemorrhagic stroke with left ventricular assist devices. J Heart Lung Transplant 2017;36(6):673–83.
15. Koval CE, Thuita L, Moazami N, et al. Evolution and impact of drive-line infection in a large cohort of continuous-flow ventricular assist device recipients. J Heart Lung Transplant 2014;33(11):1164–72.
16. Goldstein DJ, Naftel D, Holman W, et al. Continuous-flow devices and percutaneous site infections: clinical outcomes. J Heart Lung Transplant 2012;31(11):1151–7.
17. Aslam S, Darouiche RO. Role of antibiofilm-antimicrobial agents in controlling device-related infections. Int J Artif Organs 2011;34(9):752–8.
18. Padera RF. Infection in ventricular assist devices: the role of biofilm. Cardiovasc Pathol 2006;15(5):264–70.
19. Topkara VK, Dang NC, Martens TP, et al. Effect of diabetes on short- and long-term outcomes after left ventricular assist device implantation. J Heart Lung Transplant 2005;24(12):2048–53.
20. John R, Aaronson KD, Pae WE, et al. Drive-line infections and sepsis in patients receiving the HVAD system as a left ventricular assist device. J Heart Lung Transplant 2014;33(10):1066–73.
21. Yamani MH, Chuang HH, Ozduran V, et al. The impact of hypogammaglobulinemia on infection outcome in patients undergoing ventricular assist device implantation. J Heart Lung Transplant 2006;25(7):820–4.
22. Ankersmit HJ, Tugulea S, Spanier T, et al. Activation-induced T-cell death and immune dysfunction after implantation of left-ventricular assist device. Lancet 1999;354(9178):550–5.
23. Kimball PM, Flattery M, McDougan F, et al. Cellular immunity impaired among patients on left ventricular assist device for 6 months. Ann Thorac Surg 2008;85(5):1656–61.
24. Schaenman JM, Rossetti M, Korin Y, et al. T cell dysfunction and patient age are associated with poor outcomes after mechanical circulatory support device implantation. Hum Immunol 2018;79(4):203–12.
25. Dean D, Kallel F, Ewald GA, et al. Reduction in drive-line infection rates: results from the HeartMate II Multicenter Driveline Silicone Skin Interface (SSI) Registry. J Heart Lung Transplant 2015;34(6):781–9.
26. Singh A, Russo MJ, Valeroso TB, et al. Modified HeartMate II driveline externalization technique significantly decreases incidence of infection and improves long-term survival. ASAIO J 2014;60(6):613–6.
27. van Rijen M, Bonten M, Wenzel R, et al. Mupirocin ointment for preventing Staphylococcus aureus infections in nasal carriers. Cochrane Database Syst Rev 2008;(4):CD006216.
28. Kusne S, Mooney M, Danziger-Isakov L, et al. An ISHLT consensus document for prevention and management strategies for mechanical circulatory support infection. J Heart Lung Transplant 2017;36(10):1137–53.
29. Bejko J, Toto F, Gregori D, et al. Left ventricle assist devices and driveline's infection incidence: a single-centre experience. J Artif Organs 2018;21(1):52–60.
30. Martin BJ, Luc JGY, Maruyama M, et al. Driveline site is not a predictor of infection after ventricular assist device implantation. ASAIO J 2017. [Epub ahead of print].
31. Krabatsch T, Drews T, Potapov E, et al. Different surgical strategies for implantation of continuous-flow VADs-Experience from Deutsches Herzzentrum Berlin. Ann Cardiothorac Surg 2014;3(5):472–4.
32. Maltais S, Anwer LA, Tchantchaleishvili V, et al. Left lateral thoracotomy for centrifugal continuous-flow left ventricular assist device placement: an analysis from the mechanical circulatory support research network. ASAIO J 2017. [Epub ahead of print].
33. Stahovich M, Sundareswaran KS, Fox S, et al. Reduce driveline trauma through stabilization and exit site management: 30 days feasibility results from the multicenter RESIST study. ASAIO J 2016;62(3):240–5.
34. Cagliostro B, Levin AP, Fried J, et al. Continuous-flow left ventricular assist devices and usefulness of a standardized strategy to reduce drive-line infections. J Heart Lung Transplant 2016;35(1):108–14.
35. Aslam S, Dan J, Topik A, et al. Decrease in driveline infections with change in driveline management protocol. VAD J 2016;2:1–13.
36. Wus L, Manning M, Entwistle JW 3rd. Left ventricular assist device driveline infection and the frequency of dressing change in hospitalized patients. Heart Lung 2015;44(3):225–9.
37. Stulak JM, Maltais S, Cowger J, et al. Prevention of percutaneous driveline infection after left ventricular assist device implantation: prophylactic antibiotics are not necessary. ASAIO J 2013;59(6):570–4.
38. Kim J, Feller ED, Chen W, et al. FDG PET/CT imaging for LVAD associated infections. JACC Cardiovasc Imaging 2014;7(8):839–42.

39. Levy DT, Minamoto GY, Da Silva R, et al. Role of gallium SPECT-CT in the diagnosis of left ventricular assist device infections. ASAIO J 2015;61(1):e5–10.

40. Rybak MJ, Lomaestro BM, Rotschafer JC, et al. Vancomycin therapeutic guidelines: a summary of consensus recommendations from the infectious diseases Society of America, the American Society of Health-system Pharmacists, and the Society of infectious diseases Pharmacists. Clin Infect Dis 2009; 49(3):325–7.

41. Husain S, Sole A, Alexander BD, et al. The 2015 International Society for Heart and Lung Transplantation Guidelines for the management of fungal infections in mechanical circulatory support and cardiothoracic organ transplant recipients: executive summary. J Heart Lung Transplant 2016;35(3): 261–82.

42. Ament PW, Bertolino JG, Liszewski JL. Clinically significant drug interactions. Am Fam Physician 2000; 61(6):1745–54.

43. Poston RS, Husain S, Sorce D, et al. LVAD bloodstream infections: therapeutic rationale for transplantation after LVAD infection. J Heart Lung Transplant 2003;22(8):914–21.

44. Schulman AR, Martens TP, Russo MJ, et al. Effect of left ventricular assist device infection on post-transplant outcomes. J Heart Lung Transplant 2009;28(3):237–42.

45. Toda K, Yonemoto Y, Fujita T, et al. Risk analysis of bloodstream infection during long-term left ventricular assist device support. Ann Thorac Surg 2012; 94(5):1387–93.

46. Monkowski DH, Axelrod P, Fekete T, et al. Infections associated with ventricular assist devices: epidemiology and effect on prognosis after transplantation. Transpl Infect Dis 2007;9(2):114–20.

47. Quader MA, Wolfe LG, Kasirajan V. Heart transplantation outcomes in patients with continuous-flow left ventricular assist device-related complications. J Heart Lung Transplant 2015;34(1):75–81.

48. Topkara VK, Kondareddy S, Malik F, et al. Infectious complications in patients with left ventricular assist device: etiology and outcomes in the continuous-flow era. Ann Thorac Surg 2010;90(4): 1270–7.

Continuous-Flow Left Ventricular Assist Device–Related Gastrointestinal Bleeding

Ju H. Kim, MD[a], Donald F. Brophy, PharmD, MSc[b],
Keyur B. Shah, MD[c],*

KEYWORDS

- Left ventricular assist device • Gastrointestinal bleed • Angiodysplasia • Octreotide

KEY POINTS

- Gastrointestinal bleeding is the most common complication following continuous-flow left ventricular assist device (LVAD) placement.
- Causes underlying LVAD-related gastrointestinal bleeding are multifactorial, including acquired von Willebrand syndrome and abnormal angiogenesis.
- Management of gastrointestinal bleeding requires a multidisciplinary approach incorporating device manipulation, endoscopic evaluation, and pharmacologic therapy.
- Further studies on the impact of continuous-flow physiology are needed to minimize the morbidity associated with LVAD-related bleeding.

INTRODUCTION

Continuous-flow (CF) left ventricular assist device (LVAD) therapy for patients with advanced heart failure continues to increase both as a bridge to transplant (BTT) and as destination therapy (DT) for those with contraindications to heart transplant. Recent analysis of the Interagency Registry for Mechanically Assisted Circulatory Support (INTERMACS) showed that, of the more than 20,000 implants of LVADs that have been reported to the registry since 2006, most are CF devices.[1] CF LVADs increase bleeding risk by activating the coagulation pathway because of imperfect hemocompatibility and by activating circulating platelets because of supraphysiologic shear stress created by the impeller. As a result, patients are committed to lifelong antiplatelet and antithrombotic therapy, further increasing bleeding risk. Nonsurgical bleeding, mainly from the gastrointestinal (GI) tract, complicates LVAD therapy with significant morbidity. LVAD-related GI bleeding (GIB) is presently defined by INTERMACS as clinical evidence of GIB, including melena, hematochezia, hematemesis, or rectal bleeding occurring greater than 7 days postimplantation and requiring transfusion of 1 or more units of packed red blood cells (PRBCs).[2]

Disclosures: None (J.H. Kim, D.F. Brophy); K.B. Shah, consultant for Medtronic.
[a] Advanced Heart Failure and Transplant, Methodist DeBakey Cardiology Associates, Houston Methodist Hospital, 6550 Fannin Street, Smith Tower, Suite 1901, Houston, TX 77030, USA; [b] Department of Pharmacotherapy and Outcomes Science, Virginia Commonwealth University School of Pharmacy, PO Box 980533, Richmond, VA 23298, USA; [c] Advanced Heart Failure and Transplant, Pauley Heart Center, Virginia Commonwealth University, 1200 East Broad Street, PO Box: 980204, Richmond, VA 23298-0036, USA
* Corresponding author.
E-mail address: keyur.shah@vcuhealth.org

cardiology.theclinics.com

Abbreviations	
ADAMTS-13	A disintegrin and metalloproteinase with a thrombospondin type 1 motif, member 13
AVM	Arteriovenous malformation
AVWS	Acquired von Willebrand syndrome
BTT	Bridge to transplant
CF LVAD	Continuous-flow left ventricular assist device
cGMP	Cyclic guanosine monophosphate
DT	Destination therapy
GIB	Gastrointestinal bleeding
HMvWF	High-molecular-weight multimers of von Willebrand factor
INR	International Normalized Ratio
INTERMACS	Interagency Registry for Mechanically Assisted Circulatory Support
PRBCs	Packed red blood cells
TRACE	The Study of Reduced Anti-coagulation/Anti-platelet Therapy in Patients with the HeartMate II LVAS
VEGF	Vascular endothelial growth factor
VKA	Vitamin K antagonist

EPIDEMIOLOGY

Bleeding risk caused by LVAD therapy has increased compared with the first-generation pulsatile devices. Current CF LVADs are associated with a 3-fold higher risk for GIB compared with pulsatile LVADs.[3] GIB affects 15% to 30% of patients with an LVAD and 40% of those who have had GIB have a recurrence.[4] The cumulative risk of GIB has been reported as 21%, 27%, and 31% at 1, 3, and 5 years, respectively.[5] A meta-analysis of 1839 LVAD patients found a 23% pooled prevalence of GIB.[6] GIB also accounts for approximately one-third of all hospital readmissions after LVAD implantation[7] and is associated with extended hospital stays.[8] Those admitted for an LVAD-related GIB often require an average of 2 to 4 units of PRBCs per admission,[9] which can subsequently affect the chances of a successful heart transplant because of sensitization.[10] Patients with poor global outcomes, defined as a composite of death, poor quality of life, recurrent heart failure hospitalizations, or thromboembolic complications such as stroke, were more likely to have higher rates of GIB over the first year after LVAD implantation.[11] In smaller analyses, GIB

has been associated with increased risks for device thrombosis and increased mortality.[4,12]

RISK FACTORS

Numerous risk factors have been reported to be associated with LVAD-related GIB. One consistent risk factor across all studies is older age. An analysis of the Healthcare Cost and Utilization Project – Nationwide Inpatient Sample database found that LVAD patients more than 65 years of age had an adjusted odds of GIB that was 20.5 times greater than those less than 65 years of age.[3] An analysis of more than 900 HeartMate II LVAD patients implanted as both BTT and DT found that age greater than 65 years was associated with an increased risk of bleeding.[13] Smaller cohort studies have also shown that older patients are more likely to have GIB. A single-center analysis of 214 patients who received a CF LVAD found that those patients who experienced GIB were older than those who did not (60.5 vs 55 years, $P = .003$).[14] An analysis of 1149 CF-LVAD patients across multiple centers found that survival free of GIB at 1 year was lower in patients more than 70 years of age compared with younger counterparts (58% vs 69%, $P<.01$).[15] Moreover, recurrent GIB has been seen more commonly in older patients.[16]

History of GIB before LVAD implantation has been implicated as a risk factor for LVAD-related GIB, albeit inconsistently. A retrospective analysis of 101 patients comprising predominantly patients implanted with a HeartMate II as DT found that a previous history of GIB was an independent predictor (odds ratio [OR], 22.7; 95% confidence interval [CI], 2.2–228.6; $P = .008$).[16] However, a separate meta-analysis of CF-LVAD patients found that a prior history of GIB was not a significant risk factor (OR, 2.22; 95% CI, 0.83–5.96).[6]

Diminished pulsatility in CF devices has also been hypothesized as a significant risk factor for GIB. In 2009, a retrospective review comparing pulsatile flow versus CF LVADs found that the GIB event rate for CF-LVAD recipients was nearly 10 times higher.[17] A retrospective analysis of all HeartMate II LVAD patients used the pulsatility index (PI), calculated as the difference between maximum flow and minimum flow divided by the average flow over a 15-second interval multiplied by 10, to evaluate its effect on GIB. Lower PI and older age (64 vs 57 years; $P = .004$) were associated with GIB in this cohort.[18] In contrast, a different study found no differences in LVAD speed or PI between those with and without GIB.[16]

PATHOPHYSIOLOGY

The exact pathogenesis underlying CF-LVAD–related GIB remains elusive. However, factors attributable to both patient and device are thought to contribute to the increased risk in bleeding. Anticoagulation increases the risk of GIB; however, the median International Normalized Ratio (INR) at the time of the first GIB in one study was reported to be 2.4 ± 1.4.[19] A meta-analysis found multiple additional studies that reported a therapeutic or subtherapeutic INR at the time of bleed.[6] Moreover, compared with patients requiring therapeutic anticoagulation after cardiac valve replacements, CF-LVAD recipients experienced significantly higher rates of GIB (18% vs 4%; $P<.001$) despite insignificant differences in INR (2.3 ± 1.3 LVAD vs 3.3 ± 2.2; $P =$ NS) at the time of the bleed,[20] suggesting that additional factors are contributory. Although multifactorial in cause, research suggests that abnormalities in the hematologic system and vascular signaling, induced by reduced pulse pressure and sheer stress, may contribute to bleeding events in LVAD patients, as discussed later and outlined in **Fig. 1**.

Angiodysplasia

Similar to Heyde syndrome with severe aortic stenosis, the reduced pulse pressure induced by CF LVADs is thought to lead to decreased intraluminal pressure that triggers an increase in sympathetic tone, causing smooth muscle relaxation and dilatation of the mucosal veins leading to development of arteriovenous malformations (AVMs).[9,21] Moreover, the diminished pulsatility and potential hypoxia from relative hypoperfusion of the gut may also result in angiogenesis via induction of angiopoietin-2 (Ang-2), vascular endothelial growth factor (VEGF), and tumor necrosis factor (TNF).[22,23] Despite these hypothesized associations between reduced pulsatility and the formation of AVMs, exact mechanisms underlying this phenomenon are unclear and remain an active area of research.

Recently reported autopsy-based data suggest that LVAD-associated angiodysplasia may represent a distinct form of its own, unlike age-related angiodysplasia. Using small bowel obtained from deceased human donors, cows, and sheep supported with CF LVAD, significantly greater intestinal vascularity and abnormal vascular architecture were noted after LVAD support.[24] These findings were reported to be in contrast with those seen in age-related angiodysplasia, which is commonly seen in the colon, not the small bowel.[24]

There is also emerging evidence that CF-LVAD support is associated with hypervascularity in the

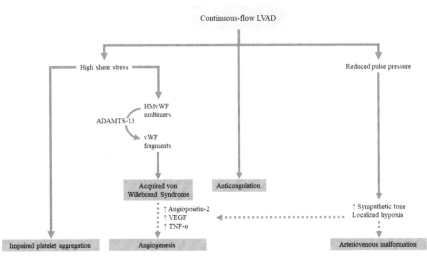

Fig. 1. Proposed multifactorial mechanisms underlying CF-LVAD–related GIB. In addition to therapeutic anticoagulation, CF physiology leads to high shear stress and reduced pulse pressure. High shear stress on the blood traversing the ventricular assist device leads to impaired platelet aggregation and loss of HMvWF multimers. These multimers may also be destroyed via enzymatic breakdown by ADAMTS-13. The resultant AVWS may affect endothelial proliferation and cause abnormal angiogenesis via angiopoietin-2 and vascular endothelial growth factor (VEGF) signaling. Reduced pulse pressure and diminished pulsatility are thought to increase sympathetic tone and cause localized hypoxia, resulting in arteriovenous malformation. This condition may also result in angiogenesis via induction of angiopoietin-2, VEGF, and tumor necrosis factor (TNF). ADAMTS-13, a disintegrin and metalloproteinase with a thrombospondin type 1 motif, member 13; HMvWF, high-molecular-weight von Willebrand factor; vWF, von Willebrand factor.

nasal mucosa, which may be representative of the mucosal changes in the GI tract inflicted by CF LVADs.[25] As the investigators note, a simultaneous connection could not be made between the presence of nasal hypervascularity and the GI AVMs. However, the findings of this pilot study merit further investigation to determine their significance.

Acquired von Willebrand Syndrome

The pathophysiology underlying acquired von Willebrand syndrome (AVWS) in CF-LVAD patients is thought to be caused by increased clearance of high-molecular-weight multimers of von Willebrand factor (HMvWF) caused by exposure to increased shear stress as blood traverses the LVAD.[26,27] Loss of HMvWF impairs platelet binding to sites of exposed collagen on injured endothelium, which increases the risk of bleeding.[28] Degradation of von Willebrand factor (vWF) may occur from shear stress as well as via an enzymatic breakdown by a disintegrin and metalloproteinase with a thrombospondin type 1 motif, member 13 (ADAMTS-13).[29] A retrospective review of 102 CF-LVAD patients found that concentrations of HMvWF decreased 30% ± 14% with HeartMate II and 34% ± 13% with the HeartWare ventricular assist device.[30]

Although the role of vWF in hemostasis is well known, vWF may be an important factor in regulating angiogenesis. As elegantly reviewed by Randi and Laffan,[31] vWF regulates endothelial proliferation and angiogenesis via multiple pathways. One is through its control of the VEGF receptor-2 signaling pathway in conjunction with its inhibitory effect on Ang-2, a vascular growth factor.[31] Increases in levels of Ang-2 and its associated higher CF-LAVD–related bleeding risk[22] may be mediated by AVWS. Moreover, levels of cyclic guanosine monophosphate (cGMP), a downstream effector of vWF with an important role in platelet activation, are increased in CF-LVAD patients.[32] Higher cGMP levels were associated with CF-LVAD–related GIB events and inversely correlated with the PI in HeartMate II patients.[32] These findings represent an exciting area of research defining the role of vWF in the pathogenesis of LVAD-related GIB with important clinical implications.

MANAGEMENT

Current management of LVAD-related GIB requires a multidisciplinary approach including both pharmacologic and nonpharmacologic strategies. In an emergency medicine setting, a thorough history and physical examination should guide initial testing, hemodynamic assessment, and appropriate resuscitation. Although retrospective studies have associated increased LVAD pulsatility with reduced incidence of GIB, a speed reduction treatment strategy has not been prospectively validated. It is reasonable to consider manipulation of the LVAD speed to increase pulsatility or adjustments in antiplatelet or anticoagulation strategies; however, this must be weighed against the increased risk of inadequate left ventricular unloading precipitating heart failure as well as device thrombosis.[33] It is imperative to consult with a gastroenterologist to perform an endoscopic evaluation for diagnostic and potentially therapeutic purposes. An anesthesiologist familiar with LVAD physiology may help minimize periprocedural complications such as sedation-related hypotension and device malfunction.[34] Consultation with a clinical pharmacist can provide valuable insight into culprit medications, drug-drug or drug-disease interactions, and various pharmacotherapeutic options.

Endoscopy

In patients presenting with GIB, the initial evaluation involves identification of the severity and location of the bleeding source. An endoscopic evaluation and intervention remains the mainstay of therapy. Bleeding can occur anywhere along the entire GI tract. Notably, bleeding rates were highest in the upper GI tract (48%; 95% CI, 39%–57%), followed by the lower GI tract (22%; 95% CI, 16%–31%), and small bowel (15%; 95% CI, 8%–25%). In 19% to 22% of patients, the source of bleeding is not found.[6,19] Esophagogastroduodenoscopy has the highest yield in locating the source of bleeding.[6] When lesions with active bleeding or stigmata of recent bleeding are identified, endoscopic treatment with argon plasma coagulation, contact coagulation, hemostatic clips, or epinephrine injection can be successful in achieving hemostasis in nearly all of the cases.[35–37] If no lesion is found, colonoscopy and/or video capsule endoscopy (VCE) may be indicated.[38] Retrospective analyses of LVAD patients with obscure GIB found that the diagnostic yield of VCE is 33% to 40%.[39,40] Although VCE may improve localization of the bleeding source, device-assisted enteroscopy, including balloon enteroscopy, may have superior yield and efficacy for treatment in CF-LVAD patients. In a single-center study, using device-assisted enteroscopy early, within 24 hours of presentation with GIB, led to significant decreases in the number of transfusions and days to treatment.[41]

PHARMACOLOGIC THERAPY
Anticoagulation

There are no data to guide optimal management of anticoagulation in patients with CF LVADs who present with GIB. Anticoagulation and/or anti-platelet dose reduction is commonly done as part of the initial management of an active bleed. However, it is unclear whether this strategy improves outcomes because it may increase the risk of thromboembolic complications.

The Study of Reduced Anti-coagulation/Anti-platelet Therapy in Patients with the HeartMate II LVAS (TRACE) was a multicenter, observational study conducted both in the United States and Europe designed to assess the impact of reduced antithrombotic therapy in patients with a HeartMate II LVAD. Reduced antithrombotic therapy was defined as aspirin only, vitamin K antagonist (VKA) only, or no antithrombotic use. In the US arm (US-TRACE), this strategy was used in 82% of patients in response to a bleeding episode. In those managed with VKA only, the median INR was 1.85 compared with 1.1 in those managed with aspirin or no antithrombotic therapy. The median aspirin dose was 81 mg daily. Despite the less intense antithrombotic regimen, 43% of patients experienced an episode of major bleeding within 1 year and GIB accounted for 66% of these episodes.[42] In those who had a GIB, there was no difference in the event rates between those managed with VKA only (13%) versus aspirin only (14%) versus no antithrombotic used (15%).[42]

The European arm of the TRACE study (TRACE-EU) examined a different patient population. Instead of reducing antithrombotic therapy in response to a bleeding episode, the European patients were managed on monotherapy with a VKA as a standard of care. A 2-year analysis of these data suggested that anticoagulation with a VKA with a target INR of 2 to 3 without antiplatelet therapy is feasible and maintains low rates of thrombotic complications.[43]

Individual centers may develop protocols based on local experience and preference depending on the INR at time of bleeding, the number of bleeding episodes, and any pertinent comorbidities that necessitate antithrombotic therapy.[44]

Octreotide

Octreotide is a synthetic analogue of somatostatin, a peptide secreted by the gastric and intestinal mucosa that has a predominantly inhibitory effect in the GI tract. Octreotide has been used as an option to treat various GI indications, including GIB caused by acquired angiodysplasia.[45,46] Its effect on improving GIB is mediated by splanchnic vasoconstriction, improved platelet aggregation, increased vascular resistance, and inhibition of angiogenesis via VEGF and basic fibroblast growth factor inhibition.[47] However, data supporting the use of octreotide in CF-LVAD–related GIB are limited largely to case reports with no clear consensus regarding benefit (**Table 1**).

In an early single-center, retrospective review of both pulsatile-flow and CF-LVAD recipients, 10 episodes of GIB were identified, all in the CF-LVAD cohort. These patients were treated with interruption in antithrombotic therapy, addition of proton pump inhibitors, and octreotide administered either continuously at 25 µg/min, subcutaneously at 100 µg twice daily, or 10-mg intramuscular injections monthly with improvement in bleeding.[48] However, in a retrospective analysis of a predominantly DT cohort with a 22.8% incidence of GIB, 13 patients were identified who had received octreotide. This study reported no significant differences in the number of PRBC transfusions, rebleeding rates, lengths of hospital stay, or all-cause mortality.[16] Another case series of 116 patients with CF LVAD predominantly implanted as DT found 7 patients with recurrent GIB refractory to conventional therapy, including endoscopy, addition of proton pump inhibitors, and reduction of anticoagulation and antiplatelet therapy. Two of these patients were treated with octreotide 20 mg depot monthly and 5 received 50 µg subcutaneously twice daily for 3 months. No differences in hospitalizations caused by GIB, number of PRBCs transfused, or number of endoscopic procedures were found between 3 months before and after octreotide administration. Only after removing 1 patient deemed to be a nonresponder because of continued bleeding from a gastric antral vascular ectasia did the group find a trend toward fewer blood transfusions and fewer endoscopic procedures and readmissions caused by GIB.[49]

In contrast, several case reports have shown significant improvements in VAD-related GIB with octreotide. A HeartMate II patient with a history of atrial fibrillation who had no bleeding complications while on chronic anticoagulation developed recurrent GIB after LVAD placement. The bleeding continued despite reductions in pump speed and reduction in antithrombotic therapy. He remained free of bleeding after the addition of octreotide 100 µg subcutaneously twice daily followed by a 20-mg intramuscular depot injection before discharge.[50] A Jarvik 2000 recipient with intractable GIB caused by severe gastric angiodysplasia was successfully treated with octreotide with no bleeding reported

Table 1
Studies on the effect of octreotide on continuous-flow left ventricular assist device–related gastrointestinal bleeding

Study	Patient Population	Design	Outcomes	Limitations
Hayes et al,[48] 2010	N = 5, Jarvik 2000 (2, BTT), HVAD (2, BTT), VentrAssist (1, DT)	Octreotide given as either 25 µg/min infusion, 100 µg SC BID, or 10 mg IM monthly	Bleeding controlled in all 5 patients with no reported adverse outcomes	Retrospective analysis
Aggarwal et al,[16] 2012	N = 13, HeartMate II, DT (93%)	Analysis of outcomes between those with GIB who received octreotide vs those who did not	No significant difference in number of PRBC transfusions, rebleeding rates, lengths of stay, or all-cause mortality	Retrospective analysis
Rennyson et al,[50] 2013	N = 1, HeartMate II, BTT	Octreotide 100 µg SC BID then 20 mg IM depot at discharge	No bleeding for 6 mo, tolerated full anticoagulation for TIA until transplant	Single case report
Coutance et al,[51] 2014	N = 1, Jarvik 2000, DT	Octreotide 100 µg TID then 30 mg SC monthly	No bleeding at 23 mo	Single case report
Dang et al,[52] 2014	N = 1, HVAD, BTT	Octreotide 100 µg SC BID followed by 20 mg IM monthly	Free from GIB for 8 wk	Single case report, limited follow-up
Loyaga-Rendon et al,[49] 2015	N = 7, DT (71%)	Seven patients with recurrent GIB treated with octreotide 50 µg SC BID × 3 mo or 20 mg IM monthly	No difference in number of transfusions, endoscopic procedures, or GIB-related readmissions	Small case series
Malhotra et al,[54] 2017	N = 10, HeartMate II	Phase I study with octreotide 20 mg IM monthly × 4 mo	Depot formulation of octreotide seemed safe and well tolerated without GIB	Small case series, limited follow-up
Shah et al,[53] 2017	N = 51, HeartMate II, DT (50%)	Octreotide IM depot (67%) or daily SC injection (33%)	Octreotide associated with significantly less rebleeding	Retrospective analysis, comparison with a historical control group

Abbreviations: BID, bis in die (twice a day); DT, destination therapy; HVAD, HeartWare ventricular assist device; IM, intramuscular; SC, subcutaneous; TIA, transient ischemic attack.

at 23 months.[51] A HeartWare LVAD patient with recurrent GIB refractory to reductions in pump speed and antithrombotic therapy remained free from bleeding for 8 weeks after the initiation of octreotide 100µg subcutaneously twice daily followed by 20-mg intramuscular injections monthly.[52] Moreover, a retrospective multicenter analysis that compared 51 patients who had received octreotide for secondary prevention of CF-LVAD–related GIB with a historical control group of 240 patients from the HeartMate II clinical trials found that the octreotide-treated group had a significantly lower rate of rebleeding (24% vs 43%; $P = .04$).[53]

The safety and tolerability of octreotide were evaluated in a phase I study of 10 patients with HeartMate II LVAD who received octreotide 20 mg intramuscularly every 4 weeks for 16 weeks. After a follow-up of 28 weeks, none of the patients experienced GIB or any significant adverse effects related to the medication.[54] Additional prospective, randomized controlled trials are needed to clarify the role of octreotide in CF-LVAD–related GIB. However, based on the current literature, it seems to be a safe, well-tolerated option for those patients with bleeding refractory to conventional therapy.

Thalidomide

The mechanisms of action underlying thalidomide remain unclear. Initially prescribed as a sedative and used for its antiemetic properties in morning sickness, it was found to be teratogenic and taken off of the market worldwide in the 1960s. However, after its antiangiogenic properties were discovered in the 1990s, thalidomide is now used in various inflammatory and malignant conditions.[55]

Postulated to inhibit VEGF and basic fibroblast growth factor, thalidomide has also been used in treatment of GIB caused by angiodysplasia. In one case series, 7 patients with chronic bleeding angiodysplasias that failed endoscopic treatment were treated with thalidomide, initially 50 mg daily and increased weekly by 50 mg daily to either 200 mg daily or development of side effects. Three of the patients who tolerated treatment for 6 months did not require any blood transfusions. However, the other 4 patients were unable to tolerate the drug because of side effects, including fatigue, peripheral neuropathy, and severe rash leading to its discontinuation. These patients had a return of transfusion requirements to pretreatment levels.[56] A randomized trial for the treatment of recurrent bleeding from GI angiodysplasias showed that the group treated with thalidomide 100 mg daily for 4 months had a significantly higher percentage of patients whose bleeding episodes decreased by more than half in the first year of follow-up.[57]

Based on these data, a man with recurrent CF-LVAD–related GIB caused by AVMs refractory to argon plasma laser coagulation was treated with thalidomide. In addition to decreasing his LVAD pump speed to increase pulsatility and lowering his INR goal, he was treated with thalidomide 50 mg twice daily. The patient did not have a recurrence of GIB or evidence of thrombosis for 1 year of follow-up after starting thalidomide.[58] A follow-up case series from the same group using the same dosing strategy described 8 patients in whom GIB was either reduced or stopped with thalidomide use. However, thalidomide had to be discontinued in 2 patients because of symptomatic neuropathy.[59] Another case series reported on 11 patients with CF-LVAD–related GIB refractory to conventional interventions who were treated with thalidomide 50 mg daily. Only 1 patient had recurrence of GIB during thalidomide therapy. Adverse effects included somnolence, constipation, and neuropathy that affected 2 patients. The investigators reported an overall lower rate of adverse events (45.5% vs 76.8% by Draper and colleagues[59] in 2015), citing the lower dose of thalidomide used in a population with a lower body

mass index as a possible explanation. In addition, another group reported a case series of 4 patients with recurrent CF-LVAD–related GIB with no identified angiodysplasia or AVM who were treated with thalidomide 50 mg daily with resolution of bleeding.[60,61]

Although the optimal dosing of thalidomide for the treatment of CF-LVAD–related GIB remains unclear, data from these small case series argue for identifying the lowest effective dose in those who respond with improvements in bleeding. Careful monitoring of adverse effects, patient counseling on the importance of avoiding pregnancy, and risk stratification for thromboembolism are necessary in the use of thalidomide for this indication.

Angiotensin Inhibition

Angiotensin II has been implicated in AVM-related GIB via activation of transforming growth factor-beta and VEGF pathways that induce angiogenesis.[62] Moreover, angiotensin II signaling via the angiotensin type 1 receptor induces Ang-2, promoting angiogenesis.[63] Therefore, one group hypothesized that angiotensin II inhibition with angiotensin-converting enzyme inhibitors (ACEIs) or angiotensin receptor blockers (ARBs) would disrupt angiogenesis and decrease the development of angiodysplasias in patients with CF LVADs. A retrospective analysis of 131 patients with a CF LVAD found that, of the 31 patients who did not receive ACEIs or ARBs, the rate of AVM-related GIB was 29% versus 9% in those who were treated with ACEIs or ARBs.[64] ACEI or ARB therapy was associated with a reduced risk for all-cause GIB (OR, 0.29; 95% CI, 0.12–0.72) and AVM-related GIB (OR, 0.23; 95% CI, 0.07–0.71).[64] The same group later reported a 69% reduction in post-LVAD implant risk of major GIB and 76% reduction in risk of AVM-related GIB in patients who received 30 consecutive days of angiotensin-converting enzyme or angiotensin receptor blocker postimplantation.[65] Although limited by its small sample size and retrospective nature, further studies on this commonly prescribed staple of heart failure pharmacotherapy may shed light on its potential for decreasing CF-LVAD–related GIB caused by angiodysplasia.

Danazol

Danazol, a weak androgen, has been used in cases of refractory GIB caused by von Willebrand disease. In a case series, 3 patients with AVWS who continued to have GIB despite vWF concentrate replacement, endoscopic ablations, or bowel resection were treated with danazol, initiated at 100 mg daily with titration up to 500 mg daily, with improvement in reduction of transfusion requirements.[66] Based on these observations, danazol was hypothesized to be efficacious also for CF-LVAD–related GIB. In a case report, a patient with a history of GIB caused by AVMs before HeartMate II LVAD implantation and multiple postimplantation hospitalizations for GIB from AVMs refractory to conventional methods was treated with danazol 200 mg twice daily for 49 days. During and after therapy with danazol, the patient did not require any blood transfusions or hospitalizations for GIB during the 9 months of follow-up.[67] Adverse effects in these studies included worsening renal function limiting continued use of danazol as well as drug-induced liver toxicity necessitating discontinuation.[66,67]

Desmopressin

Desmopressin is the synthetic analogue of vasopressin. In AVWS, desmopressin increases factor VIII and vWF concentrations for a short period of time.[68] It is approved for patients with bleeding secondary to AVWS or hemophilia A. Only 1 case report is currently available in which inhaled desmopressin 150 μg inhaled in 1 nostril 3 d/wk was used to control LVAD-related GIB. For the following 6 months, the patient had significant improvements in bleeding with no additional transfusions or hospital readmissions for bleeding.[69]

SUMMARY

Our limited grasp of the effects of CF physiology is reflected in the persistently high rates of GIB that complicate CF-LVAD therapy. Its multifactorial cause requires a multidisciplinary approach in management, including device adjustment, endoscopic evaluation, and adjunct pharmacologic therapy. Definitive treatment of LVAD-related GIB seems to be heart transplant,[14] which is unavailable to the DT population. Therefore, further investigations into the physiologic effects of diminished pulsatility, roles of key proteins such as vWF, as well as markers of angiogenesis such as Ang-2 merit close attention. Strategies for individualized bleeding and thrombotic risk assessments will be beneficial to determine the optimal intensity of anticoagulation. Randomized controlled studies are needed to validate or refute effects on both primary and secondary prevention of GIB for all pharmacotherapeutic options reviewed in this article.

REFERENCES

1. Kirklin JK, Pagani FD, Kormos RL, et al. Eighth annual INTERMACS report: special focus on framing the impact of adverse events. J Heart Lung Transplant 2017;36(10):1080–6.
2. Interagency Registry for Mechanically Assisted Circulatory Support. Appendix A - Adverse event definitions. Available at: http://www.uab.edu/medicine/intermacs/images/protocol_5.0/appendix_a/AE-Definitions-Final-02-4-2016.docx.
3. Joy PS, Kumar G, Guddati AK, et al. Risk factors and outcomes of gastrointestinal bleeding in left ventricular assist device recipients. Am J Cardiol 2016;117(2):240–4.
4. Stulak JM, Lee D, Haft JW, et al. Gastrointestinal bleeding and subsequent risk of thromboembolic events during support with a left ventricular assist device. J Heart Lung Transplant 2014;33(1):60–4.
5. Stulak JM, Davis ME, Haglund N, et al. Adverse events in contemporary continuous-flow left ventricular assist devices: a multi-institutional comparison shows significant differences. J Thorac Cardiovasc Surg 2016;151(1):177–89.
6. Draper KV, Huang RJ, Gerson LB. GI bleeding in patients with continuous-flow left ventricular assist devices: a systematic review and meta-analysis. Gastrointest Endosc 2014;80(3):435–46.e1.
7. Hasin T, Marmor Y, Kremers W, et al. Readmissions after implantation of axial flow left ventricular assist device. J Am Coll Cardiol 2013;61(2):153–63.
8. Li F, Hinton A, Chen A, et al. Left ventricular assist devices impact hospital resource utilization without affecting patient mortality in gastrointestinal bleeding. Dig Dis Sci 2017;62(1):150–60.
9. Demirozu ZT, Radovancevic R, Hochman LF, et al. Arteriovenous malformation and gastrointestinal bleeding in patients with the HeartMate II left ventricular assist device. J Heart Lung Transplant 2011;30(8):849–53.
10. Holley CT, Harvey L, Roy SS, et al. Gastrointestinal bleeding during continuous-flow left ventricular assist device support is associated with lower rates of cardiac transplantation. ASAIO J 2015;61(6):635–9.
11. Fendler TJ, Nassif ME, Kennedy KF, et al. Global outcome in patients with left ventricular assist devices. Am J Cardiol 2017;119(7):1069–73.
12. Jabbar HR, Abbas A, Ahmed M, et al. The incidence, predictors and outcomes of gastrointestinal bleeding in patients with left ventricular assist device (LVAD). Dig Dis Sci 2015;60(12):3697–706.
13. Boyle AJ, Jorde UP, Sun B, et al. Pre-operative risk factors of bleeding and stroke during left ventricular assist device support: an analysis of more than 900 HeartMate II outpatients. J Am Coll Cardiol 2014;63(9):880–8.

14. Patel SR, Oh KT, Ogriki T, et al. Cessation of continuous flow left ventricular assist device-related gastrointestinal bleeding after heart transplantation. ASAIO J 2017;64(2):191–5.

15. Kim JH, Singh R, Pagani FD, et al. Ventricular assist device therapy in older patients with heart failure: characteristics and outcomes. J Card Fail 2016; 22(12):981–7.

16. Aggarwal A, Pant R, Kumar S, et al. Incidence and management of gastrointestinal bleeding with continuous flow assist devices. Ann Thorac Surg 2012;93(5):1534–40.

17. Crow S, John R, Boyle A, et al. Gastrointestinal bleeding rates in recipients of nonpulsatile and pulsatile left ventricular assist devices. J Thorac Cardiovasc Surg 2009;137(1):208–15.

18. Wever-Pinzon O, Selzman CH, Drakos SG, et al. Pulsatility and the risk of nonsurgical bleeding in patients supported with the continuous-flow left ventricular assist device HeartMate II. Circ Heart Fail 2013;6(3):517–26.

19. Goldstein DJ, Aaronson KD, Tatooles AJ, et al. Gastrointestinal bleeding in recipients of the HeartWare ventricular assist system. JACC Heart Fail 2015;3(4):303–13.

20. Shrode CW, Draper KV, Huang RJ, et al. Significantly higher rates of gastrointestinal bleeding and thromboembolic events with left ventricular assist devices. Clin Gastroenterol Hepatol 2014;12(9):1461–7.

21. Suarez J, Patel CB, Felker GM, et al. Mechanisms of bleeding and approach to patients with axial-flow left ventricular assist devices. Circ Heart Fail 2011; 4(6):779–84.

22. Tabit CE, Chen P, Kim GH, et al. Elevated angiopoietin-2 level in patients with continuous-flow left ventricular assist devices leads to altered angiogenesis and is associated with higher nonsurgical bleeding. Circulation 2016;134(2):141–52.

23. Truby LK, Topkara VK. Angiopoietin-2: marker or mediator of angiogenesis in continuous-flow left ventricular assist device patients? J Thorac Dis 2016; 8(11):3042–5.

24. Kang J, Hennessy-Strahs S, Kwiatkowski P, et al. Continuous-flow LVAD support causes a distinct form of intestinal angiodysplasia. Circ Res 2017; 121(8):963–9.

25. Patel SR, Madan S, Saeed O, et al. Association of nasal mucosal vascular alterations, gastrointestinal arteriovenous malformations, and bleeding in patients with continuous-flow left ventricular assist devices. JACC Heart Fail 2016;4(12):962–70.

26. Uriel N, Pak SW, Jorde UP, et al. Acquired von Willebrand syndrome after continuous-flow mechanical device support contributes to a high prevalence of bleeding during long-term support and at the time of transplantation. J Am Coll Cardiol 2010;56(15): 1207–13.

27. Crow S, Chen D, Milano C, et al. Acquired von Willebrand syndrome in continuous-flow ventricular assist device recipients. Ann Thorac Surg 2010; 90(4):1263–9 [discussion: 1269].

28. Klovaite J, Gustafsson F, Mortensen SA, et al. Severely impaired von Willebrand factor-dependent platelet aggregation in patients with a continuous-flow left ventricular assist device (HeartMate II). J Am Coll Cardiol 2009;53(23):2162–7.

29. Bartoli CR, Restle DJ, Zhang DM, et al. Pathologic von Willebrand factor degradation with a left ventricular assist device occurs via two distinct mechanisms: mechanical demolition and enzymatic cleavage. J Thorac Cardiovasc Surg 2015;149(1): 281–9.

30. Meyer AL, Malehsa D, Bara C, et al. Acquired von Willebrand syndrome in patients with an axial flow left ventricular assist device. Circ Heart Fail 2010; 3(6):675–81.

31. Randi AM, Laffan MA. Von Willebrand factor and angiogenesis: basic and applied issues. J Thromb Haemost 2017;15(1):13–20.

32. Grosman-Rimon L, Tumiati LC, Fuks A, et al. Increased cyclic guanosine monophosphate levels and continuous-flow left-ventricular assist devices: implications for gastrointestinal bleeding. J Thorac Cardiovasc Surg 2016;151(1):219–27.

33. Maltais S, Kilic A, Nathan S, et al. PREVENtion of HeartMate II pump thrombosis through clinical management: the PREVENT multi-center study. J Heart Lung Transplant 2017;36(1):1–12.

34. Mathis MR, Sathishkumar S, Kheterpal S, et al. Complications, risk factors, and staffing patterns for noncardiac surgery in patients with left ventricular assist devices. Anesthesiology 2017;126(3): 450–60.

35. Elmunzer BJ, Padhya KT, Lewis JJ, et al. Endoscopic findings and clinical outcomes in ventricular assist device recipients with gastrointestinal bleeding. Dig Dis Sci 2011;56(11):3241–6.

36. Meyer MM, Young SD, Sun B, et al. Endoscopic evaluation and management of gastrointestinal bleeding in patients with ventricular assist devices. Gastroenterol Res Pract 2012;2012:630483.

37. Dakik HK, McGhan AA, Chiu ST, et al. The diagnostic yield of repeated endoscopic evaluation in patients with gastrointestinal bleeding and left ventricular assist devices. Dig Dis Sci 2016;61(6): 1603–10.

38. Cushing K, Kushnir V. Gastrointestinal bleeding following LVAD placement from top to bottom. Dig Dis Sci 2016;61(6):1440–7.

39. Amornsawadwattana S, Nassif M, Raymer D, et al. Video capsule endoscopy in left ventricular assist device recipients with obscure gastrointestinal bleeding. World J Gastroenterol 2016;22(18): 4559–66.

40. Zikos TA, Pan J, Limketkai B, et al. Efficacy of video capsule endoscopy in the management of suspected small bowel bleeding in patients with continuous flow left ventricular assist devices. Gastroenterol Res 2017;10(5):280–7.

41. Sarosiek K, Bogar L, Conn MI, et al. An old problem with a new therapy: gastrointestinal bleeding in ventricular assist device patients and deep overtube-assisted enteroscopy. ASAIO J 2013;59(4):384–9.

42. Katz JN, Adamson RM, John R, et al. Safety of reduced anti-thrombotic strategies in HeartMate II patients: a one-year analysis of the US-TRACE study. J Heart Lung Transplant 2015;34(12):1542–8.

43. Netuka I, Litzler PY, Berchtold-Herz M, et al. Outcomes in HeartMate II patients with no antiplatelet therapy: 2-year results from the European TRACE study. Ann Thorac Surg 2017;103(4):1262–8.

44. Guha A, Eshelbrenner CL, Richards DM, et al. Gastrointestinal bleeding after continuous-flow left ventricular device implantation: review of pathophysiology and management. Methodist Debakey Cardiovasc J 2015;11(1):24–7.

45. Lamberts SW, van der Lely AJ, de Herder WW, et al. Octreotide. N Engl J Med 1996;334(4):246–54.

46. Brown C, Subramanian V, Wilcox CM, et al. Somatostatin analogues in the treatment of recurrent bleeding from gastrointestinal vascular malformations: an overview and systematic review of prospective observational studies. Dig Dis Sci 2010;55(8):2129–34.

47. Dasgupta P. Somatostatin analogues: multiple roles in cellular proliferation, neoplasia, and angiogenesis. Pharmacol Ther 2004;102(1):61–85.

48. Hayes HM, Dembo LG, Larbalestier R, et al. Management options to treat gastrointestinal bleeding in patients supported on rotary left ventricular assist devices: a single-center experience. Artif Organs 2010;34(9):703–6.

49. Loyaga-Rendon RY, Hashim T, Tallaj JA, et al. Octreotide in the management of recurrent gastrointestinal bleed in patients supported by continuous flow left ventricular assist devices. ASAIO J 2015;61(1):107–9.

50. Rennyson SL, Shah KB, Tang DG, et al. Octreotide for left ventricular assist device-related gastrointestinal hemorrhage: can we stop the bleeding? ASAIO J 2013;59(4):450–1.

51. Coutance G, Saplacan V, Belin A, et al. Octreotide for recurrent intestinal bleeding due to ventricular assist device. Asian Cardiovasc Thorac Ann 2014;22(3):350–2.

52. Dang G, Grayburn R, Lamb G, et al. Octreotide for the management of gastrointestinal bleeding in a patient with a HeartWare left ventricular assist device. Case Rep Cardiol 2014;2014:826453.

53. Shah KB, Gunda S, Emani S, et al. Multicenter evaluation of octreotide as secondary prophylaxis in patients with left ventricular assist devices and gastrointestinal bleeding. Circ Heart Fail 2017;10(11). https://doi.org/10.1161/CIRCHEARTFAILURE.117.004500.

54. Malhotra R, Shah KB, Chawla R, et al. Tolerability and biological effects of long-acting octreotide in patients with continuous flow left ventricular assist devices. ASAIO J 2017;63(3):367–70.

55. Franks ME, Macpherson GR, Figg WD. Thalidomide. Lancet 2004;363(9423):1802–11.

56. Kamalaporn P, Saravanan R, Cirocco M, et al. Thalidomide for the treatment of chronic gastrointestinal bleeding from angiodysplasias: a case series. Eur J Gastroenterol Hepatol 2009;21(12):1347–50.

57. Ge ZZ, Chen HM, Gao YJ, et al. Efficacy of thalidomide for refractory gastrointestinal bleeding from vascular malformation. Gastroenterology 2011;141(5):1629–37.e1-4.

58. Ray R, Kale PP, Ha R, et al. Treatment of left ventricular assist device-associated arteriovenous malformations with thalidomide. ASAIO J 2014;60(4):482–3.

59. Draper K, Kale P, Martin B, et al. Thalidomide for treatment of gastrointestinal angiodysplasia in patients with left ventricular assist devices: case series and treatment protocol. J Heart Lung Transplant 2015;34(1):132–4.

60. Seng BJJ, Teo LLY, Chan LL, et al. Novel use of low-dose thalidomide in refractory gastrointestinal bleeding in left ventricular assist device patients. Int J Artif Organs 2017;40(11):636–40.

61. Chan LL, Lim CP, Lim CH, et al. Novel use of thalidomide in recurrent gastrointestinal tract bleeding in patients with left ventricular assist devices: a case series. Heart Lung Circ 2017;26(10):1101–4.

62. Ferrari G, Cook BD, Terushkin V, et al. Transforming growth factor-beta 1 (TGF-beta1) induces angiogenesis through vascular endothelial growth factor (VEGF)-mediated apoptosis. J Cell Physiol 2009;219(2):449–58.

63. Otani A, Takagi H, Oh H, et al. Angiotensin II induces expression of the Tie2 receptor ligand, angiopoietin-2, in bovine retinal endothelial cells. Diabetes 2001;50(4):867–75.

64. Houston BA, Schneider AL, Vaishnav J, et al. Angiotensin II antagonism is associated with reduced risk for gastrointestinal bleeding caused by arteriovenous malformations in patients with left ventricular assist devices. J Heart Lung Transplant 2017;36(4):380–5.

65. Converse M, Sobhanian M, Mardis A, et al. Impact of angiotensin II inhibitors on the incidence of gastrointestinal bleeds after left ventricular assist device placement. J Heart Lung Transplant 2017;36(4):S150.

66. Botero JP, Pruthi RK. Refractory bleeding from intestinal angiodysplasias successfully treated with danazol in three patients with von Willebrand disease. Blood Coagul Fibrinolysis 2013;24(8):884–6.

67. Schettle SD, Pruthi RK, Pereira NL. Continuous-flow left ventricular assist devices and gastrointestinal bleeding: potential role of danazol. J Heart Lung Transplant 2014;33(5):549–50.

68. Auerswald G, Kreuz W. Haemate P/Humate-P for the treatment of von Willebrand disease: considerations for use and clinical experience. Haemophilia 2008; 14(Suppl 5):39–46.

69. Hollis IB, Chen SL, Chang PP, et al. Inhaled desmopressin for refractory gastrointestinal bleeding in a patient with a HeartMate II left ventricular assist device. ASAIO J 2017;63(4):e47–9.

Neurologic Events in Continuous-Flow Left Ventricular Assist Devices

Ajay Kadakkal, MD[a], Samer S. Najjar, MD[b],*

KEYWORDS

- LVAD • Mechanical circulatory support • Neurologic events • Ischemic stroke • Hemorrhagic stroke
- Hypertension

KEY POINTS

- Stroke remains a common complication in the era of continuous-flow left ventricular assist devices (LVADs) therapy.
- Both ischemic and hemorrhagic stroke influence survival and quality of life after LVAD therapy.
- Risk factors for stroke include age, sex, hypertension, and infection.
- Further studies are urgently needed to help prevent neurologic complications, alleviate residual deficits, and improve clinical outcomes.

INTRODUCTION

With the burgeoning population of advanced systolic heart failure, continuous-flow (CF) left ventricular assist devices (LVADs) have emerged as a durable and effective therapy to increase survival and improve quality of life.[1,2] Mechanical circulatory support (MCS) is now an accepted therapy both as a bridge to heart transplantation and as destination therapy.[3,4]

In the last decade, the technology has advanced from pulsatile to CF-LVADs. CF-LVAD pumps are smaller and have demonstrated greater durability than pulsatile LVADs.[5–7] Nonetheless, durable CF-LVADs still have a high burden of medical complications, both perioperatively and during long-term follow-up. These complications most commonly include infections, pump malfunction, arrhythmias, heart failure, bleeding, and thrombotic events.[8,9] Of those, neurologic events, both ischemic and hemorrhagic, stand out as the most-feared complications, as they have the greatest adverse impact on quality of life, disability, candidacy for heart transplantation, and caregiver burden.[10,11] Additionally, neurologic events are the leading cause of mortality for patients on long-term LVAD support.[12] In this article, the authors review the incidence and prevalence of neurologic events in patients with durable CF-LVADs and discuss their risk factors and their impact on clinical outcomes.

NEUROLOGIC EVENTS

Neurologic events may be clinically silent, whereby suspicious lesions are found on a brain imaging study, in the absence of any past or present clinical neurologic symptoms. Alternatively, patients may present with new focal (or diffuse) neurologic symptoms. If these symptoms completely resolve within 24 hours, and no new

Disclosure Statement: S.S. Najjar reports receiving institutional research support from Medtronic and Abbott.
[a] Advanced Heart Failure Program, MedStar Heart and Vascular Institute, MedStar Washington Hospital Center, 110 Irving Street, Northwest Room 1F-1222, Washington, DC 20010, USA; [b] Advanced Heart Failure Program, MedStar Heart and Vascular Institute, MedStar Washington Hospital Center, 110 Irving Street, Northwest Room 1F-1219, Washington, DC 20010, USA
* Corresponding author.
E-mail address: Samer.S.Najjar@MedStar.net

lesions are noted on brain imaging, they are termed a transient ischemic attack (TIA). Otherwise, they are labeled as a cerebrovascular accident (CVA) or a stroke. CVAs are classified as ischemic or hemorrhagic events. The latter could be a primary hemorrhagic event or could be a complication of an ischemic CVA with transformation into a hemorrhagic CVA.

A variety of scoring models have been used to describe the severity of the stroke or the extent of disability. In the MCS field, the modified Rankin Scale is the instrument that is most commonly used to assess the degree of disability and dependence of patients who have had a stroke (**Table 1**), particularly in research studies. The modified Rankin Scale is typically measured several months after the neurologic event, to evaluate the residual neurologic deficits from the stroke. The pivotal multicenter studies of axial and centrifugal devices have used a modified Rankin Scale of greater than 3 to denote a disabling stroke (ie, inability to walk without assistance).

Interestingly, ischemic CVAs in patients with LVADs seem to have a predilection for the right cerebral hemisphere. In a single-center retrospective analysis of 317 patients who received an LVAD between 2000 and 2011 (pulsatile and CF-LVADs), 46 neurologic events were documented, of which 27 (59%) occurred in the right hemisphere and 13 (28%) in the left hemisphere; 3 were bilateral and 3 were in the vertebrobasilar territory.[13] This geographic preference is hypothesized to be due to the anatomy of the aortic arch and to the

surgical anastomosis of the outflow graft to the aorta, which could preferentially direct embolic material toward the brachiocephalic trunk. Indeed, a computational fluid dynamic model showed that the alteration of the location of the anastomosis of the LVAD outflow cannula as well as its angle of incidence can reduce the risk of thromboembolic events in an experimental model.[14]

INCIDENCE/PREVALENCE

Several studies have evaluated the incidence and prevalence of neurologic events in patients with CF-LVADs. These studies include the pivotal studies of the axial and centrifugal flow pumps as well as single and multicenter retrospective reviews of institutions and registries. Event rates are often expressed as events per patient year (eppy) to account for the differing follow-up time of the patients, which influences the exposure risk.

In a retrospective review of 230 patients who were implanted with a HeartMate II (Abbott Corp, Abbott Park IL) at a single center, Harvey and colleagues[15] observed a neurologic event rate of 0.064 eppy, of which 19 (48.7%) were embolic and 20 (51.3%) were hemorrhagic. **Table 2** summarizes the neurologic event rates in the landmark trials that led to the approval of the HeartMate II device for bridge to transplantation, destination therapy, and in the early postapproval commercial experience (as gleaned from the Interagency Registry for Mechanically Assisted Circulatory Support [INTERMACS] registry). The rate of ischemic strokes ranged between 0.03 eppy and 0.09 eppy. The rate of hemorrhagic strokes ranged between 0.01 and 0.05 eppy.

Table 3 summarizes the neurologic event rates in the pivotal trials in Europe and the United States that led to the approval of the HVAD (Medtronic Inc, Minneapolis, MN) for bridge to transplantation and in the US continued access protocol. The rate of ischemic stroke ranged between 0.04 eppy and 0.17 eppy. The rate of hemorrhagic stroke ranged between 0.07 eppy and 0.11 eppy.

Several landmark studies have compared the risk of stroke between axial and centrifugal flow devices.[16–18] Notably, the ENDURANCE clinical trial randomly assigned 446 patients with advanced heart failure to receive a HeartMate II or an HVAD CF-LVAD in a 1:2 ratio. Rogers and colleagues[18] observed that the incidence of stroke (both ischemic and hemorrhagic) was significantly higher in the group that received the centrifugal pump. Of 149 patients who received a HeartMate II, 18 patients had 19 neurologic events (0.09 eppy), of which 12 were ischemic (0.06 eppy) and 7 were hemorrhagic (0.03 eppy). Of 296

Table 1 Modified Rankin scale	
No symptoms	0
No significant disability: able to perform all usual activities and duties	1
Slight disability: unable to perform all previous activities but can independently manage own affairs without assistance	2
Moderate disability: requires assistance but able to walk independently	3
Moderate severe disability: unable to walk without assistance, unable to complete ADLs without assistance	4
Severe disability: bedridden, incontinent, required constant nursing care	5
Death	6

Abbreviation: ADLs, activities of daily living.

Data from van Swieten JC, Koudstaal PJ, Visser MC, et al. Interobserver agreement for the assessment of handicap in stroke patients. Stroke 1988;19:604–60; and Rankin L. Cerebral vascular accidents in patients over the age of 60. II. Prognosis. Scott Med J 1957;2:200–15.

Table 2
Neurologic events (HeartMate II)

	BTT[7]	BTT[43]	BTT[44]	DT[45]	DT[46]	BTT + DT[30]	DT[18]
N	281	169	1496	281	247	956	148
Follow-up	182 pt-y	142 pt-y	1082 pt-y	498 pt-y	386 pt-y	1715 pt-y	296 pt-y
Date of Publication	2009	2011	2011	2012	2013	2014	2017
Ischemic CVA (eppy)	0.09	0.06	0.06	0.05	0.03	0.04	0.06
Hemorrhagic CVA (eppy)	0.05	0.01	0.02	0.03	0.05	0.05	0.03

The neurologic eppy in the pivotal trials of the HeartMate II device for both bridge to transplant and destination therapy.
Abbreviations: BTT, bridge to transplant; DT, destination therapy.

patients who received a HeartWare, 88 patients experienced 117 neurologic events (0.29 eppy), of which 70 were ischemic (0.17 eppy) and 47 were hemorrhagic (0.11 eppy). In the subsequent ENDURANCE Supplemental trial, which included a blood pressure management protocol for the HVAD arm, the overall neurologic rate (stroke and TIA) in patients who received an HVAD was reduced by 24.7%, including an impressive 50% reduction in the rate of hemorrhagic strokes.[19]

More recently, in the MOMENTUM 3 clinical trial whereby 361 patients with advanced heart failure were randomly assigned to receive a HeartMate II or a HeartMate III (Abbott Corp, Abbott Park IL) CF-LVAD, Mehra and colleagues[17] initially reported that the incidence of stroke did not significantly differ between the 2 devices (7.9% vs 10.9% respectively) at 6 months. However, in the longer-term 2-year follow-up, the overall stroke rate was significantly lower in the centrifugal flow cohort than the axial flow cohort (10.1% vs 19.2%; hazard ratio, 0.47; $P = .02$).[20] Of 189 patients who received a HeartMate III, 19 had 22 strokes (14 were ischemic and 8 were hemorrhagic). Of 172 patients who received a HeartMate II, 33 had 43 strokes (26 were ischemic and 17 were hemorrhagic).[20]

Neurologic events were also compared between axial and centrifugal devices in a bridge-to-transplant cohort of 497 patients who received

an implant at centers participating in the Mechanical Circulatory Support Research Network. A total of 16% of patients who received a HeartMate II had a neurologic event, compared with 19% of patients who received an HVAD. The event rate for ischemic CVA (but not hemorrhagic CVA) was significantly lower for HeartMate II than HVAD (0.071 eppy vs 0.157 eppy) in univariate analysis. However, this difference was no longer statistically significant in adjusted multivariable models.[21]

The largest report of neurologic events to date includes 7112 patients in the INTERMACS registry who received a CF-LVAD between May 2012 and March 2015. During a median follow-up of 9.79 months, Acharya and colleagues[22] reported that 752 (10.57%) patients had at least 1 stroke (0.123 eppy), of which 447 (51.38%) were ischemic and 423 (48.62%) were hemorrhagic. Only 143 strokes (16.4%) occurred within 2 weeks of implant.

CLINICAL OUTCOMES

The reason neurologic events are one of the most dreaded complications of an LVAD is because of their potential adverse (sometimes dramatic) impact on quality of life. Obviously, the greater the residual deficit after a neurologic event (ie, higher modified Rankin Scale), the greater the severity of the functional compromise and its

Table 3
Neurologic events (HeartWare)

	BTT[2]	BTT[6]	BTT[4]	BTT[28]	DT[18]
N	50	140	322	382	297
Follow-up	48 pt-y	89 pt-y	305 pt-y	407 pt-y	594 pt-y
Date of Publication	2011	2012	2013	2015	2017
Ischemic (eppy)	0.04	0.11	0.09	0.06	0.17
Hemorrhagic (eppy)	0.08	0.09	0.09	0.07	0.11

The neurologic eppy in the pivotal trials of the HeartWare device as bridge to transplant therapy.
Abbreviations: BTT, bridge to transplant; DT, destination therapy.

associated debility and loss of independence.[23] Furthermore, the sequelae of neurologic events often result in additional burdens being imposed on patients' support system, including family members and caregivers.

Neurologic events may also compromise patients' candidacy for heart transplantation. For example, among patients in the INTERMACS registry who received an implanted LVAD as a bridge-to-transplantation strategy, those who had a stroke had a much lower rate of transplantation than those who did not (15.57% vs 33.33%).[22]

Importantly, stroke has also been shown to adversely affect survival. In the INTERMACS registry of CF-LVADs that were implanted between 2008 and 2014, stroke was the leading primary cause/mode of death.[8] This finding is further emphasized in an analysis of the US Nationwide Inpatient Sample database for the years 2007 to 2011. The incidence of ischemic stroke and hemorrhagic stroke in patients with LVADs increased patients' in-hospital mortality by 4- and 18-fold, respectively.[24] Similarly, in an analysis of administrative claims data between 2005 and 2013 from acute care hospitals in 3 states, stroke in LVAD patients was a strong and independent predictor of subsequent in-hospital mortality (hazard ratio 6.1).[25] Furthermore, in a more recent single-center study of 301 patients with CF-LVAD who were followed for a median of 376 days, the in-hospital mortality for hemorrhagic stroke was higher than ischemic stroke (59% vs 28%).[23]

Interestingly, the risk of stroke has been observed to have a bimodal distribution, with the highest risk immediately after the implant and then again approximately 1 year later. This finding was observed in a single-center study of 402 patients who received a CF-LVAD, with a median follow-up of approximately 1 year, which showed the overall incidence of stroke was 17% (0.14 eppy). The novel finding of this study, however, was that the mortality from stroke also followed a similar bimodal distribution, with the highest risk immediately after the implant and then again 9 to 12 months later. In multivariable analysis, stroke that occurred after discharge from the hospital (but not stroke that occurred during the hospitalization for LVAD implantation) was an independent predictor of mortality. Both hemorrhagic stroke that occurred during the implant hospitalization and hemorrhagic stroke that occurred after discharge from the hospital were independent predictors of mortality.[10] Similarly, Harvey and colleagues[15] reported the mortality rate for patients with a HeartMate II CF-LVAD who had a stroke was 2-fold greater than the mortality rate for patients who remained free of stroke. In this study, the survival rate for hemorrhagic stroke was numerically lower than the survival rate for ischemic stroke (60% vs 77% at 12 months, 39% vs 58% at 24 months); but this was not statistically significant.

In the INTERMACS registry, 13% of patients with a stroke had an additional neurologic event. One-month survival after the first stroke was 63.6%; 6-month survival was 50.9%; 12-month survival was 43.7%.[22] Those with a hemorrhagic stroke had a significantly worse survival than those with an ischemic stroke (**Fig. 1**).

RISK FACTORS

Several risk factors have been evaluated as predictors of stroke, including both modifiable and

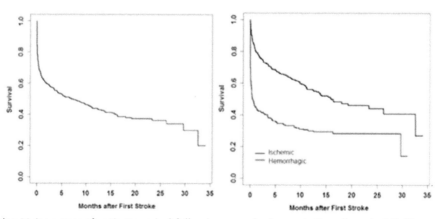

Fig. 1. Kaplan-Meier curves of patient survival following neurologic event: Overall survival (*left*); survival stratified by stroke type (ischemic or neurologic). Patients with hemorrhagic stroke had a significantly lower survival than those with ischemic stroke (*P*<.001). (*From* Acharya D, Loyaga-Rendon R, Morgan CJ, et al. INTERMACS analysis of stroke during support with continuous-flow left ventricular assist devices: risk factors and outcomes. JACC Heart Fail 2017;5(10):706; with permission.)

nonmodifiable risk factors. There are conflicting data on atrial fibrillation[21,26–28] and diabetes mellitus.[29,30] In this section, the authors focus on age, sex, blood pressure, and infection/inflammation.

Sex

Several studies found that women seem to be at an increased risk of neurologic events,[22,25,31,32] particularly hemorrhagic strokes.[25,33] In an analysis of 956 patients who received a HeartMate II and survived to discharge, female sex was an independent predictor of both ischemic stroke (hazard ratio 1.88) and hemorrhagic stroke (hazard ratio 1.94). In the INTERMACS registry of US patients, female sex was an independent predictor of overall stroke (hazard ratio 1.51), ischemic stroke (hazard ratio 1.46), and hemorrhagic stroke (hazard ratio 1.65).[22] However, in the European Registry for Patients with Mechanical Circulatory Support, which is an online database that collects data on patients with LVADs from 50 European and non-European centers (in 15 countries), there was no difference in the event rate of ischemic or hemorrhagic strokes between men and women among 966 patients (15.6% women) who were followed for a median of 1.26 years.[34] Similarly, Coffin and colleagues[21] did not find sex to be an independent predictor of neurologic events.

Age

The impact of age on neurologic events has been evaluated in 497 patients who received a CF-LVAD as a bridge to transplant. Coffin and colleagues[21] found that age was an independent predictor of neurologic events (hazard ratio 1.3). In 956 patients who received a HeartMate II LVAD and who survived to discharge, Boyle and colleagues[30] stratified them into those older than and younger than 65 years of age. They found younger age to be an independent predictor of hemorrhagic stroke but not ischemic stroke. Female sex was the only other independent predictor of hemorrhagic stroke, indicating that women younger than 65 years who received a CF-LVAD were at the highest risk of a hemorrhagic CVA.[30]

Infection

Infection also seems to confer an increased risk of neurologic events. A single-center study of 307 patients who received an LVAD (of which 140 received a CF-LVAD), postoperative infection was an independent predictor of neurologic events.[35] In another single-center study of 230 patients with a HeartMate II CF-LVAD, those who had postoperative sepsis had a higher risk of stroke.[15] Additionally, in a single-center retrospective analysis of 87 patients with the HeartMate II CF-LVAD, those who had a blood stream infection had an 8-fold greater risk of hemorrhagic or ischemic neurologic events (P = .001) and a greater than 20-fold risk of hemorrhagic CVA (P = .03).[36] Similarly, in a cohort of 164 Japanese patients with LVADs, Yoshioka and colleagues[37] reported that bacteremia was an independent risk factor for hemorrhagic stroke (hazard ratio 2.36). This same group also reported that patients with CF-LVAD who had LVAD-related infections had a higher number of cerebral microbleeds as assessed by brain MRI.

Blood Pressure

The CVA risk factor that has received the most attention is blood pressure. It is well known that both axial and centrifugal CF-LVADs are afterload dependent. However, centrifugal flow devices are more sensitive to alterations in afterload than axial flow devices, because of the differing pressure-flow relationships between the two types of pumps.[38] Thus, for a given change in blood pressure the centrifugal pumps are likely to experience a greater change in flow. The importance of blood pressure management is underscored in a study of 96 patients who received a CF-LVAD and remained on support for greater than 30 days. Lampert and colleagues[39] noted that those who were not on antihypertensive medications had a significantly higher chance of having a neurologic event.

Nassif and colleagues[40] stratified 275 patients from a single center who received a CF-LVAD and who were followed for a mean of 16 months into 2 groups based on whether their blood pressure 48 hours before discharge was greater than or less than the median systolic blood pressure of 100 mm Hg. Stroke was observed in 16% of those whose systolic blood pressure was greater than the mean but in only 7% of those whose systolic blood pressure was less than 100 mm Hg. In multivariable analysis, a systolic blood pressure greater than 100 mm Hg was associated with a 2.5-fold higher risk of stroke (P = .022). When systolic blood pressure was analyzed as a continuous variable, there was a 19% increase in the risk of stroke for every 5-mm Hg increase in systolic blood pressure (P = .02).[40]

In an analysis of 382 patients who received an HVAD CF-LVAD as part of the ADVANCE trial and continued access protocol, Teuteberg and colleagues[28] observed a prevalence of 6.8% of ischemic CVAs and 8.4% of hemorrhagic CVAs. In univariate analysis, ischemic neurologic events were associated with aspirin dose (≤81 mg), mean arterial pressure (MAP) greater than 90 mm Hg, history of atrial fibrillation, age greater than 56 years, and white race. However, in multivariable analysis, only low aspirin dosage and atrial fibrillation remained as independent predictors of ischemic CVAs. In univariate analysis, hemorrhagic neurologic events were associated with aspirin dose (<81 mg), MAP greater than 90 mm Hg, pump speed (>2750), time in therapeutic range (<40%), and international normalized ratio (INR) greater than 3.0. However, in multivariable analysis, only hypertension, low aspirin dosage, and an INR greater than 3.0 remained independent predictors of hemorrhagic CVAs.

Interestingly, Teuteberg and colleagues[28] then surveyed the blood pressure practices at the 30 centers where these patients were implanted with the HVAD. They found that 8 of them had established protocols for strict monitoring of and aggressive management of blood pressure. At these sites, there was a significantly lower occurrence of a MAP greater than 100 mm Hg. Importantly, the prevalence of hemorrhagic CVAs at these 8 sites was significantly lower than the prevalence at the other sites (1.8% vs 9.3%), and the rate of hemorrhagic CVAs tended to be lower (0.02 eppy vs 0.08 eppy, $P = .07$). There were no differences in the prevalence or the rate of ischemic CVAs between centers that did and those that did not follow a blood pressure protocol.

The importance of blood pressure control was further underscored in the findings from the ENDURANCE clinical trial. Although the main finding of the trial was that the HVAD was noninferior to the HeartMate II with respect to the primary end point of survival free from disabling stroke or device removal (for failure or malfunction), there was an important difference in the rate of neurologic events. Patients who received the HVAD had a significantly higher risk of stroke compared with those who received the HeartMate II pump (29.7% vs 12.1%) and a significantly lower rate of freedom from stroke (85.0% vs 65.2% at 2 years). In a post hoc analysis that stratified patients who received the HVAD according to their blood pressure, those whose mean blood pressure was lower than 90 mm Hg had a lower frequency of strokes, particularly hemorrhagic strokes.

These insights into the important impact of blood pressure as a risk factor for neurologic events led to the design of the ENDURANCE Supplemental trial. Similar to ENDURANCE, this was a randomized clinical study whereby patients with advanced heart failure who were not eligible for heart transplantation were randomized 2:1 to receive the HVAD versus the HeartMate II device.

However, patients who received an HVAD in the ENDURANCE Supplemental trial were required to perform ambulatory blood pressure monitoring, a stipulation that was not present in the original ENDURANCE trial. Implementation of this blood pressure protocol resulted in a 24.7% reduction in overall neurologic events, including a 50% reduction in the rate of hemorrhagic strokes.[19] This finding lends strong support to the concept that optimizing blood pressure control may lower the risk of neurologic (particularly hemorrhagic) events in patients with the HVAD CF-LVAD. As mentioned earlier, in the MOMENTUM 3 trial, patients who received a HeartMate III device had significantly lower neurologic events when compared with the HeartMate II. In contrast to the findings of the ENDURANCE trial, no correlation was found with regard to blood pressure control between the coaxial flow cohort and centrifugal flow cohort. The findings of the ENDURANCE and MOMENTUM 3 clinical trials suggest that the differences in stroke rates among these 3 pumps is not only related to centrifugal or axial flow. Further study and longer-term follow-up is needed to differentiate whether coaxial flow or centrifugal flow significantly impact stroke rates independent of other variables, including pump design, anticoagulation regimen, blood pressure control, and other baseline risk factors as mentioned in this section.[20]

MANAGEMENT

Currently there is no standardized protocol for the management of neurologic events. Treatment strategies for the most part are institution specific. Computed tomography imaging of the brain should be obtained as soon possible to help classify patients into hemorrhagic or ischemic events, as management strategies differ between the two groups.

In the case of a hemorrhagic event, prompt neurosurgical consideration should be considered and a decision about reversal of anticoagulation and the choice of reversing agent (eg, prothrombin complex concentrate, fresh frozen plasma, desmopressin, vitamin K, platelet transfusions) should be made. The optimal timing of when to resume antiplatelet and/or anticoagulant therapies is currently undefined.

In the case of an ischemic event, the treating team will also need to make a decision about discontinuation of antiplatelet and anticoagulant agents, based in part on the risk of hemorrhagic conversion. Systemic tissue plasminogen activator, which has shown benefit in acute embolic strokes in the general population, has not been widely studied in the LVAD population. Thrombolytics may be less efficacious in patients with CF-LVAD, as some embolic strokes in these patients may be due to thrombi that formed within the CF-LVAD, which are composed of fibrin and denatured proteins that may be less readily responsive to thrombolysis. Furthermore, patients with CF-LVAD are at a higher risk for hemorrhagic transformation because of the concomitant use of anticoagulants, known acquired von-Willebrand factor deficiency due to shear stress, and possibly high rates of hemorrhagic conversions in the subset of patients whose are infected or who have bacteremia. On the other hand, endovascular stroke therapy has shown promise in selected individuals presenting with acute ischemic strokes.[41]

The authors think that the management of LVAD patients with strokes is best accomplished in a multidisciplinary team approach. Beyond advanced heart failure cardiologists, surgeons, and LVAD coordinators, the team should include (but is not limited to) stroke specialists, neurosurgeons (in the case of a hemorrhagic CVA), intensivists, and rehabilitation experts.[42] Physical, occupational, and speech therapy are a critical part of the recovery and rehabilitation process.

SUMMARY

The incidence and prevalence of neurologic events after implantation of a CF-LVAD remain unacceptably high, particularly given the adverse and often dramatic impact that these complications have on quality of life, disability, and survival as well as the burden on caregivers and family members. There is a pressing need to identify additional modifiable risk factors that could help lower the risk of CVA and to develop best practice guidelines for the clinical management of strokes to mitigate the extent of their damage and neurologic injury. Further understanding of the pathogenesis and the pathophysiology of both ischemic and hemorrhagic events is sorely needed to help devise novel strategies that could lower these event rates and ideally prevent them. These strategies could include design alterations to the pump that could lower its thrombogenicity or improve the pump-patient interface, surgical refinement of the location or angle of the outflow graft guided by insights gleaned from computational flow dynamics, personalized management of antithrombotic and anticoagulation regimen, and so forth.

Ultimately, neurologic events remain one of the main barriers that impede further acceptance of this technology by the general cardiology and medical community. Furthermore, they are one of the major (and legitimate) contributing obstacles that stand in the way of expanding this technology to earlier stages of heart failure.

REFERENCES

1. Rose EA, Gelijns AC, Moskowitz AJ, et al. Long-term use of a left ventricular assist device for end-stage heart failure. N Engl J Med 2001;345(20):1435–43.
2. Strueber M, O'Driscoll G, Jansz P, et al. Multicenter evaluation of an intrapericardial left ventricular assist system. J Am Coll Cardiol 2011;57(12):1375–82.
3. Strueber M, Larbalestier R, Jansz P, et al. Results of the post-market registry to evaluate the heartware left ventricular assist system (ReVOLVE). J Heart Lung Transplant 2014;33(5):486–91.
4. Slaughter MS, Pagani FD, McGee EC, et al. HeartWare ventricular assist system for bridge to transplant: combined results of the bridge to transplant and continued access protocol trial. J Heart Lung Transplant 2013;32(7):675–83.
5. Miller LW, Pagani FD, Russell SD, et al. Use of a continuous-flow device in patients awaiting heart transplantation. N Engl J Med 2007;357(9):885–96.
6. Aaronson KD, Slaughter MS, Miller LW, et al. Use of an intrapericardial, continuous-flow, centrifugal pump in patients awaiting heart transplantation. Circulation 2012;125(25):3191–200.
7. Pagani FD, Miller LW, Russell SD, et al. Extended mechanical circulatory support with a continuous-flow rotary left ventricular assist device. J Am Coll Cardiol 2009;54(4):312–21.
8. Kirklin JK, Naftel DC, Pagani FD, et al. Seventh INTERMACS annual report: 15,000 patients and counting. J Heart Lung Transplant 2015;34(12):1495–504.
9. Najjar SS, Slaughter MS, Pagani FD, et al. An analysis of pump thrombus events in patients in the HeartWare ADVANCE bridge to transplant and continued access protocol trial. J Heart Lung Transplant 2014;33(1):23–34.
10. Frontera JA, Starling R, Cho SM, et al. Risk factors, mortality, and timing of ischemic and hemorrhagic stroke with left ventricular assist devices. J Heart Lung Transplant 2017;36(6):673–83.
11. Cho SM, Moazami N, Frontera JA. Stroke and intracranial hemorrhage in heartmate ii and heartware left ventricular assist devices: a systematic review. Neurocrit Care 2017;27(1):17–25.
12. Kirklin JK, Pagani FD, Kormos RL, et al. Eighth annual INTERMACS report: special focus on framing the impact of adverse events. J Heart Lung Transplant 2017;36(10):1080–6.
13. Kato TS, Ota T, Schulze PC, et al. Asymmetric pattern of cerebrovascular lesions in patients after left ventricular assist device implantation. Stroke 2012;43(3):872–4.

14. Osorio AF, Osorio R, Ceballos A, et al. Computational fluid dynamics analysis of surgical adjustment of left ventricular assist device implantation to minimise stroke risk. Comput Methods Biomech Biomed Engin 2013;16(6):622–38.

15. Harvey L, Holley C, Roy SS, et al. Stroke after left ventricular assist device implantation: outcomes in the continuous-flow era. Ann Thorac Surg 2015; 100(2):535–41.

16. Lalonde SD, Alba AC, Rigobon A, et al. Clinical differences between continuous flow ventricular assist devices: a comparison between HeartMate II and HeartWare HVAD. J Card Surg 2013;28(5): 604–10.

17. Mehra MR, Naka Y, Uriel N, et al. A fully magnetically levitated circulatory pump for advanced heart failure. N Engl J Med 2017;376(5):440–50.

18. Rogers JG, Pagani FD, Tatooles AJ, et al. Intrapericardial left ventricular assist device for advanced heart failure. N Engl J Med 2017;376(5):451–60.

19. Milano CA, Rogers JG, Tatooles AJ, et al. The treatment of patients with advanced heart failure ineligible for cardiac transplantation with the HeartWare ventricular assist device: results of the ENDURANCE supplement trial. J Heart Lung Transplant 2017; 36(4):S10.

20. Mehra MR, Goldstein DJ, Uriel N, et al. Two-year outcomes with a magnetically levitated cardiac pump in heart failure. N Engl J Med 2018. https://doi.org/10.1056/NEJMoa1800866.

21. Coffin ST, Haglund NA, Davis ME, et al. Adverse neurologic events in patients bridged with long-term mechanical circulatory support: a device-specific comparative analysis. J Heart Lung Transplant 2015;34(12):1578–85.

22. Acharya D, Loyaga-Rendon R, Morgan CJ, et al. INTERMACS analysis of stroke during support with continuous-flow left ventricular assist devices: risk factors and outcomes. JACC Heart Fail 2017;5(10): 703–11.

23. Willey JZ, Gavalas MV, Trinh PN, et al. Outcomes after stroke complicating left ventricular assist device. J Heart Lung Transplant 2016;35(8):1003–9.

24. Shahreyar M, Bob-Manuel T, Khouzam RN, et al. Trends, predictors and outcomes of ischemic stroke and intracranial hemorrhage in patients with a left ventricular assist device. Ann Transl Med 2018; 6(1):5.

25. Parikh NS, Cool J, Karas MG, et al. Stroke risk and mortality in patients with ventricular assist devices. Stroke 2016;47(11):2702–6.

26. Enriquez AD, Calenda B, Gandhi PU, et al. Clinical impact of atrial fibrillation in patients with the HeartMate II left ventricular assist device. J Am Coll Cardiol 2014;64(18):1883–90.

27. Stulak JM, Deo S, Schirger J, et al. Preoperative atrial fibrillation increases risk of thromboembolic events after left ventricular assist device implantation. Ann Thorac Surg 2013;96(6):2161–7.

28. Teuteberg JJ, Slaughter MS, Rogers JG, et al. The HVAD left ventricular assist device: risk factors for neurological events and risk mitigation strategies. JACC Heart Fail 2015;3(10):818–28.

29. Morgan JA, Brewer RJ, Nemeh HW, et al. Stroke while on long-term left ventricular assist device support: incidence, outcome, and predictors. ASAIO J 2014;60(3):284–9.

30. Boyle AJ, Jorde UP, Sun B, et al. Pre-operative risk factors of bleeding and stroke during left ventricular assist device support: an analysis of more than 900 HeartMate II outpatients. J Am Coll Cardiol 2014; 63(9):880–8.

31. Morris AA, Pekarek A, Wittersheim K, et al. Gender differences in the risk of stroke during support with continuous-flow left ventricular assist device. J Heart Lung Transplant 2015;34(12):1570–7.

32. Hsich EM, Naftel DC, Myers SL, et al. Should women receive left ventricular assist device support?: findings from INTERMACS. Circ Heart Fail 2012;5(2): 234–40.

33. Bogaev RC, Pamboukian SV, Moore SA, et al. Comparison of outcomes in women versus men using a continuous-flow left ventricular assist device as a bridge to transplantation. J Heart Lung Transplant 2011;30(5):515–22.

34. Magnussen C, Bernhardt AM, Ojeda FM, et al. Gender differences and outcomes in left ventricular assist device support: the European registry for patients with mechanical circulatory support. J Heart Lung Transplant 2018;37(1):61–70.

35. Kato TS, Schulze PC, Yang J, et al. Pre-operative and post-operative risk factors associated with neurologic complications in patients with advanced heart failure supported by a left ventricular assist device. J Heart Lung Transplant 2012;31(1):1–8.

36. Aggarwal A, Gupta A, Kumar S, et al. Are blood stream infections associated with an increased risk of hemorrhagic stroke in patients with a left ventricular assist device? ASAIO J 2012;58(5):509–13.

37. Yoshioka D, Sakaniwa R, Toda K, et al. Relationship between bacteremia and hemorrhagic stroke in patients with continuous-flow left ventricular assist device. Circ J 2018;82(2):448–56.

38. Moazami N, Fukamachi K, Kobayashi M, et al. Axial and centrifugal continuous-flow rotary pumps: a translation from pump mechanics to clinical practice. J Heart Lung Transplant 2013;32(1):1–11.

39. Lampert BC, Eckert C, Weaver S, et al. Blood pressure control in continuous flow left ventricular assist devices: efficacy and impact on adverse events. Ann Thorac Surg 2014;97(1):139–46.

40. Nassif ME, Tibrewala A, Raymer DS, et al. Systolic blood pressure on discharge after left ventricular assist device insertion is associated with

subsequent stroke. J Heart Lung Transplant 2015; 34(4):503–8.

41. Al-Mufti F, Bauerschmidt A, Claassen J, et al. Neuro-endovascular interventions for acute ischemic strokes in patients supported with left ventricular assist devices: a single-center case series and review of the literature. World Neurosurg 2016;88: 199–204.

42. Willey JZ, Demmer RT, Takayama H, et al. Cerebrovascular disease in the era of left ventricular assist devices with continuous flow: risk factors, diagnosis, and treatment. J Heart Lung Transplant 2014;33(9): 878–87.

43. Starling RC, Naka Y, Boyle AJ, et al. Results of the post-U.S. Food and Drug Administration-approval study with a continuous flow left ventricular assist device as a bridge to heart transplantation: a prospective study using the INTERMACS (interagency

registry for mechanically assisted circulatory support). J Am Coll Cardiol 2011;57(19):1890–8.

44. John R, Naka Y, Smedira NG, et al. Continuous flow left ventricular assist device outcomes in commercial use compared with the prior clinical trial. Ann Thorac Surg 2011;92(4):1406–13 [discussion: 1413].

45. Park SJ, Milano CA, Tatooles AJ, et al. Outcomes in advanced heart failure patients with left ventricular assist devices for destination therapy. Circ Heart Fail 2012;5(2):241–8.

46. Jorde UP, Kushwaha SS, Tatooles AJ, et al. Results of the destination therapy post-food and drug administration approval study with a continuous flow left ventricular assist device: a prospective study using the INTERMACS registry (interagency registry for mechanically assisted circulatory support). J Am Coll Cardiol 2014;63(17):1751–7.

Antithrombotic Strategies and Device Thrombosis

Paul A. Gurbel, MD[a],*, Palak Shah, MD, MS[b], Shashank Desai, MD[b], Udaya S. Tantry, PhD[c]

KEYWORDS

- Device thrombosis • Antithrombotic therapy • Platelets • Warfarin • Aspirin • Bleeding

KEY POINTS

- Device thrombosis, thromboembolic events, and bleeding are major adverse events that contribute to the morbidity of left ventricular assist device (LVAD) therapy.
- Current guidelines for antithrombotic therapy are largely based on results of device trials that did not randomize patients to a particular antithrombotic strategy.
- Thrombotic and bleeding events often occur in the same patient over time and challenge the identification of optimal antithrombotic therapy strategies.
- Advances in antithrombotic therapy may result from randomized trials that embed laboratory assays that blueprint hemostasis pathways in LVAD patients.
- Emerging studies are attempting to link specific assay results to the occurrence of thrombotic and bleeding events that may also facilitate personalization of antithrombotic therapy.

INTRODUCTION

Left ventricular assist devices (LVADs) with continuous-flow pumps have emerged as a main therapeutic strategy during the last decade in patients with advanced refractory heart failure (HF). These LVADs are used as either a bridge to transplant (BTT) or destination therapy (DT) in patients who are considered ineligible for transplantation. Currently, the most widely used continuous-flow pump models include the HeartMate II (HMII) device (Abbott Laboratories, Abbott Park, IL) that uses an axial pump design as well as the HVAD (Medtronic, Minneapolis, MN) and the HeartMate 3 (Abbott Laboratories, Abbott Park, IL) that both use a centrifugal flow pump design. Because of the improved pump design and treatment strategies, newer-generation continuous-flow devices are associated with enhanced survival, functional capacity, and quality of life. With either strategy, the duration of expected VAD support continues to increase. However, the annual rate of device thrombosis along with infection, gastrointestinal bleeding, and stroke still remains high and

Disclosure: Dr P.A. Gurbel received consultant/speaker fees from Bayer, Merck, Janssen, New Haven Pharmaceuticals, UptoDate, Medicure, and World Medical; grant support from National Institutes of Health, Bayer, Janssen, Haemonetics, Merck, Idorsia, Instrumentation Labs, and Amgen; and patents in the area of personalized antiplatelet therapy and interventional cardiology. Dr U.S. Tantry received consultation fees from Medicure, UptoDate. Dr P. Shah received grant support from the American Heart Association and Enduring Hearts through a Scientist Development Grant, as well as Merck, Medtronic, and Haemonetics. Dr S. Desai reports no disclosures.
^a Interventional Cardiology and Cardiovascular Medicine Research, Inova Center for Thrombosis Research and Drug Development, Inova Heart and Vascular Institute, 3300 Gallows Road, Falls Church, VA 22042, USA; ^b Heart Failure and Transplantation, Inova Heart and Vascular Institute, 3300 Gallows Road, Falls Church, VA 22042, USA; ^c Inova Center for Thrombosis Research and Drug Development, Inova Heart and Vascular Institute, 3300 Gallows Road, Falls Church, VA 22042, USA
* Corresponding author.
E-mail address: Paul.Gurbel@inova.org

cardiology.theclinics.com

significantly influences morbidity and mortality among these patients.[1]

Optimal antithrombotic therapy is very critical in patients treated with LVADs, because device thrombosis is strongly influenced by both platelet function and coagulation. The International Society for Heart and Lung Transplantation's (ISHLT) guidelines recommend antiplatelet therapy with aspirin and anticoagulation with warfarin in patients treated with LVADs.[2] These recommendations are based on opinions and protocols mandating these agents in clinical device trials but not on strong evidence from adequately powered randomized trials. Moreover, there are specific manufacturer recommendations for anticoagulation and antiplatelet therapy that differ from society guidelines.[3,4] In this article, the authors discuss multiple risk factors associated with device thrombosis, limitations of current antithrombotic therapy strategies, and future directions.

PATHOPHYSIOLOGY OF DEVICE THROMBOSIS

The underlying pathophysiology of device thrombosis is multifactorial and can be related to patient management (antiplatelet/anticoagulant therapy), patient characteristics, surgical implant technique, and device engineering. Device thrombosis is characterized by the development of thrombus/clot within the flow path of the pump, including the titanium inflow cannula, within the pump housing, on the rotor, or in the outflow graft. Thrombus can either originate in the pump itself or migrate from the left atrium/ventricle or from right-sided cardiac chambers through a septal defect and lodge into the pump components. Consequences

of device thrombosis range from small thrombi formation without any clinical consequences to device malfunction with life-threatening hemodynamic impairment, cardiogenic shock, and death. Additional complications include peripheral thromboembolism, transient ischemic attack, and ischemic stroke with or without hemorrhagic complications.

Signs of device thrombosis include recurrent HF signs and symptoms, hemoglobinuria (tea-colored urine), along with laboratory markers of hemolysis, such as lactate dehydrogenase (LDH) levels greater than 2.5 times the upper limit of laboratory normal, a plasma free-hemoglobin concentration greater than 40 mg/dL, hemoglobinuria, anemia, or an elevated bilirubin level.[1,5–7] Of these findings, elevated LDH levels have been shown to be strongly correlated with hemolysis due to device thrombosis.[5] Power spikes and/or falsely elevated device flows (if clot on rotor) or flow reduction (if clot occluding inflow cannula) may be seen, but the sensitivity of these measures on interrogation is low.[6]

Two types of pump thrombi have been described: acute catastrophic red thrombi that predominantly consist of red cells trapped in the fibrin mesh. Red thrombus typically is soft and usually forms at the inlet and outlet stators. It may be associated with blood stasis due to flow conditions, ingested clot, or inadequate anticoagulation. White thrombi are rich in platelets with debris in fibrin mesh that typically forms over time. White thrombus generation depends on turbulent blood flow and heat generation and forms on the pump surface[8] (**Fig. 1**).

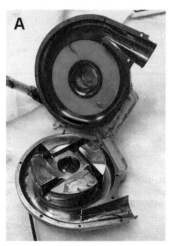
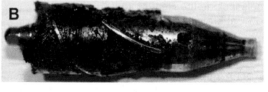

Fig. 1. White and red clot in the setting of device thrombosis. (*A*) White clot is rich in platelets with a fibrin mesh that typically forms overtime. (*B*) Red clot is rich in red blood cells that may be associated with blood stasis due to low-flow conditions, ingested clot, or inadequate anticoagulation.

PREVALENCE OF DEVICE THROMBOSIS

Initial continuous-flow LVAD studies used aggressive antithrombotic protocols with early initiation of heparin, warfarin, and aspirin. The bleeding event rates with the initial LVAD studies were high, with 65% of patients requiring a reoperation or blood transfusion.[9] Subsequent analyses of earlier LVAD studies suggested that less aggressive anticoagulation strategies on short-term follow-up were associated with less bleeding without an increased hazard of thrombotic events.[10,11] The field adopted less intensive anticoagulation and antiplatelet strategies that might have contributed to an increased risk for device thrombosis. Starling and colleagues[12] reported a rapid increase in the 3-month incidence of thrombosis of HMII from 2.2% before March 2011 to 8.4% afterward. This report was followed by a detailed analysis of the Interagency Registry for Mechanically Assisted Circulatory Support's (INTERMACS) database of 6910 patients that reported a 6-fold increase in rates of device thrombosis between 2011 and 2012.[13] The later implant year, younger age, higher creatinine, larger body mass index, white race, left ventricular ejection fraction greater than 20%, and higher LDH level at 1 month were correlated with device thrombosis based on the INTERMACS analysis of the HMII device.[13,14] Regarding HVAD, a mean arterial pressure greater than 90 mm Hg, aspirin dose of 81 mg or less, international normalized ratio (INR) of 2 or less, and INTERMACS profile level 3 or greater (ie, less sick) at implant were reported as risk factors for device thrombosis.[15] Fortunately, heightened attention to monitoring LDH and recognizing early hemolysis before pump thrombosis has been attributed to a decrease in the prevalence of device thrombosis after 2014.[16] A predefined strategy for surgical implantation (pump fixation to the diaphragm, optimal inflow cannula positioning), perioperative anticoagulation (heparinization and warfarin within 48 hours), and follow-up management (recommended LVAD speed >9000 rpm, blood pressure <90 mm Hg) was shown to reduce the incidence of confirmed device thrombosis with HMII from 8.4% to 2.9% at 3 months.[12,17] Thus, in addition to the VAD technology and patient condition at the time of VAD implantation, clinical management of VAD patients plays a significant role in the development of thrombosis.

MECHANISM OF DEVICE THROMBOSIS

Multiple pump-, patient- and management-related risk factors have been implicated in the bleeding and thrombotic complications of LVAD therapy (**Fig. 2**).[1] The primary mechanism of device thrombosis has been attributed to hemocompatibility and shear stress. Platelets and the coagulation system are activated when blood components come in contact with device surfaces. This activation leads to thrombus generation within the device followed by turbulent blood flow and increased shear stress that further activates platelets and propagates thrombus formation.[18] At present, the relative contribution of platelet- and thrombin-dependent pathways for thrombus formation and bleeding in LVAD patients is not fully characterized. Indicators of hypercoagulability, sustained elevations in markers of thrombin generation (thrombin/antithrombin complex and prothrombin fragments 1 and 2), and elevated serum fibrinogen concentrations have been reported in HMII patients.[19,20] Some but not all studies have demonstrated elevated expression of platelet activation markers, such as p-selectin, CD41, CD63, and platelet microparticles, following LVAD implantation.[21–27] Finally, using the platelet activation state (PAS) assay, it has been shown that device thrombosis was associated with altered PAS values.[28]

Loss of high-molecular-weight multimers of von Willebrand factor (HMvWF) observed following LVAD implantation may be due to LVAD-induced nonphysiologic high shear stress. Loss of HMvWF may impair binding to the injured endothelial surface and may predispose patients to an increased risk for bleeding.[29–31] Shedding of platelet surface receptors, such as glycoprotein (GP) Ibα, GP VI, and GP IIb/IIIa, has been shown in patients with LVAD and has been associated with an elevated risk of bleeding. Oxidative stress– and abnormal shear stress–induced LVAD thrombosis may be responsible for platelet receptor shedding (**Fig. 3**).[32–36] These markers may assist in discriminating thrombotic and bleeding risks.

STANDARD ANTITHROMBOTIC THERAPY AFTER LEFT VENTRICULAR ASSIST DEVICE

Patients receiving an LVAD are inherently high-risk patients with multiple medical comorbidities in addition to imbalanced hemostatic characteristics. Moreover, current continuous-flow devices are made of thrombogenic surfaces that may predispose the risk for early thrombosis, subsequent hemolysis, and device malfunction. There are inherent limitations in the ability to accurately detect thrombus early within the pump given the varying flow characteristics and design elements. Finally, the same patient may experience both bleeding and thrombotic events over the course

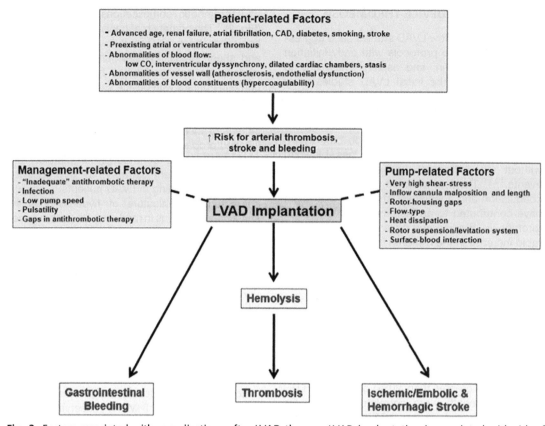

Fig. 2. Factors associated with complications after LVAD therapy. LVAD implantation is associated with risk of gastrointestinal bleeding, hemolysis/thrombosis, and stroke. These risks are related to patient, management, and pump factors. CAD, coronary artery disease; CO, cardiac output. (*From* Shah P, Tantry US, Bliden KP, et al. Bleeding and thrombosis associated with ventricular assist device therapy. J Heart Lung Trans 2017;36(11):1165; with permission.)

of time, indicating temporal changes in hemostatic risk factors. Both bleeding and thrombotic events are also influenced by a relative response to various antithrombotic agents.

The current choice of antithrombotic therapy and its intensity depends on patient characteristics, including device type, extent of thrombotic and bleeding risks, and institutional preference (**Table 1**). Patients treated with an LVAD may need surgical procedures that require bridging of anticoagulation. In these cases, heparin or antiplatelet therapies are the main choices to mitigate the risk of thrombosis. Extra precaution should be taken regarding periprocedural timing of withdrawal of warfarin, initiation of parenteral anticoagulation, and restarting oral anticoagulation to avoid excessive bleeding complications. Guidelines recommend 81 to 325 mg aspirin daily as an oral antiplatelet agent and defer to manufacturer recommendation for additional antiplatelet therapy.[2] For HMII, 81 mg daily plus 75 mg dipyridamole twice daily is recommended by the manufacturer, as the latter strategy was used in the

clinical trials of HMII.[3] The HVAD manufacturer primarily recommends 325 mg daily aspirin for all patients based on the interim observation of the ADVANCE (Evaluation of the HeartWare Left Ventricular Assist Device for the Treatment of Advanced Heart Failure) trial, which showed that with an INR of 2 to 3 and 325 mg daily aspirin was associated with less device thrombosis as compared with 81 mg daily aspirin.[4,15]

ANTITHROMBOTIC MANAGEMENT OF PUMP THROMBOSIS

The most conservative management of device thrombosis is aggressive anticoagulation with warfarin and oral antiplatelet therapy with aspirin. Goldstein and colleagues[37] have proposed an algorithm for the diagnosis and management of a suspected thrombosis with a stepwise approach to guide diagnosis and treatment according to clinical presentation. Intensified short-term parenteral anticoagulant with heparin and/or antiplatelet therapy may provide effective protection against

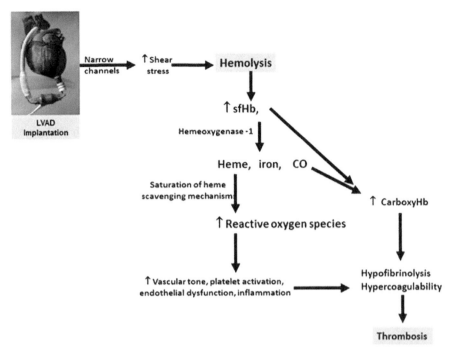

Fig. 3. Mechanism of hemolysis-induced thrombosis following LVAD Implantation. LVAD-induced shear force results in hemolysis and release of free hemoglobin. Because of the saturation of heme scavenging mechanisms, there is an elevation of reactive oxygen species (ROS). ROS induce hypercoagulability by increasing vascular tone, platelet activation, endothelial dysfunction, and inflammation. At the same time elevated levels of carboxyhemoglobin in blood results in hypofibrinolysis and hypercoagulability. The net summation of these hemolysis effects is an increased risk for thrombosis. CarboxyHb, carboxy hemoglobin; CO, carbon monoxide; sfHb, serum free hemoglobin. (*From* Shah P, Tantry US, Bliden KP, et al. Bleeding and thrombosis associated with ventricular assist device therapy. J Heart Lung Trans 2017;36(11):1167; with permission.)

thrombotic events and subsequent severe device malfunction if the thrombosis is diagnosed early. Power spikes and laboratory identification of hemolysis may be helpful in this scenario. Direct thrombin inhibitors (DTIs), such as argatroban and bivalirudin, may also be considered. Unlike heparin, which predominantly binds to free thrombin, DTIs inhibit both free and clot-bound thrombin. However, because of insufficient evidence, these agents are not used widely. To maximize the antithrombotic effect and to minimize bleeding complications, the intravenous anticoagulants should be monitored regularly to maintain the target activated partial thromboplastin time. Several case reports and small studies reported conflicting results with respect to the benefits of intensified antiplatelet therapy with GP IIb/IIIa inhibitors. Although there are some initial favorable responses reported in early care reports, larger case series reported a high risk of bleeding outweighing the benefits of GP IIb/IIIa inhibitors associated with LVAD therapy.[38] Augmented antithrombotic therapy for device thrombosis has been reported to be associated with a nearly

50% success rate; there are many incidences of recurrent hemolysis, peripheral thromboembolism including stroke, or worsening pump thrombosis.[1]

Similarly, multiple conflicting reports have been published regarding the efficacy of thrombolytic therapy for device thrombosis. These agents have been administered both systemically and directly within the left ventricle. In an analysis from the HVAD Bridge to Transplant ADVANCE Trial, among 19 patients treated with tissue plasminogen activator (tPA; systemic: n = 8, intraventricular: n = 7, and unreported: n = 4), resolution of pump thrombosis was demonstrated in 6 of the 8 patients treated with systemic tPA and in 4 of the 7 patients who received intraventricular tPA. In addition, an 82% success rate was reported in patients treated with tPA plus dual antiplatelet therapy as compared with only 37% with triple therapy of heparin, eptifibatide, and tPA. In another report, 4 of the 5 patients treated with systemically administered fibrinolytics had successful resolution of suspected pump thrombosis.[39] Similarly, other case reports have demonstrated that intravascular use of tPA

Table 1
Recommendation for anticoagulant and antiplatelet therapy in patients treated with left ventricular assist devices

HeartMate II	
ISHLT's guidelines for HMII patients on heparin	1. There should be complete reversal of heparin after cardiopulmonary bypass/leaving OR. 2. Consider aspirin at ICU admission, within 24 h. 3. Administer IV heparin or alternative anticoagulation with aPTT goal (40–60 s), if there is no evidence of bleeding on POD1–POD2. 4. Start warfarin (INR [2.0–3.0]) and aspirin (81–325 mg daily) after removal of chest tubes on POD2–POD3.

Manufacturer	1. Before leaving the OR, completely reverse the anticoagulation.
	2. Optional: After implantation, as early as possible, administer 10% LMW dextran at 25 mL/h (this step is optional until the benefit of dextran administration is further delineated).
	3. Begin IV heparin after 12–24 h or when chest tube drainage is <50 mL/h:
	  • Initially titrate to aPTT of 45–50 for 24 h (1.2–1.4 times control).
	  • After 24 h increase heparin and titrate to aPTT 50–60 (1.4–1.7 times control).
	  • After another 24 h, increase heparin and titrate to PTT 55–65 (1.5–1.8 times control).
	  • On POD2–POD3, initiate aspirin 81–100 mg QD and dipyridamole 75 mg TID.
	  • On POD 3–POD5, once there is no evidence of bleeding and the chest tubes have been removed, begin warfarin (overlapping with the heparin). Discontinue heparin after obtaining an acceptable, stable INR. The INR should be maintained in the range of 2.0–3.0.
	  • Maintain patients throughout support on aspirin, dipyridamole, and warfarin.
	Conditions requiring possible modification to anticoagulation:
	1. Sustained low pump flow states (<3.0 L/min):
	  • Consider increasing anticoagulation to upper limits of normal.
	2. Risk of bleeding:
	  • Consider increasing antiplatelet medications and decreasing heparin/warfarin (INR 1.7–2.3). Antiplatelet effect should be confirmed with laboratory studies, for example, TEG.

HVAD	

Manufacturer	1. Anticoagulation should be individualized for each patient. Start low-dose heparin at 10 units per kilogram per hour on POD1 with initial aPTT goal of 40–50 s and gradually increase the heparin dosage to maintain the aPTT of 50–60 s.
	2. The long-term oral anticoagulation strategy is warfarin and aspirin.
	3. If using aspirin alone, check aspirin responsiveness with a reliable assay (eg, VerifyNow) to establish the dose or to select an alternative medication.
	4. Multi-antiplatelet therapy options include the following:
	  • 81 mg aspirin plus Aggrenox (25 mg aspirin plus 200 mg extended-release dipyridamole) daily
	  • 81 mg aspirin plus 75 mg clopidogrel daily
	5. For patients who are aspirin sensitive or intolerant, 75–150 mg/d clopidogrel is a viable alternative. A loading dose of 300 mg clopidogrel followed by 75 mg/d is recommended to reduce the lag time in reaching full therapeutic benefit (typically a 3–4 d lag).
	6. Warfarin should be started within POD4 and titrated to maintain an INR of 2.0–3.0.

Abbreviations: aPTT, activated partial thromboplastin time; ICU, intensive care unit; IV, intravenous; LMW, low molecular weight; OR, operating room; POD, postoperative day; PTT, partial thromboplastin time; TEG, thromboelastography.

administration was associated with successful resolution of pump thrombosis. Detailed analysis of the device log-file to analyze trends in power consumption (ie, increased power to maintain the set rotor speed) may be helpful in deciding which patients will respond to thrombolytic therapy[40,41] (**Fig. 4**). Finally, in patients who are appropriate surgical candidates, device exchange

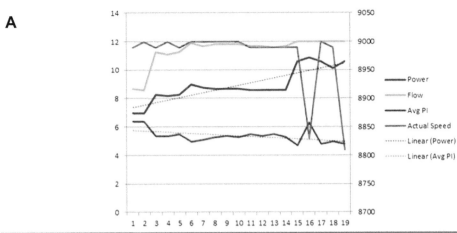

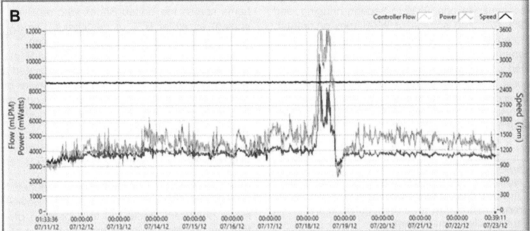

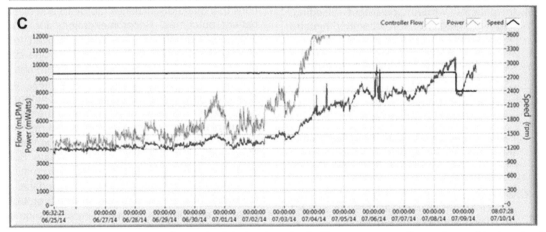

Fig. 4. Log-file analysis to assist in diagnosis of device thrombosis. The system controller can be used to download information from the device log-file that includes trends in power, flow, speed, pulsatility, and other pump parameters. Graphical analysis of linear trends in these pump parameters may assist in the diagnosis of device thrombosis. (*A*) Log-file analysis of the HMII pump that reveals uptrending power (*red line*), while at a stable speed (9000 rpm). (*B*) Acute thrombus ingestion manifests in an acute increase in power (*red line*) and calculated flow (*green line*) despite stable HVAD speed of 2600 rpm (*black line*). (*C*) Gradual buildup of thrombus on the HVAD rotor will slow increase in the power and flow, with stable speed of 2800 rpm. avg PI, average pulsatility index.

has been associated with a significant freedom from subsequent stroke or death when compared with medical therapy.[42]

In the PREVENT (PREVENtion of HeartMate II Pump Thrombosis Through Clinical Management) study, the recommended structured clinical practices, including surgical implant technique, anticoagulation strategy, and pump speed management, aimed to reduce the risk of pump thrombosis were prospectively tested (**Box 1**). In this study, 300 patients from 24 heart centers who were treated with the HMII were included. The primary end point of confirmed device thrombosis was observed in 2.9% of patients at 3 months and 4.8% at 6 months. In the study, adherence rates to key recommendations were as follows: 78% to surgical recommendations, 95% to heparin bridging, and 79% to pump speeds of 9000 rpm or greater. Moreover, full adherence to implant techniques, heparin bridging, and pump speeds was associated with a significantly lower risk of device thrombosis at 6 months (1.9% vs 8.9%; $P<.01$) and lower composite risk of suspected thrombosis, hemolysis, and ischemic stroke (5.7% vs 17.7%; $P<.01$) at 6 months.[15]

The newest-generation continuous-flow LVAD is the HeartMate 3. This device incorporates a variety of device design elements to improve the hemocompatibility of the device. The gaps between the rotor and pump housing are wider to facilitate blood flow and reduce red cell trauma and hemolysis. The pump includes a computerized pulsatility algorithm that increases and reduces the pump speed by 200 rpm every 2 seconds. Initial laboratory data suggest lower levels of hemolysis and increased preservation of HMvWF with this device.[43] This device has been studied in the Multicenter Study of MagLev Technology in Patients Undergoing Mechanical Circulatory Support Therapy with HeartMate 3 (MOMENTUM 3) trial, which randomized 1028 patients across the United States who received an implant as either BTT or destination therapy to the HMII or HeartMate 3 in a 1:1 fashion.[44] The 2-year follow-up data suggest the HeartMate 3 was associated with a lower risk of suspected device thrombosis (1.1% vs 15.7%) and lower incidence of stroke (10.1% vs 19.2%).[45] Long-term follow-up of the remainder of the cohort will help assess the true efficacy of this device.

SUMMARY

LVAD technology has dramatically reduced the mortality of patients with end-stage HF. However, major persistent limitations to expansion of the therapy are bleeding and thrombotic complications that markedly influence morbidity and overall patient outcomes. Recommendations for LVAD thrombosis prophylaxis are largely derived from clinical device trials that implement a one-size-fits-all strategy. They are also derived from observational cohorts, retrospective analyses, and expert opinion. Significant advances in antithrombotic therapy will likely only result from the design and implementation of well-constructed randomized trials that incorporate direct measurement of hemostasis pathways in individual patients. Such work that blueprints the hemostatic abnormalities in individual patients holds the promise of facilitating the personalization of antithrombotic therapy and improved net clinical outcomes. Moreover, objective serial laboratory-based assessment of thrombogenicity seems needed to balance the risk of bleeding and thrombotic complications in LVAD-treated patients. Unfortunately, there is no gold standard surrogate marker for small thrombus forming in the LVAD until it becomes near clinically apparent. Thus, much of the biological vacillations that occur in thrombogenicity cannot be accurately detected and correlated to behaviors. The clinical risk factors for

---

Box 1
PREVENtion of HeartMate II Pump Thrombosis Through Clinical Management recommendations for anticoagulation and antiplatelet management

1. In patients without persistent bleeding, begin bridging with unfractionated heparin or LMWH within 48 hours of device implantation with a goal PTT of 40 to 45 seconds in the first 48 hours, followed by titration up to PTT of 50 to 60 seconds by 96 hours. If heparin is contraindicated, consider other alternatives, including argatroban, intravenous warfarin, and bivalirudin.

2. Initiate warfarin within 48 hours to obtain a goal INR of 2.0 to 2.5 by postoperative days 5 to 7, at which time heparin therapy may be discontinued.

3. When there is no evidence of bleeding, initiate aspirin therapy (81–325 mg daily) 2 to 5 days after HMII implantation.

4. Maintain patients throughout LVAD support on aspirin and warfarin with a goal INR of 2.0 to 2.5.

Abbreviations: LMWH, low-molecular-weight heparin; PTT, partial thromboplastin time.

Adapted from Maltais S, Kilic A, Nathan S. Prevention of heartmate II pump thrombosis through clinical management: the PREVENT multi-center study. J Heart Lung Trans 2017;36(1):3; with permission.

bleeding and thrombosis have a range of associated hazards making clinical algorithms for choosing optimal antithrombotic therapy challenging. The importance of a dynamic strategy that serially assesses hemostatic pathways over time is highlighted by the fact that bleeding and thrombotic events will often occur in the same individual.

One potential future approach that has been investigated in limited cohorts is thromboelastography (TEG)-guided therapy. TEG measures the interaction between fibrin polymerization and activated platelets that occurs during the formation of a platelet-fibrin clot. TEG provides simultaneous assessment of platelet function and coagulation and, thus, may provide more comprehensive information on bleeding and thrombotic risks as compared with other currently available ex vivo assays used in the treatment of LVAD patients. On the horizon are assays, such as the PAS assay, that sensitively detect changes in platelet activation and may facilitate the personalization of antiplatelet therapy.

The newest-generation device, HeartMate 3, has been associated with lower levels of shear stress and reduced hemolysis, which should mitigate activation of platelets and the coagulation system. Early data suggest a near absence of device thrombosis, which represents a major advancement in mechanical circulatory support.

REFERENCES

1. Shah P, Tantry US, Bliden KP, et al. Bleeding and thrombosis associated with ventricular assist device therapy. J Heart Lung Transplant 2017;36:1164–73.
2. Feldman D, Pamboukian SV, Teuteberg JJ, et al. The 2013 International Society for Heart and Lung Transplantation guidelines for mechanical circulatory support: executive summary. J Heart Lung Transplant 2013;32:157–303.
3. HeartMate II. LVAS operating manual. Pleasanton (CA): Thoratec Corporation; 2007.
4. HeartWare ventricular assist system instructions for use. Miami Lakes (FL): HeartWare, Inc; 2012.
5. Shah P, Mehta VM, Cowger JA, et al. Diagnosis of hemolysis and device thrombosis with lactate dehydrogenase during left ventricular assist device support. J Heart Lung Transplant 2014;33:102–4.
6. Cowger JA, Romano MA, Shah P, et al. Hemolysis: a harbinger of adverse outcome after left ventricular assist device implant. J Heart Lung Transplant 2014;33:35–43.
7. Gavalas MV, Breskin A, Yuzefpolskaya M, et al. Discriminatory performance of positive urine hemoglobin for detection of significant hemolysis in patients with continuous-flow left ventricular assist devices. J Heart Lung Transplant 2017;36:59–63.
8. Blitz A. Pump thrombosis-A riddle wrapped in a mystery inside an enigma. Ann Cardiothorac Surg 2014;3:450–71.
9. Miller LW, Pagani FD, Russell SD, et al. Use of a continuous-flow device in patients awaiting heart transplantation. N Engl J Med 2007;357:885–96.
10. Slaughter MS, Naka Y, John R, et al. Post-operative heparin may not be required for transitioning patients with a HeartMate II left ventricular assist system to long-term warfarin therapy. J Heart Lung Transplant 2010;29:616–24.
11. Boyle AJ, Russell SD, Teuteberg JJ, et al. Low thromboembolism and pump thrombosis with the HeartMate II left ventricular assist device: analysis of out- patient anti-coagulation. J Heart Lung Transplant 2009;28:881–7.
12. Starling RC, Moazami N, Silvestry SC, et al. Unexpected abrupt increase in left ventricular assist device thrombosis. N Engl J Med 2014;370:33–40.
13. Kirklin JK, Naftel DC, Kormos RL, et al. Interagency Registry for Mechanically Assisted Circulatory Support (INTERMACS) analysis of pump thrombosis in the HeartMate II left ventricular assist device. J Heart Lung Transplant 2014;33:12–22.
14. Shah P, Birk S, Maltais S, et al. Left ventricular assist device outcomes based on flow configuration and pre-operative left ventricular dimension: an interagency registry for mechanically assisted circulatory support analysis. J Heart Lung Transplant 2017;36:640–9.
15. Najjar SS, Slaughter MS, Pagani FD, et al. An analysis of pump thrombus events in patients in the HeartWare ADVANCE bridge to transplant and continued access protocol trial. J Heart Lung Transplant 2014;33:23–34.
16. Kirklin JK, Naftel DC, Pagani FD, et al. Pump thrombosis in the Thoratec HeartMate II device: an update analysis of the INTERMACS Registry. J Heart Lung Transplant 2015;34:1515–26.
17. Maltais S, Kilic A, Nathan S, et al, PREVENT Study Investigators. PREVENtion of HeartMate II pump thrombosis through clinical management: the PREVENT multi-center study. J Heart Lung Transplant 2017;36:1–12.
18. de Biasi AR, Manning KB, Salemi A. Science for surgeons: understanding pump thrombogenesis in continuous-flow left ventricular assist devices. J Thorac Cardiovasc Surg 2015;149:667–73.
19. John R, Panch S, Hrabe J, et al. Activation of endothelial and coagulation systems in left ventricular assist device recipients. Ann Thorac Surg 2009;88:1171–9.
20. Slaughter MS, Sobieski MA, Gallagher C, et al. Fibrinolytic activation during long-term support with the HeartMate II left ventricular assist device. ASAIO J 2008;54:115–9.

21. Dewald O, Schmitz C, Diem H, et al. Platelet activation markers in patients with heart assist device. Artif Organs 2005;29:292–9.

22. Loffler C, Straub A, Bassler N, et al. Evaluation of platelet activation in patients supported by the Jarvik 2000high-rotational speed impeller ventricular assist device. J Thorac Cardiovasc Surg 2009;137:736–41.

23. Ashbrook M, Walenga JM, Schwartz J, et al. Left ventricular assist device induced coagulation and platelet activation and effect of the current anticoagulant therapy regimen. Clin Appl Thromb Hemost 2013;19:249–55.

24. Bonaros N, Mueller MR, Salat A, et al. Extensive coagulation monitoring in patients after implantation of the MicroMed Debakey continuous flow axial pump. ASAIO J 2004;50:424–31.

25. Houel R, Mazoyer E, Boval B, et al. Platelet activation and aggregation profile in prolonged external ventricular support. J Thorac Cardiovasc Surg 2004;128:197–202.

26. Slaughter MS, Sobieski MA 2nd, Graham JD, et al. Platelet activation in heart failure patients supported by the HeartMate II ventricular assist device. Int J Artif Organs 2011;34:461–8.

27. Diehl P, Aleker M, Helbing T, et al. Enhanced microparticles in ventricular assist device patients predict platelet, leukocyte and endothelial cell activation. Interact Cardiovasc Thorac Surg 2010;11:133–7.

28. Consolo F, Sferrazza G, Motolone G, et al. Platelet activation is a preoperative risk factor for the development of thromboembolic complications in patients with continuous-flow left ventricular assist device. Eur J Heart Fail 2017. https://doi.org/10.1002/ejhf.1113.

29. Geisen U, Heilmann C, Beyersdorf F, et al. Non-surgical bleeding in patients with ventricular assist devices could be explained by acquired von Willebrand disease. Eur J Cardiothorac Surg 2008;33:679–84.

30. Klovaite J, Gustafsson F, Mortensen SA, et al. Severely impaired von Willebrand factor-dependent platelet aggregation in patients with a continuous-flow left ventricular assist device (HeartMate II). J Am Coll Cardiol 2009;53:2162–7.

31. Meyer AL, Malehsa D, Bara C, et al. Acquired von Willebrand syndrome in patients with an axial flow left ventricular assist device. Circ Heart Fail 2010;3:675–81.

32. Mondal NK, Chen Z, Trivedi JR, et al. Association of oxidative stress and platelet receptor glycoprotein GPIbα and GPVI shedding during nonsurgical bleeding in heart failure patients with continuous-flow left ventricular assist device support. ASAIO J 2017. https://doi.org/10.1097/MAT.0000000000000680.

33. Hu J, Mondal NK, Sorensen EN, et al. Platelet glycoprotein Ibα ectodomain shedding and non-surgical bleeding in heart failure patients supported by continuous-flow left ventricular assist devices. J Heart Lung Transplant 2014;33:71–9.

34. Lukito P, Wong A, Jing J, et al. Mechanical circulatory support is associated with loss of platelet receptors glycoprotein Ibα and glycoprotein VI. J Thromb Haemost 2016;14:2253–60.

35. Mondal NK, Chen Z, Trivedi JR, et al. Oxidative stress induced modulation of platelet integrin α2bβ3 expression and shedding may predict the risk of major bleeding in heart failure patients supported by continuous flow left ventricular assist devices. Thromb Res 2017;158:140–8.

36. Chen Z, Mondal NK, Ding J, et al. Activation and shedding of platelet glycoprotein IIb/IIIa under non-physiological shear stress. Mol Cell Biochem 2015;409:93–101.

37. Goldstein DJ, John R, Salerno C, et al. Algorithm for the diagnosis and management of suspected pump thrombus. J Heart Lung Transplant 2013;32:667–70.

38. Doligalski CT, Jennings DL. Device-related thrombosis in continuous-flow left ventricular assist device support. J Pharm Pract 2016;29:58–66.

39. Muthiah K, Macdonald PS, Kotlyar E, et al. Thrombolysis for suspected intrapump thrombosis in patients with continuous flow centrifugal left ventricular assist device. Artif Organs 2013;37:313–22.

40. Jorde UP, Aaronson KD, Najjar SS, et al. Identification and management of pump thrombus in the heartware left ventricular assist device system: a novel approach using log file analysis. JACC Heart Fail 2015;3:849–56.

41. Stulak JM, Dunlay SM, Sharma S, et al. Treatment of device thrombus in the HeartWare HVAD: success and outcomes depend significantly on the initial treatment strategy. J Heart Lung Transplant 2015;34:1535–41.

42. Levin AP, Saeed O, Willey JZ, et al. Watchful waiting in continuous-flow left ventricular assist device patients with ongoing hemolysis is associated with an increased risk for cerebrovascular accident or death. Circ Heart Fail 2016;9(5) [pii:e002896].

43. Netuka I, Kvasnička T, Kvasnička J, et al. Evaluation of von Willebrand factor with a fully magnetically levitated centrifugal continuous-flow left ventricular assist device in advanced heart failure. J Heart Lung Transplant 2016;35:860–7.

44. Mehra MR, Naka Y, Uriel N, et al, MOMENTUM 3 Investigators. A fully magnetically levitated circulatory pump for advanced heart failure. N Engl J Med 2017;376:440–50.

45. Mehra MR, Goldstein DJ, Uriel N, et al, MOMENTUM 3 Investigators. Two-year outcomes with a magnetically levitated cardiac pump in heart failure. N Engl J Med 2018. https://doi.org/10.1056/NEJMoa1800866.

Impact of Mechanical Circulatory Support on Posttransplant Outcomes

Todd F. Dardas, MD, MS

KEYWORDS

- Heart transplant • Mechanical circulatory support • Temporary circulatory support • Artificial heart
- Survival • Risk factors • Health utility

KEY POINTS

- Mechanical circulatory support is not associated with reduced posttransplant survival in most cases.
- Significant reductions in transplant survival may occur following left ventricle assist device (LVAD) support complicated by infection, total artificial heart, and extracorporeal life support.
- Continuous-flow LVAD support is associated with an increased risk of posttransplant vasoplegia syndrome.

INTRODUCTION

Mechanical circulatory support (MCS) devices allow for myocardial recovery, serve to stabilize end-organ function before definitive therapy, act as permanent support, provide a bridge to transplant (BTT), and dramatically increase the likelihood of surviving cardiogenic shock. When used as part of a BTT strategy, MCS may extend life to the median survival of heart transplant, which is currently more than 12 years. However, MCS devices are associated with complications that may prevent transplant or reduce posttransplant survival. For those truly in need of MCS, the potential gain in survival of MCS far outweighs the alternative of waiting for a transplant unsupported. Accordingly, ventricular assist device (VAD) support at listing is present among 25% to 40% of candidates in recent series.[1,2] Experience with MCS before a transplant is growing rapidly; as more experience accumulates, the advanced heart failure community will reduce the risk of mortality and morbidity attributable to MCS. This article focuses on posttransplant outcomes specifically associated with selected MCS devices.

DURABLE DEVICES

Left Ventricular Assist Devices

Each left VAD (LVAD) generation has achieved lower mortality than prior generations, and high-quality prospective trials have established the efficacy of durable LVADs as BTT.[3–5] Declining mortality among LVAD-supported candidates (43% mortality in 2005–2006 decreasing to 8% in 2015–2016) and increasing prevalence of MCS at the time of listing (increasing from 10% to 35% prevalence between 2005–2016) suggest increasing experience and improved efficacy.[1] Mortality for status 1A registrants declined dramatically over the same time, and this decline is partly attributable to LVADs used as rescue therapy. Thus, the use of LVADs as BTT is well accepted; the advanced heart failure community is responsible for identifying and managing risk factors contributing to higher rates of posttransplant outcomes.

Disclosure: Research grant (International Society for Heart and Lung Transplantation/Medtronic).
Department of Medicine, University of Washington, 1959 Northeast Pacific Street, Box 356422, Seattle, WA 98195, USA
E-mail address: tdardas@uw.edu

Cardiol Clin 36 (2018) 551–560
https://doi.org/10.1016/j.ccl.2018.06.009
0733-8651/18/© 2018 Elsevier Inc. All rights reserved.

Posttransplant mortality

Early experience with pulsatile-flow LVADs (PF-VADs) as BTT suggested no association between LVADs and posttransplant mortality.[6–9] In the PF-VAD era, mortality was similar between VAD- and non–VAD-supported recipients after adjusting for severity of illness, donor-recipient mismatches, and cold ischemic time.[6–9] Consistent with high rates of infectious complications encountered with pulsatile devices available at the time, these reports describe a higher risk of first infection and dying of infection after transplant among PF-VAD–supported recipients.[8,9] Early comparisons between pulsatile and continuous-flow (CF) devices suggested equality between the two modalities with regard to posttransplant survival.[10]

CF devices have proven more reliable with fewer complications and improved survival compared with pulsatile devices and, accordingly, have replaced pulsatile devices as the mainstay of durable MCS. In the CF era, mortality has decreased for registrants in general and among persons initially supported with LVADs.[1,11] However, increasing survival among registrants obligatorily increases the number of prevalent registrants and exacerbates the supply-demand mismatch of donor hearts, resulting in scrutiny of even small differences in mortality as programs attempt to optimize the utility of each donor. Given the obligate need for repeat surgery and high burden of complications, posttransplant outcomes with durable LVADs will remain of great interest.

Several reports address posttransplant mortality among LVAD-supported transplant recipients when compared with unsupported recipients in the CF-VAD era and found no clinically significant difference in posttransplant mortality (**Table 1**). Weiss and colleagues[12] reported no significant increase in posttransplant mortality for persons supported with the HeartMate II (Abbott Corp, Abbott Park IL) (multivariable hazard ratio [HR] 1.22; 95% confidence interval [CI] 0.87–1.72). Dardas and colleagues[13] reported posttransplant survival for MCS and non-MCS registrants from the Organ Procurement and Transplantation Network (OPTN) registry. This report suggests an increase in posttransplant morality among persons with implantable LVADs using elective time (HR 1.2, 95% CI 0.88–1.3) and among LVADs with complications (HR 1.2, 95% CI 0.99–1.4), though neither were statistically significant when compared with a reference group of recipients supported with dual inotropes and intra-aortic balloon pumps (IABPs). Trivedi and colleagues[14] noted clinically nonsignificant differences in 3-year survival among registrants transplanted from status 1B with an LVAD using elective status 1A time (84%), status 1B

LVADs (85%) and status 1A VAD-supported patients with complications (78%, $P = .01$). Donneyong and colleagues[15] used a time-dependent Cox model with propensity matching to evaluate the effect of HeartMate II support before transplant compared with no support. When adjusted for donor, recipient, and propensity to receive LVAD support, the investigators found that 30-day (HR 1.23; 95% CI 0.79–1.95) and 30- to 365-day (HR 1.31; 95% CI 0.85–2.01) mortality rates were higher among the LVAD-supported group, though statistical significance was not met. Higher risk among LVAD-supported recipients was not seen in the large, pooled International Society of Heart Lung Transplant (ISHLT) adult heart transplant Registry analysis (sampled from 2004–2008), which demonstrated a relative risk (RR) of 1.16 (95% CI RR 0.82–1.65) for CF-VADs compared with no inotropes at transplant and an RR of 1.19 (95% CI RR 0.84–1.69) when CF-VADs were compared with those without inotropes or MCS.[16] Posttransplant mortality was not significantly increased in a modern ISHLT Registry analysis (2005–2015), which demonstrated only 2% absolute risk reduction for inotropes when compared with pretransplant CF-VAD support.[2] Although there are differing mortality signals among LVAD-bridged patients, most data suggest no decrement in survival among recipients transplanted from durable LVAD support (**Fig. 1**).

The exception is LVAD-supported patients with complications. Quader and colleagues[17] reported 14% posttransplant mortality at 1 year among those recipients with device complications and 10% mortality among recipients with CF-VADs without complications. Although these complications were not further delineated in this investigation, most reports have found a higher risk of posttransplant mortality among patients with device infections. Concern for recrudescent infections among device-supported recipients is justified given the obligate need for posttransplant immunosuppression and the high frequency of infections encountered during VAD support. Although pump-related infections may resolve with explant at transplant, resistant organisms and/or deeply seated infections at relatively impenetrable sites may not resolve or recur in the presence of immunosuppression. Reports from the CF-VAD era indicate variable signals toward increased posttransplant mortality following LVADs complicated by infection. John and colleagues[18] reported a nonsignificant decrease in 1-year survival posttransplant survival between those persons without a percutaneous lead infection (89%) when compared with those with a percutaneous lead infection (75%, $P = .07$). In

Table 1
Posttransplant survival among continuous-flow ventricular assist devices and comparator groups

Author	Source	Sample Time Frame	Group of Interest	Reference Group	Follow-up Time	HR	95% CI	KM	P Value
Nativi et al,[16] 2011	ISHLT Registry	2004–2008	CF devices	Inotropes, no VAD	4 y	1.2	0.82–1.65	—	.41
				No inotropes, no VAD	4 y	1.2	0.84–1.69	—	.32
Donneyong et al,[15] 2014	UNOS	2004–2010	HMII	All other recipients	0–30 d	1.2	0.79–1.95	—	.36
			HMII	All other recipients	30–365 d	1.3	0.85–2.01	—	.22
			HMII	All other recipients	>365 d	0.4	0.36–0.77	—	.01
Dardas et al,[13] 2012	UNOS	2005–2010	CF-VAD listed status 1A using elective time	Status 1A by dual inotropes/Swan or IABP	All available	1.2	0.88–1.3	—	.44
			CF-VAD listed status 1A with complication	Status 1A by dual inotropes/Swan or IABP	All available	1.2	0.99–1.4	—	.07
Lund et al,[2] 2017	ISHLT Registry	2005–2015	CF-VAD	All other recipients	1 y	—	—	90 vs 88%	—
Trivedi et al,[14] 2016	UNOS	2006–2013	CF-VAD listed status 1A using elective time	CF-VAD listed status 1B	3 y	—	—	84 vs 85%	.5
			CF-VAD listed status 1A with complication	CF-VAD listed status 1B	3 y	—	—	84 vs 78%	—
Weiss et al,[12] 2011	UNOS	2009–2010	HMII	All other recipients	1 y	1.2	0.87–1.72	—	.25
			CF-VAD	All other recipients	1 y	2.0	1.06–3.97	—	.03

Abbreviations: CI, confidence interval; HMII, HeartMate II LVAD; HR, hazard ratio; IABP, intra-aortic balloon pump; ISHLT, International Society of Heart Lung Transplant; KM, Kaplan-Meier product limit estimate; UNOS, United Network of Organ Sharing.

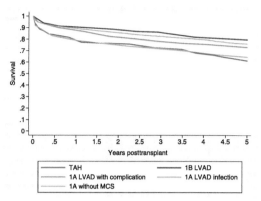

Fig. 1. Five-year posttransplant survival from studies of mechanically supported recipients. TAH, total artificial heart. (*Data from* Trivedi JR, Rajagopal K, Schumer EM, et al. Differences in status 1A heart transplantation survival in the continuous flow left ventricular assist device era. Ann Thorac Surg 2016;102(5):1512–6; and Copeland JG, Copeland H, Gustafson M, et al. Experience with more than 100 total artificial heart implants. J Thorac Cardiovasc Surg 2012;143(3):727–34; and Unpublished data from the author, status 1A transplants without mechanical circulatory support group.)

their series, the occurrence of any type of infection was not associated with worse outcomes ($P = .38$). Healy and colleagues[19] evaluated a larger series of recipients and described the effect of various status 1A complication groups on posttransplant survival (see **Fig. 1**, **Table 2**). These investigators noted that justifications for infection increased the risk of posttransplant morality when compared with justification for elective 30 days of status 1A time (1-year survival 79% vs 84%, $P = .012$).[19] These studies suggest that carefully selected persons with device-related infections can have acceptable posttransplant

Table 2		
Hazard ratios for selected left ventricular assist device complications at 10-year follow-up		
Group	HR	95% CI
Status 1A LVAD using elective time	Reference	
Thromboembolism	1.12	0.81, 1.56
Device infection	1.3	1.09, 1.56
Device malfunction	0.81	0.62, 1.06
Arrhythmia	1.24	0.76, 2.00
Other	0.95	0.68, 1.32

Data from Healy AH, Baird BC, Drakos SG. Impact of ventricular assist device complications on posttransplant survival: an analysis of the united network of organ sharing database. Ann Thorac Surg 2013;95(3):870–75.

outcomes but that reducing the prevalence of infections among VAD-supported registrants may result in incremental improvement in posttransplant survival. Although posttransplant mortality may be nominally higher among registrants with infections, this association does not disqualify these patients for transplant but certainly highlights the need to minimize complications and their effects.

Studies of transplant timing from VAD support have not provided clarity on whether an optimal time for transplant exists. The first report of transplant timing among persons with CF devices was reported by John and colleagues[18] who noted 1-year posttransplant survival of 87% among persons supported for a median of 151 days with the HeartMate II device. When examining the duration of support and effect on posttransplant outcomes, the investigators noted no significant difference between persons receiving a transplant at less than 30 days, 30 to 89 days, 90 to 179 days, and greater than 180 days at 30 days after transplant ($P = .28$) and 1-year posttransplant mortality ($P = .18$). A more modern series of patients reported by Kamdar and colleagues[20] suggested no significant difference ($P = .47$) between patients supported for less than 180 days (1-year survival 89%) and those supported for more than 180 days (1-year survival 93%). The investigators reported an effect opposite the larger series report by John and colleagues,[18] which suggests declining survival with longer support (1-year survival 84% for transplants 90–179 days vs 79% for transplants more than 365 days after implant). Colvin and colleagues[21] and Dardas and colleagues[22] evaluated transplant timing via simulation of the transplant system. Colvin and colleagues[21] found no marked change in posttransplant survival when increasing the number of elective status 1A days from 30 days to 90 days. Dardas and colleagues[22] reported fewer transplants (53% vs 51% at 5 years), higher morality (17% vs 21% at 5 years), and a higher fraction death among transplants occurring after LVAD complications (7% vs 9%). Conclusions from these studies are not definitive, as urgency for transplant, therapeutic bias, and survivor bias figure strongly into posttransplant outcomes. Randomized controlled trials in the area of timing are infeasible, and the current practice of favoring rapid transplant remains the appropriate strategy for most BTT scenarios.

The improved survival among persons in need of VAD support justifies their use for BTT. The aggregate data suggest a nonsignificant decrease in posttransplant survival among VAD-supported recipients without complications. Those persons with LVAD complications have decreased survival, but there is sufficient survival to justify transplant. The prospect of extending life for a decade or more with the provision of transplant via BTT LVAD strategies is a more valuable goal than maximizing the utility of every donor heart.

Selected posttransplant morbidities

Vasoplegia Hypotension refractory to numerous high-dose pressors with adequate cardiac output characterizes the vasoplegia syndrome (VS). Awareness of this syndrome and evidence for a strong association with MCS are increasing. The incidence of VS varies by report but may be as high as 10% to 27% after cardiac surgery.[23] VS may be more common in the CF-VAD era. Among

heart transplant recipients, VS portends a higher risk of mortality with reports of case-fatality rates of 17% to 25%.[24,25] Vasopressin deficiency, increased nitric oxide (NO) synthesis, and cytokine release contribute to initiation and maintenance of refractory vasodilation (**Fig. 2**).[23–28] Data also suggest that increases in pulsatility (generated experimentally by lower VAD speed) correlate with a paradoxic decrease in muscle sympathetic nerve activity (a surrogate for sympathetic tone).[29] This mechanism may explain the strong association between CF-VADS and VS at the time of transplant. Given the refractory nature of this condition, identifying both causation and risk factors remains of paramount interest to avoid excess morbidity and mortality.

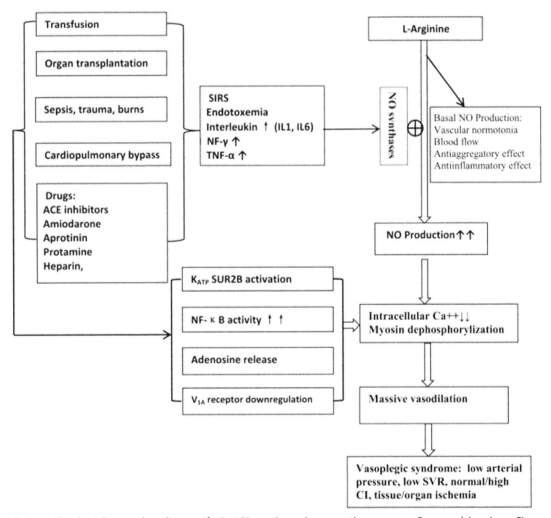

Fig. 2. Pathophysiology and mediators of VS. ACE, angiotensin-converting enzyme; Ca++, calcium ions; CI, cardiac index; CPB, cardiopulmonary bypass; IL, interleukin; K$_{ATP}$ ATP-sensitive potassium channel; NF, nuclear factor; SIRS, systemic inflammatory response syndrome; SVR, systemic vascular resistance; TNF, tumor-necrotizing factor. (*From* Liu H, Yu L, Yang L, et al. Vasoplegic syndrome: an update on perioperative considerations. J Clin Anesth 2017;40:66; with permission.)

Risk factors for VS vary between studies. However, CF-VADs as BTT are a consistent risk factor. In a recent series of 138 transplants from a single institution, Truby and colleagues[23] identified male sex (odds ratio [OR] 10.64, P = .023), body mass index (OR 1.17, P = .001), BTT LVAD (OR 3.29, P = .041), and preoperative inotrope score (OR 4.57, P = .002) as risk factors for VS. The strong association with CF-VADs is consistent with the findings of Patarroyo and colleagues,[25] who reported an OR of 2.8 (95% CI 1.1–7.4) for BTT CF-VADs among a series of 348 heart transplants. This investigation also notes an increased risk of VS attributable to thyroid disease (OR 2.7; 95% CI 1.0–7.0, P = .04), though this factor was weakly significant. Many studies associated VS with the severity of illness before transplant, which must be considered with caution, as hypotension is part of the syndrome's definition. Older data suggest a strong association between angiotensin-converting enzyme (ACE) use for vasoplegia following cardiac surgery.[30] Given this effect, many centers are attempting to minimize ACE-inhibitor (ACE-I) use before surgery. However, given the uncertainty of transplant timing and known benefits of ACE-I in heart failure treatment, randomized controlled trials are necessary to establish the harm of ACE-I cessation at arbitrary intervals before transplant.[31]

Treatment of VS is largely supportive with some sources advocating for the use of methylene blue, which inhibits NO synthase and the cyclic GMP messenger system. Although no randomized trial of incident VS treatment exists, Ozal and colleagues[32] randomized coronary artery bypass surgery patients at high risk of VS (defined as use of ACE-I, calcium channel blockers, or heparin) to methylene blue or no methylene blue. The treatment group had no VS, whereas the untreated group had a 26% incidence of VS (P<.001).[32–34] As more LVAD patients proceed to transplant, VS has the potential to become a greater issue than the other aforementioned risk factors for severe morbidity and mortality after BTT; further studies with methylene blue in this population are warranted.

Allosensitization Durable LVAD support induces allosensitization via hemolysis and frequent transfusions encountered with gastrointestinal bleeding. Allosensitization decreases the available donor pool and increases the risk of posttransplant mortality. Given the need to provide transplant to VAD-supported patients quickly after complications develop, allosensitization is equivalent to a risk factor for mortality among this population. Alba and colleagues[35] investigated HLA antibody formation among 143 CF-LVAD–supported patients. At baseline, 33% exhibited greater than 10% of panel reactive antibodies (PRAs). Sensitized patients increased to 50% of the sample after LVAD implant, and sensitization occurred against both class I and class II antigens. Risk factors for sensitization included younger age, female sex, and pre-VAD sensitization. No differences were detected in posttransplant survival in this series. Similarly, Ko and colleagues[36] reported sensitization (increase to >10% PRA among persons with <10% PRA before LVAD implant) among 23% of CF-LVAD implants (**Fig. 3**). Importantly, the increases in preformed antibody resolved in 67% of patients. The investigators also note a higher risk of acute cellular rejection and antibody-mediated rejection during follow-up among newly sensitized LVAD patients but not among newly sensitized patients without LVADs. Despite the higher rates of rejection, medium-term survival was similar between the newly sensitized group with LVADs and those without MCS. Among LVAD patients with very high levels of sensitization, mortality was 40%. Currently, there are no effective strategies for minimizing bleeding without potentially increasing the thrombosis risk in CF-VADs.[37,38] Thus, rapid treatment of bleeding sources, a high transfusion threshold, and careful management of both antiplatelet and anticoagulant agents are critical to reduce allosensitization events, as is the development of more biocompatible materials. Ultimately, short-term and long-term survival after transplant are similar for supported and unsupported recipients suggesting that allosensitization does not play a prominent role in posttransplant survival.

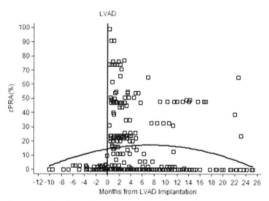

Fig. 3. Calculated PRA (cPRA) values before and after LVAD implant (*red horizontal line*). Values increased at the time of LVAD implant and then reduced, on average, thereafter (*black line*). (*From* Ko BS, Drakos S, Kfoury AG, et al. Immunologic effects of continuous-flow left ventricular assist devices before and after heart transplant. J Heart Lung Transplant 2016;35(8):1027; with permission.)

Total Artificial Heart

Biventricular support is increasing in the United States, while remaining a small segment of the durable device experience. However, persons with biventricular and isolated RV failure are among the most challenging patients to successfully support to durable devices and transplant as the result of concomitant liver and kidney dysfunction. If durable support is feasible, options for durable devices include the SynCardia Total Artificial Heart (SynCardia Systems, LLC, Tucson, AZ) and either paracorporeal or biventricular CF-VADs.

A recent query of the OPTN registry identified only 212 total artificial heart (TAH)–supported recipients.[39] TAH support shares many of the risk factors described with CF support. The introduction of a wearable, ambulatory driver for the TAH allows for improved physical rehabilitation whether in or out of the hospital, though not all patients meet the criteria for Freedom driver (SynCardia LLC) use and other morbidities, such as stroke and depression, may impinge on rehabilitation efforts. Renal failure and liver dysfunction can occur among TAH patients as the result of venous hypertension, despite adequate cardiac output delivered by the device. Intravascular volume and device settings must be assessed and meticulously adjusted to avoid worsening renal and liver function that may lead to delisting or a higher risk of organ failure at the time of transplant. Cheng and colleagues[39] reported a 24% prevalence of renal failure or dialysis after TAH transplants.

Posttransplant survival among TAH patients is decreased when compared with persons without MCS and to those supported with CF-LVADs (see **Fig. 1**). The force of mortality is greatest in the perioperative phase with 80% survival at 1 year as compared with 88% to 93% 1-year survival among other transplant recipients.[40] Graft failure and sepsis early after transplant are common and mirror the cause of death among persons with ongoing TAH support suggesting that end-organ function may be more difficult to restore with transplant alone and that infections may be harder to identify and treat during TAH support.[41] In modern series, median posttransplant survival is 6 to 7 years following TAH support, which is among the lowest posttransplant survival of devices discussed in this article.[39,40] When compared with biventricular VADs (paracorporeal, pulsatile, and CF–biventricular assist device [BiVAD] configurations), posttransplant survival was greater for the BiVAD group compared with the TAH group empirically; but no differences were found after adjusting for confounders (TAH HR 1.29, $P = .1$).[39] Median survival with BiVADs

exceeds 8 years.[39] As discussed for durable LVADs, any decrease in posttransplant survival attributable to TAH support or BiVAD support must be considered against the very high mortality without support as long as meaningful posttransplant survival is achieved. However, TAH survival is far less than the current median survival of 12 years; whether these transplants represent reasonable use of donor hearts is debatable.

TEMPORARY CIRCULATORY SUPPORT

The development of the TandemHeart (CardiacAssist, Inc, Pittsburgh, PA), Impella (Abiomed, Danvers, MA), and miniaturized extracorporeal life support (ECLS) devices allows for temporary circulatory support of left ventricular (LV) and right ventricular (RV) failure via more direct ventricular unloading. These devices are commonly used to evaluate the trajectory of end-organ function to assess the feasibility of durable support or transplant. Therefore, many patients supported with these devices had recent and severe end-organ dysfunction and are at an increased risk for end-organ decompensation after transplant. However, if end-organ function is improved and perfusion maintained, these devices offer additional perfusion when compared with optimal medical therapy alone.

TandemHeart

The TandemHeart offers LV and RV unloading via inflow proximal to the LV or RV and outflow above the semilunar valves. Unloading at the level of the left atrium or inferior vena cava/superior vena cava offers substantial ventricular unloading. These devices are complicated by the need for relative immobility to maintain inflow cannula position (left-sided support) or outflow cannula position (right-sided support) and require heparinization. Hemolysis is rare with the TandemHeart.[42,43] A query of the OPTN registry revealed 35 patients with TandemHeart at the time of transplant with 90-day survival of 88% (95% CI 71%–95%) and 1-year survival of 84% (95% CI 66%–93%, Dardas TF, unpublished data, 2018). Thus, limited data suggest that TandemHeart before transplant results in no incremental decrease in posttransplant survival among carefully selected patients.

Impella

The Impella family of devices offers a rapidly implantable temporary MCS option. The intraventricular inflow and outflow above the aortic or pulmonic valve may allow for greater ventricular unloading than IABPs, extracorporeal membrane oxygenation (ECMO), or TandemHeart. These devices require relatively large sheaths or surgical conduits for delivery, heparinization, and are subject to hemolysis and, less commonly, mechanical failure. Placement of Impella devices via an axillary or subclavian approach is feasible and may allow for meaningful physical therapy before transplant.[44,45]

Reports of BTT success after long periods of Impella support exist.[46] A query of the OPTN registry, identified 55 transplants with previous Impella with 90-day survival of 91% (95% CI 79%–96%) and 1-year survival of 88% (95% CI 76%–95%, unpublished data). Placement of the Impella in the axillary or subclavian artery may allow for ambulation and physical therapy. As randomized experiences with larger Impella devices grows, more data will become available to assess whether Impella devices are superior to IABP and other forms of temporary circulatory support.

Extracorporeal Life Support

ECMO or ECLS can support critical cardiogenic shock as a bridge to transplant, durable MCS, or recovery. ECLS can provide support for left- and right-sided failure but requires large cannulae, which predispose patients to significant bleeding, infections, and embolic complications. Although attractive for its ability to offer full circulatory support and oxygenation, ultimately, the high burden of complications limit the use of ECLS as a reliable bridge to transplant. A recent meta-analysis of ECMO complications documents the high incidence of complications that may preclude transplant (**Fig. 4**).[47] Consistent with these highly morbid complications, numerous concerns were raised during the development of the new heart allocation system as to whether ECLS-supported candidates should have access to the highest urgency tier of the new system.[48] The probability of death after 30 days of ELCS support is 24%. Posttransplant survival after ECLS is 76% at 1 year, and posttransplant dialysis occurred in 24% of persons not on dialysis before transplant (unpublished data). These values may underrepresent posttransplant mortality in this population. Regardless, ECLS-supported candidates were afforded tier 1 urgency for 2 weeks in the new allocation system. After this time, urgency is subject to Regional Review Board approval. For programs, ECLS use will remain a resource-intensive mode of circulatory support that must be applied early in the course of cardiogenic shock and maintained by expert teams of providers. As time on ECLS accumulates, teams will need to carefully assess whether transplant remains beneficial.

SUMMARY

MCS continues to develop and serves a critical role in the treatment armamentarium for persons with cardiogenic shock. Posttransplant survival among persons supported with durable LVADs is equivalent to patients receiving a transplant without MCS, whereas temporary MCS and biventricular MCS have lower but acceptable posttransplant survival when compared with waiting unsupported. Caution is appropriate when considering transplant of MCS patients supported with CF-LVADs complicated by infections and those with either TAH or ECLS support. However, for most patients supported with MCS, transplant remains a positive outcome and a means to end the burden of MCS. Case-by-case evaluation of the prospect for reasonable posttransplant survival is necessary among these high-risk populations.

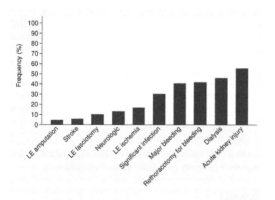

Fig. 4. Major complications during ECLS. LE, lower extremity. (*Adapted from* Cheng R, Hachamovitch R, Kittleson M. Complications of extracorporeal membrane oxygenation for treatment of cardiogenic shock and cardiac arrest: a meta-analysis of 1866 adult patients. Ann Thorac Surg 2014;97(2):614; with permission.)

REFERENCES

1. Colvin M, Smith JM, Hadley N, et al. OPTN/SRTR 2016 annual data report: heart. Am J Transplant 2018;18(Suppl 1):291–362.
2. Lund LH, Khush KK, Cherikh WS, et al. The registry of the international society for heart and lung transplantation: thirty-fourth adult heart transplantation report-2017; focus theme: allograft ischemic time. J Heart Lung Transplant 2017;36(10):1037–46.
3. Pagani FD, Miller LW, Russell SD, et al. Extended mechanical circulatory support with a continuous-flow rotary left ventricular assist device. J Am Coll Cardiol 2009;54(4):312–21.
4. Aaronson KD, Slaughter MS, Miller LW, et al. Use of an intrapericardial, continuous-flow, centrifugal

pump in patients awaiting heart transplantation. Circulation 2012;125(25):3191–200.

5. Mehra MR, Naka Y, Uriel N, et al. A fully magnetically levitated circulatory pump for advanced heart failure. N Engl J Med 2017;376(5):440–50.

6. Frazier OH, Rose EA, McCarthy P, et al. Improved mortality and rehabilitation of transplant candidates treated with a long-term implantable left ventricular assist system. Ann Surg 1995;222(3):327–36 [discussion: 336–8].

7. Massad MG, McCarthy PM, Smedira NG, et al. Does successful bridging with the implantable left ventricular assist device affect cardiac transplantation outcome? J Thorac Cardiovasc Surg 1996;112(5):1275–81 [discussion: 1282–3].

8. Patlolla V, Patten RD, Denofrio D, et al. The effect of ventricular assist devices on post-transplant mortality an analysis of the United network for organ sharing thoracic registry. J Am Coll Cardiol 2009;53(3):264–71.

9. Jaski BE, Kim JC, Naftel DC, et al. Cardiac transplant outcome of patients supported on left ventricular assist device vs. intravenous inotropic therapy. J Heart Lung Transplant 2001;20(4):449–56.

10. Klotz S, Stypmann J, Welp H, et al. Does continuous flow left ventricular assist device technology have a positive impact on outcome pretransplant and posttransplant? Ann Thorac Surg 2006;82(5):1774–8.

11. Schulze PC, Kitada S, Clerkin K, et al. Regional differences in recipient waitlist time and pre- and posttransplant mortality after the 2006 United Network for organ sharing policy changes in the donor heart allocation algorithm. JACC Heart Fail 2014;2(2):166–77.

12. Weiss ES, Allen JG, Arnaoutakis GJ, et al. Creation of a quantitative recipient risk index for mortality prediction after cardiac transplantation (IMPACT). Ann Thorac Surg 2011;92(3):914–21 [discussion: 921–2].

13. Dardas T, Mokadam NA, Pagani F, et al. Transplant registrants with implanted left ventricular assist devices have insufficient risk to justify elective organ procurement and transplantation network status 1A time. J Am Coll Cardiol 2012;60(1):36–43.

14. Trivedi JR, Rajagopal K, Schumer EM, et al. Differences in status 1A heart transplantation survival in the continuous flow left ventricular assist device era. Ann Thorac Surg 2016;102(5):1512–6.

15. Donneyong M, Cheng A, Trivedi JR, et al. The association of pretransplant HeartMate II left ventricular assist device placement and heart transplantation mortality. ASAIO J 2014;60(3):294–9.

16. Nativi JN, Drakos SG, Kucheryavaya AY, et al. Changing outcomes in patients bridged to heart transplantation with continuous- versus pulsatile-flow ventricular assist devices: an analysis of the registry of the International Society for Heart and Lung Transplantation. J Heart Lung Transplant 2011;30(8):854–61.

17. Quader MA, Wolfe LG, Kasirajan V. Heart transplantation outcomes in patients with continuous-flow left ventricular assist device-related complications. J Heart Lung Transplant 2015;34(1):75–81.

18. John R, Pagani FD, Naka Y, et al. Post-cardiac transplant survival after support with a continuous-flow left ventricular assist device: impact of duration of left ventricular assist device support and other variables. J Thorac Cardiovasc Surg 2010;140(1):174–81.

19. Healy AH, Baird BC, Drakos SG, et al. Impact of ventricular assist device complications on posttransplant survival: an analysis of the United network of organ sharing database. Ann Thorac Surg 2013;95(3):870–5.

20. Kamdar F, John R, Eckman P, et al. Postcardiac transplant survival in the current era in patients receiving continuous-flow left ventricular assist devices. J Thorac Cardiovasc Surg 2013;145(2):575–81.

21. Colvin M, Miranda-Herrera D, Gustafson SK, et al. Impact of increased time at the highest urgency category on heart transplant outcomes for candidates with ventricular assist devices. J Heart Lung Transplant 2016;35(3):326–34.

22. Dardas TF, Cheng RK, Mahr CM, et al. Adverse effects of delayed transplant listing among patients with implantable left ventricular assist devices. J Card Fail 2018. https://doi.org/10.1016/j.cardfail.2018.01.003.

23. Truby LK, Takeda K, Farr M, et al. Incidence and impact of on-cardiopulmonary bypass vasoplegia during heart transplantation. ASAIO J 2018;64(1):43–51.

24. Byrne JG, Leacche M, Paul S, et al. Risk factors and outcomes for 'vasoplegia syndrome' following cardiac transplantation. Eur J Cardiothorac Surg 2004;25(3):327–32.

25. Patarroyo M, Simbaqueba C, Shrestha K, et al. Preoperative risk factors and clinical outcomes associated with vasoplegia in recipients of orthotopic heart transplantation in the contemporary era. J Heart Lung Transplant 2012;31(3):282–7.

26. Fischer GW, Levin MA. Vasoplegia during cardiac surgery: current concepts and management. Semin Thorac Cardiovasc Surg 2010;22(2):140–4.

27. Levin MA, Lin H-M, Castillo JG, et al. Early on-cardiopulmonary bypass hypotension and other factors associated with vasoplegic syndrome. Circulation 2009;120(17):1664–71.

28. Liu H, Yu L, Yang L, et al. Vasoplegic syndrome: an update on perioperative considerations. J Clin Anesth 2017;40:63–71.

29. Cornwell WK 3rd, Tarumi T, Stickford A, et al. Restoration of pulsatile flow reduces sympathetic nerve activity among individuals with continuous-flow left ventricular assist devices. Circulation 2015;132(24):2316–22.

30. Boeken U, Feindt P, Mohan E, et al. Post-perfusion syndrome and disturbed microcirculation after cardiac surgery: the role of angiotensin-converting-enzyme inhibitors. Thorac Cardiovasc Surg 1999; 47(6):347–51.

31. Raja SG, Fida N. Should angiotensin converting enzyme inhibitors/angiotensin II receptor antagonists be omitted before cardiac surgery to avoid postoperative vasodilation? Interact Cardiovasc Thorac Surg 2008;7(3):470–5.

32. Ozal E, Kuralay E, Yildirim V, et al. Preoperative methylene blue administration in patients at high risk for vasoplegic syndrome during cardiac surgery. Ann Thorac Surg 2005;79(5):1615–9.

33. Mehaffey JH, Johnston LE, Hawkins RB, et al. Methylene blue for vasoplegic syndrome after cardiac operation: early administration improves survival. Ann Thorac Surg 2017;104(1):36–41.

34. Levin RL, Degrange MA, Bruno GF, et al. Methylene blue reduces mortality and morbidity in vasoplegic patients after cardiac surgery. Ann Thorac Surg 2004;77(2):496–9.

35. Alba AC, Tinckam K, Foroutan F, et al. Factors associated with anti-human leukocyte antigen antibodies in patients supported with continuous-flow devices and effect on probability of transplant and post-transplant outcomes. J Heart Lung Transplant 2015;34(5):685–92.

36. Ko BS, Drakos S, Kfoury AG, et al. Immunologic effects of continuous-flow left ventricular assist devices before and after heart transplant. J Heart Lung Transplant 2016;35(8):1024–30.

37. Kirklin JK, Naftel DC, Kormos RL, et al. Interagency registry for mechanically assisted circulatory support (INTERMACS) analysis of pump thrombosis in the HeartMate II left ventricular assist device. J Heart Lung Transplant 2014;33(1):12–22.

38. Starling RC, Moazami N, Silvestry SC, et al. Unexpected abrupt increase in left ventricular assist device thrombosis. N Engl J Med 2014;370(1):33–40.

39. Cheng A, Trivedi JR, Van Berkel VH, et al. Comparison of total artificial heart and biventricular assist device support as bridge-to-transplantation. J Card Surg 2016;31(10):648–53.

40. Copeland JG, Copeland H, Gustafson M, et al. Experience with more than 100 total artificial heart implants. J Thorac Cardiovasc Surg 2012;143(3):727–34.

41. Copeland JG, Smith RG, Arabia FA, et al. Total artificial heart bridge to transplantation: a 9-year experience with 62 patients. J Heart Lung Transplant 2004;23(7):823–31.

42. Bruckner BA, Jacob LP, Gregoric ID, et al. Clinical experience with the TandemHeart percutaneous ventricular assist device as a bridge to cardiac transplantation. Tex Heart Inst J 2008; 35(4):447–50.

43. Tempelhof MW, Klein L, Cotts WG, et al. Clinical experience and patient outcomes associated with the TandemHeart percutaneous transseptal assist device among a heterogeneous patient population. ASAIO J 2011;57(4):254–61.

44. Bansal A, Bhama JK, Patel R, et al. Using the minimally invasive impella 5.0 via the right subclavian artery cutdown for acute on chronic decompensated heart failure as a bridge to decision. Ochsner J 2016;16(3):210–6.

45. Lotun K, Shetty R, Patel M, et al. Percutaneous left axillary artery approach for Impella 2.5 liter circulatory support for patients with severe aortoiliac arterial disease undergoing high-risk percutaneous coronary intervention. J Interv Cardiol 2012;25(2):210–3.

46. Lima B, Kale P, Gonzalez-Stawinski GV, et al. Effectiveness and safety of the impella 5.0 as a bridge to cardiac transplantation or durable left ventricular assist device. Am J Cardiol 2016;117(10):1622–8.

47. Cheng R, Hachamovitch R, Kittleson M, et al. Complications of extracorporeal membrane oxygenation for treatment of cardiogenic shock and cardiac arrest: a meta-analysis of 1,866 adult patients. Ann Thorac Surg 2014;97(2):610–6.

48. Kittleson MM, Kobashigawa JA. Cardiac transplantation: current outcomes and contemporary controversies. JACC Heart Fail 2017;5(12):857–68.

Hemodynamic Pump-Patient Interactions and Left Ventricular Assist Device Imaging

Nikhil Narang, MD, Jayant Raikhelkar, MD,
Gabriel Sayer, MD, Nir Uriel, MD, MSc*

KEYWORDS

- Left ventricular assist device • Invasive hemodynamics • Echocardiography • Aortic insufficiency

KEY POINTS

- Each type of continuous-flow left ventricular assist device (cfLVAD) has a unique pressure differential to flow relationship as demonstrated by H-Q curves.
- Axial flow pumps have steeper, linear H-Q curves, resulting in less flow pulsatility, compared with centrifugal flow pumps, which have flatter H-Q curves–translating to little change in the pressure differential in response to low flows.
- The echocardiographic ramp study can be used to determine the adequate cfLVAD speed to unload the ventricle (midline intraventricular septum, intermittent aortic valve opening and minimize mitral regurgitation).
- Invasive hemodynamics, combined with echocardiography, is a useful assessment tool to best choose a speed optimize hemodynamics (CVP <12 and PCWP <18 mm Hg) and adequately unload the left ventricle.
- Three-dimensional transthoracic echocardiographicy during ramp studies can help better discern corresponding shapes of the left ventricle and right ventricle during device speed uptitration, and suggests that device position (intrapericardial vs extrathoracic) may significantly affect changes in ventricular structure and shape during speed adjustment.

INTRODUCTION

Continuous-flow left ventricular assist devices (cfLVADs) have become durable options for patients with advanced heart failure as a mode to improve both quality of life and survival, either as destination therapy or bridge to transplantation.[1,2] A patient's optimal level of hemodynamic support from LVADs may vary based on several contributing factors, such as gender, body size, volume status, presence of existing right ventricular dysfunction, and parameters determined by the clinician. Hemodynamic optimization of patients with an LVAD includes implementation of guideline-directed medical therapy with the use of diuretics, beta-blockers, angiotensin-receptor blockers/angiotensin-converting enzyme/neprilysn inhibitors, and mineralocorticoid antagonists; furthermore, the International Society of Heart and Lung Transplantation recommends

Disclosure Statement: Dr N. Uriel receives consultant fees and grant support from Abbott Healthcare and Medtronic. Dr G. Sayer receives consulting fees from Medtronic. Drs N. Narang and J. Raikhelkar have no disclosures to report.
Section of Cardiology, Department of Medicine, University of Chicago, 5841 South Maryland Avenue, Chicago, IL 60637, USA
* Corresponding author. 5841 South Maryland Avenue, MC 2016, Chicago, IL 60637.
E-mail address: nuriel@medicine.bsd.uchicago.edu

Cardiol Clin 36 (2018) 561–569
https://doi.org/10.1016/j.ccl.2018.06.013
0733-8651/18/© 2018 Elsevier Inc. All rights reserved.

that cfLVAD speeds should be adjusted to adequately unload the left ventricle, while maintaining a midline intraventricular septum along with minimizing mitral valve regurgitation (MR) plus allowing for intermittent aortic valve (AV) opening.[3] The use of echocardiography and invasive hemodynamics is imperative, and complementary clinical tools to improve the hemodynamic profile of a patient with an LVAD. This review describes the following topics: (1) normal hemodynamic characteristics of durable mechanical support, (2) methods to optimize LVAD speed, and (3) morphologic changes of both the left and right ventricle following LVAD implantation.

HEMODYNAMICS OF LEFT VENTRICULAR ASSIST DEVICES

Contemporary LVADs are classified as either axial pumps, such as the HeartMate II (Abbott, Abbott Park, IL) or centrifugal pumps, which consist of the HVAD (Medtronic, Minneapolis, Minnesota) and HeartMate 3 (Abbott, Abbott Park, IL). These devices are implanted with different techniques and have variable flow capacities, but are governed by the same principle of continuous pumping of blood out of the left ventricle (LV) throughout the cardiac cycle. Pressure-volume loops (PVLs) best demonstrate the physiologic relationship between ventricular filling and contraction in respect to external changes in loading conditions. Under normal conditions, the PVL is characterized by a trapezoidal shape with a rounded top. PVL appearance in the setting of LVAD transforms from a trapezoidal shape to a triangular shape, which is reflective of the loss of normal isovolemic periods, where systemic blood flow is not dependent on ejection through the AV[4] (**Fig. 1**). Stepwise increases in LVAD speed will coincide with similar increases in flow under static loading conditions and will cause a progressive leftward shift of the PVL, depicting increasing degrees of LV unloading. Additionally, the higher the achieved LVAD flow correlates with decreasing peak LV pressure generation and higher systemic arterial pressures, with the subsequent ventricular unloading leading to decreased pulmonary capillary wedge and left atrial pressures.

The relationships of blood flow (Q) through a cfLVAD and pressure differential (H) between the inflow and outflow cannulas (pump pressure) can best be described by the HQ curve (**Fig. 2**). The HQ curve appearance in axial versus centrifugal pump varies and ultimately reflects the differing engineered characteristics of the pump and therefore physiologic response to speed changes. At a given pump speed, pump flow decreases as the

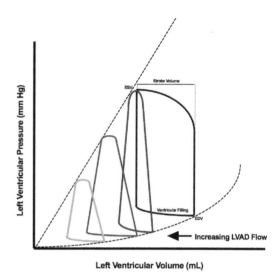

Fig. 1. Flow-dependent changes of the PVL with leftward shift representing greater LV unloading. EDV, end-diastolic volume; ESV, end-systolic volume.

pressure gradient across the inflow and outflow cannula increases. At a given pressure gradient, pump flow increases as the pump speed increases. However, intrinsic properties of the LV and the aorta in regards to pressure differential during systole and diastole will additionally impact the degree of flow changes in response to increases in pump speed. Centrifugal pumps, specifically the HVAD and HeartMate 3, operate over a wide range of flows for a very small change in pressure differential across the pump (see **Fig. 2**A).[5,6] The flat head curve for centrifugal pump is reflective of the high pump flow pulsatility inherent to the device. This results in a large dynamic range of flow of up to approximately 10 L/min for a relatively small change in pressure. From a clinical standpoint, the flat HQ curve translates to little change in the pressure differential in response to low flows, which can occur commonly in hypovolemia or even right heart failure. Therefore, relatively static pressure differentials translate to less susceptibility to increased suction during low flow conditions. In contrast, axial flow pumps (HeartMate II) have much steeper HQ curves, in which there is linear inverse relationship in flow with pump pressure differential (see **Fig. 2**B). Consequently, similar pressure differentials across the pump will produce less flow pulsatility (3–7 L/min for example) compared with the centrifugal pump design. Furthermore, the axial LVADs are more likely to generate a greater pressure differential in the setting of low flows, which may in turn trigger suction events within the LV cavity. The combined intrinsic properties of differential pump pulsatility demonstrated on the HQ

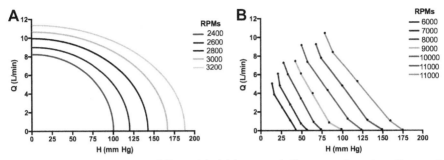

Fig. 2. Flow (Q) compared with pressure differentials (H) between inflow cannula and outflow graft at various pump speeds for (A) centrifugal pump and (B) axial flow pump.

curves along with varying ventricular and aortic loading conditions govern the complex pump-patient interactions.

LEFT VENTRICULAR ASSIST DEVICE SPEED OPTIMIZATION

A unique pump-patient interaction is present for all subtypes of patients who receive durable mechanical circulatory support. This is due to the several contributing factors that ultimately affect LVAD output, which include patient body size, gender, mean arterial pressure, volume status, intrinsic myocardial contractility, pre-LVAD implantation right ventricular (RV) function, vasoactive medications, and the presence or absence of neurohormonal blockade. Other than these factors, the clinician has the ability to alter the performance of LVAD by changing the device speed, with the goal of optimizing hemodynamics. Device speed optimization, defined as the speed in which the LV is adequately unloaded with a midline intraventricular septum with minimal MR and intermittent AV opening, can vary dramatically from patient to patient.[7]

Following LVAD implantation in the immediate postoperative period, noninvasive imaging is routinely deferred until perioperative inotropes and vasoactive drugs are weaned off to best assess the need for pump speed optimization. LVAD speed optimization, known as ramp testing, can be achieved through the use of echocardiography and invasive hemodynamics.

TWO-DIMENSIONAL AND 3-DIMENSIONAL ECHOCARDIOGRAPHIC OPTIMIZATION

Our group was the first to describe a formalized protocol for LVAD speed testing for the purpose of speed optimization and diagnosing device thrombosis.[3] In brief, before performing a ramp test, appropriate anticoagulation must be confirmed with international normalized ratio

greater than 1.8 or partial thromboplastin time greater than 60 seconds. Opening arterial pressure by Doppler during the study should be >65 mm Hg at baseline to proceed. The parasternal long-axis view is then primarily used to assess LV end-diastolic dimension (LVEDD), LV end-systolic dimension (LVESD), frequency of AV opening, degree of aortic insufficiency (AI), MR, and heart rate. Continuous-flow LVAD parameters, including power, PI (pulsatility index), and flow, are recorded at each stage. Baseline evaluation of these variables are also recorded at the given speed at presentation. For the HeartMate II devices, the device speed is then lowered to 8000 rpm and 2300 rpm for the HVAD devices. After 2 minutes of washout time, LVEDD, LVESD, degree of MR, AI, assessment of AV opening, Doppler blood pressure, and heart rate are all recorded. Pump parameters (power, PI, and flow) are also recorded during each stage. Stepwise increase in speed at intervals of 400 rpm for HeartMate II and 100 rpm for HVAD are then made; other protocols have shown 130-rpm intervals in the HVAD physiologically correlates with 400-rpm intervals in the HeartMate II.[8] The testing speed range for HeartMate II is 8000 to 12,000 rpm and 2200 to 3200 rpm for the HVAD. The protocol is complete once the upper limit speed is reached, LVEDD reaches less than 3.0 cm, suction event, or ventricular ectopic beats occur. The clinician must also pay attention to development of premature ventricular contractions, which may indicate contact of the inflow cannula with the septum. From a medical optimization standpoint, the speed is adjusted to clinically achieve a midline intraventricular septum, minimal MR, and intermittent AV opening to prevent development of AI.

Ramp testing can be used for device malfunction assessment in general and specifically for pump thrombosis. Patients with obstruction to flow, mainly pump thrombosis, had minimal change in their LVEDD size in response to speed change leading to an attenuated LVEDD slope when calculated by a linear equation (device speed on x-axis vs LVEDD on y-axis).[9] LVEDD slope of greater than -0.16 was suggestive of device thrombosis when performing echocardiographic ramp testing. Performing a ramp test in patients with HVADs was not associated with linear LVEDD reduction in response to speed changes as seen with the HeartMate II pumps.[10,11]

Recently, our group investigated ventricular structural changes in 31 patients (19 with Heart-Mate II and 12 with HVAD) who underwent hemodynamic ramp studies during which 3D transthoracic echocardiographic (TTE) imaging was performed to determine how device speed changes influence global LV and RV geometry.[12] End-diastolic and systolic volumes using 3D TTE were calculated at each stage during prespecified ramp protocol. In addition, 3D endocardial surface analysis was performed to define LV conicity and sphericity. It has been previously described that adverse remodeling leads to more spherical LV shapes from chronic volume overload in patients with severe mitral regurgitation due to mitral valve prolapse, with postsurgical function improvements occurring as represented by change to more normal, conical shape.[13] Three-dimensional TTE RV shape analysis was described in the form of free-wall and septal curvature in response to speed changes. Zero curvature indicated a flat surface, whereas the more positive or negative values signify more convexity or concavity of the surface, respectively, from the perspective of a reference point outside of the right ventricle. For the HeartMate II cohort, LV volumes decreased by (127 ± 78 mL; $P<.01$) and became more conical with increasing speeds. RV volumes increased significantly only at highest speeds (stage IV) with an average difference of 60 ± 68 mL between highest and lowest stage ($P<.01$); RV septal shape on average also became more convex (bulging into the LV) at the highest speed setting when compared with the lowest speed setting. For the HVAD cohort, LV volumes similarly decreased when comparing the lowest and highest speeds (51 ± 38 mL, $P<.01$); however, the changes in shape were more global than the longitudinal changes seen with HeartMate II. With regard to the RV, there was a non–statistically significant increase in RV volumes in response to the increase in speed. In addition, there was no change in RV septal or free-wall curvature. Schematics depicting 3D ventricular geometry with respect to pump type are shown in **Fig. 3**.

It can be postulated that differential changes in 3D TTE-derived ventricular shape may be attributed to pump position. The HeartMate II device is located in the subdiaphragmatic space and results in inferior displacement of the LV apex, whereas the intrathoracic-placed HVAD resides within the LV apex and results in less apical deformation. This is likely the same with the newer HeartMate 3 device, which is located in the intrathoracic position, although studies are lacking in changes in 3D ventricular geometry for this more contemporary pump.

INVASIVE HEMODYNAMIC OPTIMIZATION

An additional aspect to medical optimization of the patient with an LVAD is combining echocardiography and invasive hemodynamics to better improve a patient's hemodynamic profile given the complex interactions between native heart physiology and pump characteristics. We followed the original study of noninvasive ramp testing with a second analysis of LVAD speed adjustment combined with invasive hemodynamics obtained during a right heart catheterization (RHC).[14]

Patients with an LVAD were evaluated in the outpatient setting for a simultaneous echocardiographic and hemodynamic ramp test. Baseline central venous pressure (CVP), pulmonary artery pressure, pulmonary capillary wedge pressure (PCWP), Fick cardiac output (CO), and cardiac index are measured. The same steps for speed uptitration are made as previously described, with 2-minute washout periods following speed changes. At each speed interval, right heart pressures, heart rate, Doppler blood pressure, and echocardiographic images are obtained. At the conclusion of the assessment, the clinician chooses the speed that best achieves hemodynamic optimization, defined as a PCWP less than 18 mm Hg and CVP less than 12 mm Hg, with the secondary goals of intermittent AV opening and minimal MR.

In ambulatory outpatients, baseline hemodynamics revealed that only 43% of patients with an LVAD had a CVP and PCWP within the specified normal range.[14] Following the conclusion of invasive hemodynamic ramp testing, 56% of patients achieved normalization of both CVP and PCWP. The hemodynamic profiles of the overall cohort represented by CVP and PCWP are best characterized in **Fig. 4**. The dashed line in the baseline panel in **Fig. 4** equates to a CVP-to-PCWP ratio of 0.63, for which ratios greater than this cut point may suggest right heart failure. There were no significant differences in baseline hemodynamics between pump types. Furthermore, reduction in PCWP was determined to be speed-dependent and flow-dependent instead of device-dependent, and was similar as well

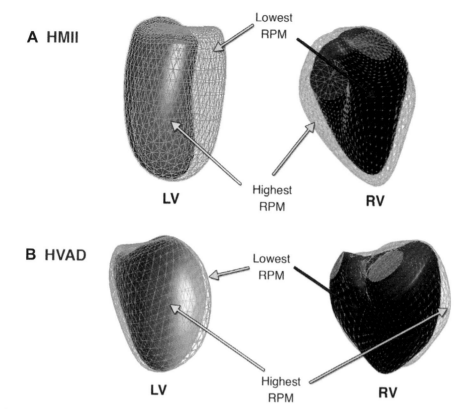

Fig. 3. Three-dimensional endocardial surfaces of the LV (*orange*) and RV (*red*) were obtained at the lowest (*gray outline*) and highest revolutions per minute (RPM) for both the axial flow pump (*A*) and centrifugal flow pump (*B*). (*From* Addetia K, Uriel N, Maffessanti F, et al. 3D morphologic changes in LV and RV during LVAD ramp studies. JACC Cardiovasc Imaging 2017;11(2 Pt 1):159–69; with permission.)

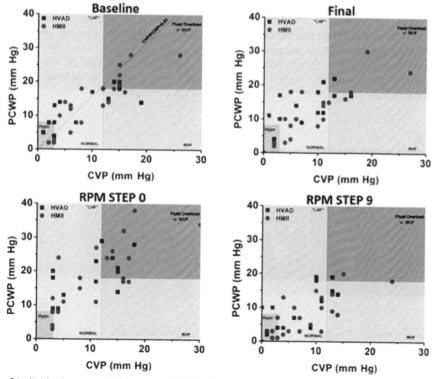

Fig. 4. Plot of individual patients' CVP versus PCWP at baseline, highest LVAD speed, and final measurement; 5 zones are described including normal, left heart failure (LHF), fluid overload, right heart failure (RHF), and hypovolemia (Hypo). (*From* Uriel N, Sayer G, Addetia K, et al. Hemodynamic ramp tests in patients with left ventricular assist devices. JACC Heart Fail 2016;4(3):213; with permission.)

between pumps. Small sample regression analysis from other centers following ramp testing demonstrated that speed adjustments of 400 rpm in the HeartMate II were equivalent to a 130-rpm adjustment in the HVAD, corresponding to a relative increase in CO of 0.3 L/min.[8] In this study, improvement in 6-minute walk distance following hemodynamic ramp optimization was observed, although long-term outcomes and data on other performance indices following ramp studies remains to be seen.

A similar hemodynamic ramp protocol was tested by our group in a contemporary HeartMate 3 cohort.[15] Consistent with our prior findings, speed optimization was able to normalize CVP and PCWP in 50% of patients with abnormal hemodynamics at baseline. All of these hemodynamic studies demonstrate a wide range of baseline hemodynamics with differing responses to speed changes, suggesting a significant benefit in performing speed optimization with the aid of simultaneous invasive hemodynamics.

Given that invasive hemodynamic assessment is not always readily available and inherent procedural risks are present due to chronic anticoagulation, Doppler echocardiographic assessment also may be used when evaluating filling pressures for the LVAD patient. Estep and colleagues[16] performed simultaneous RHC and TTEs on 50 consecutive patients with HeartMate II devices at a baseline speed of 9000 rpm. They derived a multifaceted algorithm based on this cohort incorporating TTE-derived mitral inflow velocities, right atrial and systolic pulmonary pressure estimation, and indexed left atrial volume, which demonstrated considerable diagnostic accuracy in identifying patients with PCWP greater than 15 mm Hg with an area under the curve of 0.89 ($P<.0001$). These data support using TTE in beyond measurement of ventricular dimensions, assessment of MR, and AV closure when optimizing LVAD patients.

Current studies are under way to assess speed optimization on clinical outcome. The HVAD RAMP IT UP trial,[17] which is a randomized study of invasive hemodynamic speed optimization versus standard of care, and other single-center experiences. The American Society of Echocardiography has recently published guidelines on appropriate use of LVAD ramp testing to better ascertain presence of device thrombosis, difficult-to-manage RV failure, or when a patient requires speed optimization in addition to medical therapy titration for signs and symptoms of clinical heart failure.[18]

NOVEL ASSESSMENT OF AORTIC INSUFFICIENCY

De novo AI has a prevalence of approximately 25% in the first year following cfLVAD implantation and if left untreated, can lead to progressive heart failure symptoms.[19,20] The pathophysiologic mechanism is thought to arise from valve commissure and leaflet degradation due to the lack of regular AV opening following cfLVAD implantation.[21] Furthermore, continuous LV unloading leads to valvular shear stress and an average increase in transvalvular pressure load by 25% and duration of the pressure load by 20% compared with normal circulatory physiology. Progressive AI may also lead to RV

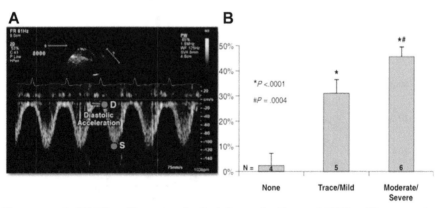

Fig. 5. (A) Measurement of LVAD outflow cannula diastolic acceleration and LVAD outflow cannula systolic-to-diastolic peak velocity ratio (S/D) using pulse wave Doppler. (B) AI severity measured by a novel mean RF compared with standard transthoracic echocardiography grading using a combination of vena contracta (VC) and visual estimation. (*Adapted from* Grinstein J, Kruse E, Sayer G, et al. Accurate quantification methods for aortic insufficiency severity in patients with LVAD: role of diastolic flow acceleration and systolic-to-diastolic peak velocity ratio of outflow cannula. JACC Cardiovasc Imaging 2016;9(6):641–51; with permission.)

dysfunction and whether it reduces survival is unclear.[22,23]

Given the lack of a true diastolic phase in LVADs, traditional echocardiographic modalities of AI quantification including vena contracta, proximal isovelocity surface area, deceleration time, and regurgitation fraction (RF) may all not be applicable to durable continuous-flow mechanical circulatory support devices. Our group investigated the accuracy of traditional modalities of AI quantification compared with novel methods, including direct calculation of aortic RF plus 2 Doppler-based indices: outflow cannula diastolic acceleration time and outflow cannula systolic-to-diastolic (S/D) peak velocity ratio.[24] Simultaneous RHC and TTEs were performed as part of ramp testing for LVAD optimization. Novel aortic RF was calculated by subtracting the venous return to the right side of the heart obtained by RHC via the Fick method from the total left-sided systemic flow measurement using TTE (full derivation in publication by Grinstein and colleagues[24]). Based on the continuity equation, total left-sided systemic flow is equal to right-sided venous return unless an intracardiac shunt or AI is present. For the 2 additional new methods of AI quantification, a modified right-

sided parasternal window was used to acquire the pulse wave Doppler signal of the outflow graft of the LVAD cannula, with the diastolic acceleration measured as the slope from the start to end of diastole (**Fig. 5**A). The S/D ratio was defined by peak systolic velocity divided by peak diastolic velocity of the pulsed wave Doppler signal of the LVAD outflow cannula.

Traditional qualitative RF assessment underestimated the degree of AI when compared with the novel aortic RF, as mean novel aortic RF for qualitatively moderate or greater AI was 45.8% ± 3.6%, lying within the higher range of RF for moderate AI (**Fig. 5**B). In addition, novel aortic RF correlated better with PCWP. Significant AI increases left ventricular end-diastolic volume, as was observed by the moderately strong correlation between PCWP and the novel aortic RF. The S/D ratio and outflow cannula diastolic acceleration correlated strongly with regurgitant fraction (R = 0.91 and 0.94, respectively) and PCWP (R = 0.82 and 0.65, respectively) as seen in **Fig. 6**. Moderate to severe AI as calculated correlated with a proposed S/D ratio with estimated S/D cut point of less than or equal to 1.1 associated with novel aortic RF of 50%. Similarly, an

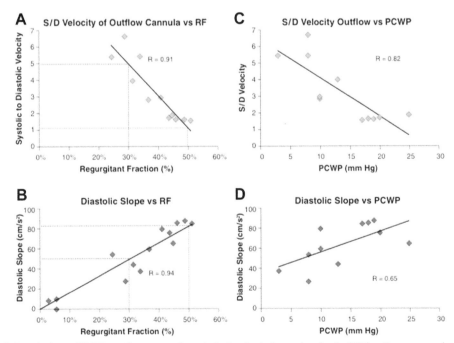

Fig. 6. (*A*) Correlation of LVAD outflow cannula systolic-to-diastolic peak velocity (S/D) ratio compared with RF for patients with trace or greater AI. (*B*) Correlation of LVAD outflow cannula diastolic acceleration compared with RF. (*C*) Correlation of LVAD outflow cannula S/D ratio compared with PCWP for patients with trace or greater AI. (*D*) Correlation of LVAD outflow cannula diastolic acceleration compared with PCWP. (*From* Grinstein J, Kruse E, Sayer G, et al. Accurate quantification methods for aortic insufficiency severity in patients with LVAD: role of diastolic flow acceleration and systolic-to-diastolic peak velocity ratio of outflow cannula. JACC Cardiovasc Imaging 2016;9(6):647; with permission.)

estimated diastolic slope acceleration cut point of 82 cm/s^2 was associated with moderate to severe AI by novel aortic RF. These new Doppler indices demonstrated stronger correlation with PCWP compared with vena contracta and can be acquired in most patients with adequate acoustic windows. Furthermore, these novel parameters were shown to be more sensitive in detecting patients at risk for worse outcomes.[25]

Patients with AI have higher PCWP, CVP, and lower pulmonary artery pulsatility index[26] then patients without AI. These data further question the mechanism of AI in the LVAD population. Does RV failure lead to reduced flow from the RV to the LV, and as such reduce the frequency of AV opening, leading aortic cusps fusion and AI? Or, does AI causing fluid overload and increased PCWP and RV afterload result in RV failure? The exact mechanism is still unknown and further studies are needed to elucidate the pathophysiology. Timely assessment of AI may be important to identify those patients who will benefit from AV replacement via surgery, transcatheter AV replacement, or AV closure.

SUMMARY

Durable LVAD support is a viable therapy for patients with end-stage heart failure as either a bridge to transplant or bridge to destination therapy. Our understanding of the complex "pump-patient" relationship has grown tremendously since the introduction of these devices more than 20 years ago. The combination of both imaging and invasive hemodynamics is crucial to understand the individual effect of LVADs on specific patient populations. Using those methods already has demonstrated the importance in device troubleshooting and medical optimization of the patient. Further prospective studies are needed to further elucidate the durable long-term effects of these protocols and true utility as part of daily practice.

REFERENCES

1. Miller LW, Pagani FD, Russell SD, et al, HeartMate II Clinical Investigators. Use of a continuous-flow device in patients awaiting heart transplantation. N Engl J Med 2007;357(9):885–96.
2. Slaughter MS, Rogers JG, Milano CA, et al, HeartMate II Investigators. Advanced heart failure treated with continuous-flow left ventricular assist device. N Engl J Med 2009;361(23):2241–51.
3. Uriel N, Morrison KA, Garan AR, et al. Development of a novel echocardiography ramp test for speed optimization and diagnosis of device thrombosis in continuous-flow left ventricular assist devices: the Columbia ramp study. J Am Coll Cardiol 2012; 60(18):1764–75.
4. Burkhoff D, Sayer G, Doshi D, et al. Hemodynamics of mechanical circulatory support. J Am Coll Cardiol 2015;66(23):2663–74.
5. Chung BB, Sayer G, Uriel N. Mechanical circulatory support devices: methods to optimize hemodynamics during use. Expert Rev Med Devices 2017; 14(5):343–53.
6. Moazami N, Fukamachi K, Kobayashi M, et al. Axial and centrifugal continuous-flow rotary pumps: a translation from pump mechanics to clinical practice. J Heart Lung Transplant 2013;32(1):1–11.
7. Feldman D, Pamboukian SV, Teuteberg JJ, et al, International Society for Heart, Lung Transplantation. The 2013 International Society for Heart and Lung Transplantation guidelines for mechanical circulatory support: executive summary. J Heart Lung Transplant 2013;32(2):157–87.
8. Shah P, Badoe N, Phillips S, et al. Unrecognized left heart failure in LVAD recipients: the role of routine invasive hemodynamic testing. ASAIO J 2018; 64(2):183–90.
9. Nahumi N, Jorde U, Uriel N. Slope calculation for the LVAD ramp test. J Am Coll Cardiol 2013;62(22): 2149–50.
10. Uriel N, Levin AP, Sayer GT, et al. Left ventricular decompression during speed optimization ramps in patients supported by continuous-flow left ventricular assist devices: device-specific performance characteristics and impact on diagnostic algorithms. J Card Fail 2015;21(10):785–91.
11. Sauer AJ, Meehan K, Gordon R, et al. Echocardiographic markers of left ventricular unloading using a centrifugal-flow rotary pump. J Heart Lung Transplant 2014;33(4):449–50.
12. Addetia K, Uriel N, Maffessanti F, et al. 3D morphological changes in LV and RV during LVAD ramp studies. JACC Cardiovasc Imaging 2017. https:// doi.org/10.1016/j.jcmg.2016.12.019.
13. Maffessanti F, Caiani EG, Tamborini G, et al. Serial changes in left ventricular shape following early mitral valve repair. Am J Cardiol 2010;106(6): 836–42.
14. Uriel N, Sayer G, Addetia K, et al. Hemodynamic ramp tests in patients with left ventricular assist devices. JACC Heart Fail 2016;4(3):208–17.
15. Uriel N, Adatya S, Maly J, et al. Clinical hemodynamic evaluation of patients implanted with a fully magnetically levitated left ventricular assist device (HeartMate 3). J Heart Lung Transplant 2017;36(1): 28–35.
16. Estep JD, Vivo RP, Cordero-Reyes AM, et al. A simplified echocardiographic technique for detecting continuous-flow left ventricular assist device malfunction due to pump thrombosis. J Heart Lung Transplant 2014;33(6):575–86.

17. ClinicalTrials.gov. Identifier NCT03021239: impact of hemodynamic ramp test-guided HVAD RPM and medication adjustments on exercise tolerance and quality of life (Ramp-it-Up). National Library of Medicine 2016. Available at: https://clinicaltrials.gov/ct2/show/study/NCT03021239?term=hvad+ramp+it+up&rank=1. Accessed March 27, 2018.

18. Stainback RF, Estep JD, Agler DA, et al, American Society of Echocardiography. Echocardiography in the management of patients with left ventricular assist devices: recommendations from the American Society of Echocardiography. J Am Soc Echocardiogr 2015;28(8):853–909.

19. Jorde UP, Uriel N, Nahumi N, et al. Prevalence, significance, and management of aortic insufficiency in continuous flow left ventricular assist device recipients. Circ Heart Fail 2014;7(2):310–9.

20. Cowger J, Pagani FD, Haft JW, et al. The development of aortic insufficiency in left ventricular assist device-supported patients. Circ Heart Fail 2010; 3(6):668–74.

21. Mudd JO, Cuda JD, Halushka M, et al. Fusion of aortic valve commissures in patients supported by a continuous axial flow left ventricular assist device. J Heart Lung Transplant 2008;27(12): 1269–74.

22. Toda K, Fujita T, Domae K, et al. Late aortic insufficiency related to poor prognosis during left ventricular assist device support. Ann Thorac Surg 2011; 92(3):929–34.

23. Cowger JA, Aaronson KD, Romano MA, et al. Consequences of aortic insufficiency during long-term axial continuous-flow left ventricular assist device support. J Heart Lung Transplant 2014;33(12): 1233–40.

24. Grinstein J, Kruse E, Sayer G, et al. Accurate quantification methods for aortic insufficiency severity in patients with LVAD: role of diastolic flow acceleration and systolic-to-diastolic peak velocity ratio of outflow cannula. JACC Cardiovasc Imaging 2016;9(6): 641–51.

25. Grinstein J, Kruse E, Sayer G, et al. Novel echocardiographic parameters of aortic insufficiency in continuous-flow left ventricular assist devices and clinical outcome. J Heart Lung Transplant 2016; 35(8):976–85.

26. Sayer G, Sarswat N, Kim GH, et al. The hemodynamic effects of aortic insufficiency in patients supported with continuous-flow left ventricular assist devices. J Card Fail 2017;23(7):545–51.

Ambulatory Ventricular Assist Device Patient Management

Tonya Elliott, MSN, RN, CCTC, CHFN[a],
Lori G. Edwards, MSN, RN[b],*

KEYWORDS

- Ambulatory care guidelines • Infection guidelines • End-of-life care

KEY POINTS

- As patients survive longer on durable left ventricular assist device (LVAD) support, it is critical for programs to develop a platform for the care of patients with a ventricular assist device (VAD) in the outpatient setting.
- Understanding the patient pump interface and developing expertise in monitoring this population will maximize patient outcomes.
- The purpose of expert, focused, routine outpatient surveillance of this population is to facilitate the integration of pulseless, electrically dependent VAD patients into the community.

THE EVOLUTION OF OUTPATIENT VENTRICULAR ASSIST DEVICE CARE

This article describes strategies, protocols, and resources necessary to care for the ambulatory ventricular assist device (VAD) patient population. Historical milestones and innovations over the past 20 years in mechanical circulatory support (MCS) technology resulted in an expansion of the number of patients with a VAD and the length of time supported living in the community. In September 1998, the Food and Drug Administration (FDA) made a ground-breaking decision and permitted patients with a Heart Mate XVE (Thoratec, Pleasanton, CA) and Novacor (Novacor, Berkley, CA) to be discharged from the hospital.[1] These first-generation, volume-displacement pumps were implanted and had wearable external accessories allowing for untethered operation for a

couple of hours on the same set of batteries. Patients were able to perform activities of daily living while supported on these devices, making discharge to home possible while awaiting transplantation. This single action by the FDA forced VAD programs to shift resources and modify protocols, as VAD teams prepared the community for the technology and outpatient clinics for follow-up care. Before 1998, patients with a VAD were relegated to life in the hospital until transplant. Discharging patients with a VAD to their home environments was associated with a positive impact on patient quality of life.[2]

The REMATCH[3] trial then transformed the treatment paradigm for advanced heart failure by allowing VADs to be implanted in patients who are not transplant candidates, called destination therapy (DT). VADs are now used in the treatment

Disclosure Statement: Authors have no financial relationships to disclose.
[a] MCS Program, MedStar Heart and Vascular Institute, 110 Irving Street, Northwest, Washington, DC 20010, USA; [b] Advanced Heart Failure/Mechanical Circulatory Support, INOVA Fairfax Hospital, 3300 Gallows Road, Falls Church, VA 22042, USA
* Corresponding author.
E-mail address: Lori.edwards@inova.org

Cardiol Clin 36 (2018) 571–581
https://doi.org/10.1016/j.ccl.2018.06.014
0733-8651/18/© 2018 Elsevier Inc. All rights reserved.

of advanced heart failure, expanding the indications for implant and therefore the number of possible candidates. Between August 1985 and February 1991, 34 patients at 7 different medical centers were treated with the 1000 IP LVAD as a bridge to transplantation.[4] All but 1 of the patients were male, and their ages ranged from 17 to 62 years.[4] The evolution of second-generation and third-generation LVADs with continuous flow (CF) technologies (including the HeartMate II, HVAD, and HeartMate 3) further expanded LVAD candidacy to include patients with smaller body surface areas, such as women and children.[5] In the HeartMate II clinical trials, patients with a body surface area as low as 1.5 m^2 could be enrolled and the cohort was 20% female. The HeartWare bridge to transplant (BTT) and DT studies enrolled patients as small as 1.2 m^2 with female representation of 20% to 28%.[6]

As programs grow and implant a more diverse cohort of patients, consideration for intrapersonal issues that concern patients of all genders and cultures must be taken into account. Psychosocial factors, such as adaptation to the equipment, coping with changes in body image and lifestyle, and managing perceived loss of independence need to be addressed by the multidisciplinary team (inclusive of psychology or social work) perioperatively and on an ongoing basis during follow-up visits.[7]

Finally, as patients survive longer on durable LVAD support, it is critical for programs to develop a platform for the care of patients with a VAD in the outpatient setting. CF physiology created pulseless patients with unique infectious, neurologic, and hematologic complications. Understanding the patient pump interface and developing expertise in monitoring this population will maximize outcomes and is the goal of the care of the ambulatory patient population. Collaboration of MCS staff with other specialists is imperative for care coordination and management of non-VAD surgical interventions and medical complications encountered while on device support.[8] The purpose of expert, focused, routine outpatient surveillance of this population is to facilitate the integration of pulseless, electrically dependent patients with a VAD into the community. To accomplish this goal, the multidisciplinary team must promote quality of life, maintain equipment integrity, optimize VAD support, and monitor for common VAD-related complications. Additionally, this long-term monitoring must include ensuring viability as a heart transplant candidate for BTT patients, consideration for patients implanted as DT to become transplantable, and monitor for possible recovery.

DISCHARGE READINESS

Discharge activities are carefully orchestrated by implanting VAD programs to empower patients to care for themselves successfully in the community. VAD programs mobilize a multidisciplinary team to maximize patients' rehabilitation and assimilations into the community while minimizing the possibility of complications.[9] Personnel involved, but not limited to, include occupational and physical therapists, infectious disease specialists, VAD coordinators, heart failure attendings, cardiac surgeons, pharmacists, nutritionists, financial coordinator, social workers, family members, and patients.

Patients and caregivers need to demonstrate competency managing VAD equipment, alarm response, and dressing change procedures before discharge. These are all topics that can and should be reviewed frequently during early return visits based on patient and caregiver needs.[10] VAD programs are required to provide patients and community stakeholders with emergency contact information and have a plan for responding to VAD emergencies. Patients and caregivers must rehearse calling the emergency notification system to demonstrate familiarity with the step before discharge.

An assessment of the home environment is important for patient safety and success at home. Assessments ensure presence of a grounded and reliable electricity supply as well as telephone services. The local electrical providers are notified by some implanting centers that customers are dependent on electricity.[9] Patients need to be able to communicate via telephone for emergencies. Key aspects of contingency plans developed for outpatient LVADs include ensuring an uninterrupted electricity supply, a plan for extended power outages, maintaining access to a working telephone, and understanding the limitation of LVAD battery life.[11]

Educating Prehospital Providers

Before discharge, VAD teams notify local emergency medical service (EMS) providers that a potentially pulseless, electrically dependent patient with a VAD lives in their first due vicinity. EMS VAD field guides developed in 2010 contain information and pictures to assist with troubleshooting equipment issues.[12,13] VAD equipment can be labeled with the implanting center emergency contact and VAD model.[13,14] Transporting patients with a VAD back to the implanting center is preferable, as implanting centers know their patients best and have equipment and expert training in monitoring and managing VAD emergencies. Each device has unique characteristics that need to be considered when developing a transport plan that is fixed wing or ground transport.[14] Additionally, prehospital providers need to bring patients' back-up equipment, batteries and controller, for replacement should the batteries drain or primary controller malfunction.[14]

Chest Compressions in Ventricular Assist Devices

Unconscious patients with a VAD pose an assessment, intervention challenge, as they are usually pulseless and therefore Advanced Cardiac Life Support algorithms do not direct providers in this scenario. The American Heart Association recently released a scientific statement directing providers when to administer chest compressions in patients with a VAD.[15] During circulation assessment, providers are directed to listen to the chest for pump hum indicating a working pump. Should signs of adequate perfusion and pump function exist, then providers must explore other noncardiac etiologies of alteration in consciousness, such as stroke or abnormal blood sugar. VAD controllers announce alarms when there is a patient or equipment issue, therefore inspecting the controller screen can provide additional information when problem solving in an emergency. When perfusion is compromised, that is, mean arterial pressure (MAP) less than 50 or the VAD is not operational, chest compressions should be initiated at same depth and frequency performed in patients who are non-VAD supported[8,15] (**Fig. 1**).

MONITORING PATIENTS WITH A VENTRICULAR ASSIST DEVICE IN AN AMBULATORY SETTING

Patients implanted with VADs must be treated as patients with heart failure because VADs do not cure heart failure but move blood forward to perfuse organs and reduce symptoms.[10] Ongoing heart failure monitoring and management must continue for the duration of VAD support. Several strategies are used in the outpatient setting to quantify and qualify patients' response to the therapy.

Equipment Assessment and Ventricular Assist Device Interrogation

Equipment integrity and proper functioning of components are assessed at every clinic visit.[8] The primary equipment and back-up equipment are inspected for any damage or battery expiration. Replacement equipment is dispensed and serial numbers are documented to ensure that every component is captured in a database. In the event of a recall, all affected equipment must be sequestered as directed by the FDA.

Device interrogation is performed by connecting the controller to the system monitor and reviewing VAD parameters. Downloading data stored in controllers also may occur in clinic at routine intervals or when there is clinical suspicion of device malfunction or abnormal VAD parameters. Ongoing assessment of learning needs related to equipment, barriers to compliance, and retention of information occurs during clinic appointments.[8]

Many centers require patients to bring in all equipment from home on an annual basis for inspection and routine replacement. This annual visit time can be used to review equipment education, insurance status, power company and EMS notification, and transplant candidacy.

Functional Status and Quality of Life

Monitoring functional status and quality of life in the outpatient setting is a useful way to track individual patient improvement or decline. The collective data can be used to characterize the benefits of the therapy. Tools commonly used to quantify functional status in the outpatient setting are 6-minute walk, New York Heart Association classification, and cardiopulmonary stress tests.[16] Characterizing frailty in the advanced heart failure patient population before and after implant adds to the understanding of the impact of the therapy. Tools such as grip strength and gait speed are easily measured in outpatient settings. One of the many goals of VAD therapy is to improve quality of life for patients. It is important to measure health-related quality of life indicators at baseline (before implantation) and at regular intervals postoperatively.[5] Patient satisfaction surveys are another method to obtain feedback from patients and caregivers regarding staff, VAD units, and clinic. These results inform program leaders when developing program goals, retooling workflow, and designing staff education modules. These surveys are administered after index hospitalization and are a requirement of some payers, including the Centers for Medicare and Medicaid Services.

Right Heart Catheterization

Routine intermittent right heart catheterization monitoring provides critical information about the correlation of the VAD flow and true cardiac output along with filling pressures that guide heart failure therapy. LVAD filling is predicated on right

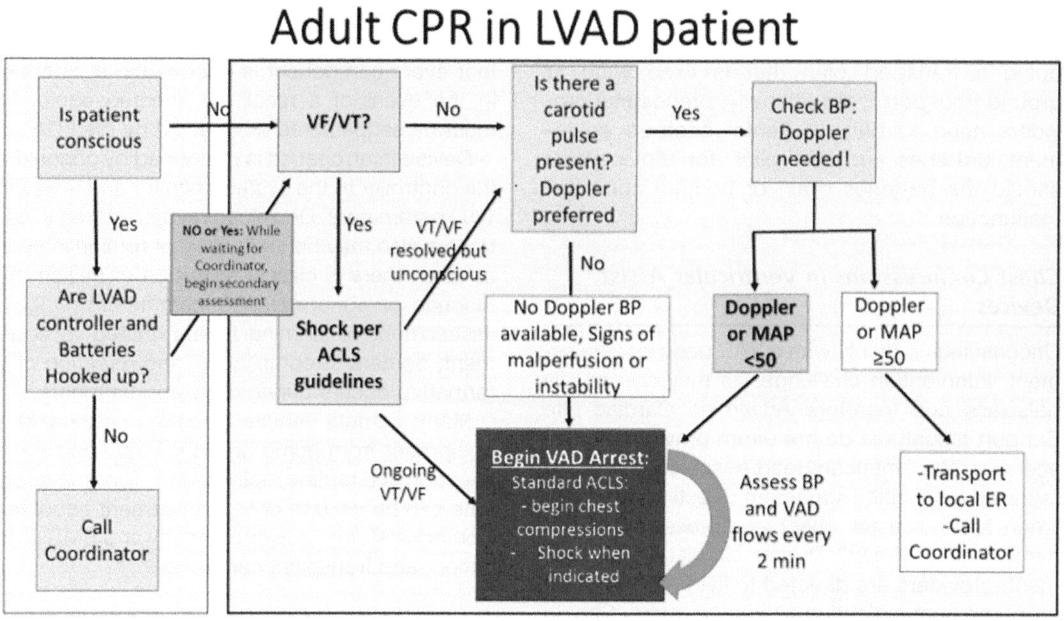

Adult CPR in LVAD patient

Fig. 1. Emergency treatment algorithm including cardiopulmonary resuscitation (CPR). ACLS, advanced cardiac life support; BP, blood pressure; ER, emergency room. (*Courtesy of* Centurion Medical Productions, Harleysville, PA.)

ventricular function and pulmonary resistance; therefore, measuring and treating these factors will optimize VAD performance.[9] For the BTT population, one of the factors that defines continued heart transplant candidacy is pulmonary vascular resistance (PVR). This parameter needs to be periodically measured and elevated PVR results need to be treated during the listing period. The 2016 International Society of Heart and Lung Transplant guidelines recommend routine right heart catheterization (RHC), annually, for the BTT patient.[17] Right ventricular (RV) failure is a leading cause of morbidity and mortality in patients with an LVAD. The Eighth Annual Interagency Registry for Mechanically Assisted Circulatory Support (INTERMACS) report reflects the devastation of early RV dysfunction, and sites it as a leading cause of early mortality.[18] Houston and colleagues[19] conducted a retrospective review of 244 RHC results to examine the effect that LVADs have on RV performance over time. Their findings suggest that the LVAD implant itself has a deleterious effect on the RV performance. RV adaptation to work actually worsens after VAD implantation. Monitoring RV function and providing targeted therapy to reduce RV workload and improve performance is a long-term goal during LVAD support.

Tehrani and colleagues[20] sought to clarify strategies for measuring cardiac output in the setting of CF VAD support. Their work led them to recommend measuring cardiac output with Fick calculation instead of thermodilution. This may require the VAD team to create protocols with the catheterization laboratory team so pulmonary artery saturation values are obtained and Fick calculations are included in routine RHC procedures and reports.

Echocardiography

Routine echocardiography (ECHO) monitoring in the ambulatory setting is necessary to ensure speed optimization and surveillance for VAD-related structural complication. Because patients with a VAD may be asymptomatic as gradual VAD-related structural changes occur, it is important to perform routine ECHOs in the outpatient setting. Educating the sonographer regarding the unique parameters and views that have to be obtained during the examination is key to getting the information from the ECHO test required to make clinical decisions.[21] It is also necessary to coordinate the team so a system monitor, to modify speeds as indicated, and a VAD-trained team member are available for the ECHO. Long-term monitoring of the aortic value is an important component of the routine surveillance ECHO, as there is a risk of developing aortic insufficiency over time.[22] This VAD-induced iatrogenic complication has been recognized for many years. Assessment of ejection fraction (EF) during routine ECHOs will identify the rare but fortunate patient who experiences myocardial recovery and may go on to explant. Optimization of neurohormonal modulation, pump speed, and constitutional factors, such as nutrition, are ingredients in the recovery recipe. When a patient with improving EF is identified, intensification of these supportive factors will improve the likelihood that explant is possible.

Infection Prevention

Drive line exit site care

Infection remains one of the vexing complications of VAD therapy. In the ambulatory setting it is usually due to trauma or contamination of the drive line exit site (DLES). Prevention of infection, especially at the DLES, is a crucial part of VAD education and care in the outpatient setting. DLES care decreases the risk of drive line infections and is a focus of outpatient monitoring and patient and caregiver education.[23] Education includes demonstration of dressing change techniques and observation of caregiver performance of sterile practice, recognition of signs and symptoms of infection, and stabilization of the drive line. Supplemental written materials reviewing these infection prevention topics are important to provide for patients and caregivers to reinforce the education once they are at home.[24] Assessment of the condition of the dressing during routine clinic appointments can provide a teaching opportunity for patients and caregivers. Routine care includes dressing changes, stabilization of the drive line, showering, and hand hygiene.

Some centers provide a DLES management system, which is a self-contained kit with all the pieces necessary to perform the dressing change (**Fig. 2**). A simple step-by-step picture guide inside the kit is a real-time tool that patients and caregivers can use during the dressing change. DLES dressing change protocols generally include proper hand hygiene, aseptic technique, cleansing with chlorhexidine, and the application of a sterile dressing. Trauma to the exit site from an accidental pull on the external components is a set up for DLES infections.[23] A stabilization device, such as a repurposed Foley or intravenous line anchor or a traditional abdominal binder will help to prevent trauma to the site. There exists variability in specific contents and frequency of DLES protocols and management systems/kits.[25] Kusne and colleagues[23] found no difference in DLES infections based on frequency of dressing change. Modifications to the DLES kit or routine may be considered during clinic visits if the skin becomes irritated by the tape or chlorhexidine. Some centers recommend sensitive skin kits/routines that eliminate chlorhexidine and use Hibiclens and normal saline.

Showering

Showering is a part of most patients' normal hygiene routine.[8] Submersion in water is never permitted in patients with a VAD with traditional drivelines exiting the abdomen. As tap water is not sterile, most VAD programs give patients permission to shower only after the DLES appears to be well approximated around the drive line. The manufacturers produce shower bags that protect the external equipment from moisture during showers. These bags can be provided to patients in the outpatient setting when it is determined that the DLES has healed sufficiently to allow for showering. It is important to teach patients and caregivers to create a routine around showering that includes changing the DLES dressing immediately after the shower.[23] Although most centers promote and provide materials to protect the DLES from water, it is impossible to make it waterproof. Wet dressings are considered soiled and require immediate attention. When a DLES becomes infected, standardized nomenclature to describe the site is useful to track response to treatment.[26]

Dental care

As part of an overall strategy to reduce pump-related infections, patients with a VAD need to follow standard recommendation for dental hygiene and visits. Oral inspections during clinic visits may be part of the routine assessment, especially for patients who required dental procedures preimplant due to poor or infected dentation. Patients need to be instructed to inform their dentists that they have a VAD and follow secondary prophylaxis recommendations.[23] If patients with a VAD require more invasive dental procedures, the preprocedure plan may also include modification of the anticoagulation plan (see anticoagulation section).

Management of Ventricular Arrhythmias

Occurrence of sustained ventricular tachycardia (VT) or ventricular fibrillation (VF) in the outpatient setting can be discovered as the result of palpitations, light headedness, an appropriate implantable cardioverter-defibrillator (ICD) shock, or VAD pump alarms due to low-flow state. Initial evaluation should include assessment of volume status electrolytes, 12-lead electrocardiogram, and effect of the arrhythmia on hemodynamic status.[27] Patients presenting with frequent suction events or complaints about fatigue should trigger an ICD interrogation to evaluate for arrhythmias.[14]

BENEFITS FOR CAREGIVERS, HOSPITALS AND PATIENTS

- Driveline Management Trays customized with exclusive Centurion dressings and securement products:
  - help lower the risk of contracting an infection with products that provide bacterial protection and long wear times
  - keep the driveline securely in place even with active patients

- provide a consistent protocol that follows the patient from the hospital, to the rehab facility, then home
- are intuitively designed to promote proper sterile technique, helping to reduce the incidence of patient complications, unscheduled nursing visits, and hospital readmissions

- Centurion's Guardian Angel Program provides clinical education designed to reinforce essential skills and behaviors for best practices to reduce LVAD complications
- Centurion custom kits are assembled with components packaged in the proper order for maximum efficiency and effectiveness
- Kits can be manufactured with latex free components and packaging

KITS CUSTOMIZED WITH CENTURION'S SECUREMENT PRODUCTS:

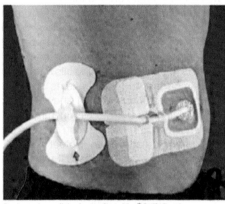

SORBAVIEW® DRESSINGS AND SORBAVIEW® SHIELD

- Provide a proven barrier against contaminants, while allowing skin to breathe freely
- Easy to apply and stay securely in place
- Feature strong adhesive that keeps dressing intact, yet is gentle and non-irritating to skin
- SorbaView SHIELD offers all the benefits of a SorbaView Dressing with built-in securement to stabilize the catheter and protect the site

FOLEY ANCHOR

- Easy to apply and remove
- Secures the driveline to the skin to prevent stress at the site
- Comfortable and safe
- Stays firmly in place, allowing for easy patient movement
- Available in two levels of patient-friendly, long-lasting adhesive

Products shown: Foley Anchor, SorbaView® SHIELD with Adhesive-free Zone, and BIOPATCH® Protective Disk with CHG*

INTUITIVELY DESIGNED KIT ENCOURAGES BEST PRACTICES

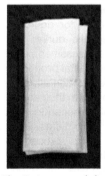 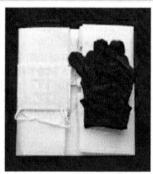 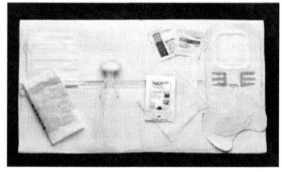

Fig. 2. Image and description of DLES management system.

Routine ICD interrogation is pivotal to reducing the risk of arrhythmias, pacing the RV to augment performance as needed, and measuring lead impedance and battery life.[8] In the absence of persistent ventricular dysrhythmias, the defibrillator function of an ICD should be turned back on postoperatively and this should be confirmed before discharge from the implant hospitalization.[4]

The ability of LVADs to maintain circulatory support independently from heart rate and atrial signals allows patients to tolerate ventricular arrhythmias, with minimal symptoms and stable hemodynamics.[28] Patients with LVADs can remain conscious while in VT or VF. VADs may be able to provide enough forward flow despite the arrhythmia to maintain consciousness and, in some cases, even adequate perfusion.[8] Treatments for VT not caused by suction event are similar to those recommended for patients without MCS, including beta blockade, antiarrhythmics, cardioversion, or defibrillation.

Most patients undergoing LVAD implantation already have previously implanted ICDs; 82% of patients in the HeartMate II trial had an ICD at the time of implant.[27] The potential benefit of ICDs in this population must be weighed against the very real risks of inappropriate shocks and device infections, a major concern in patients with LVADs, on a case-by-case basis.[27] The same issues of course apply to generator changes in patients who reach elective replacement voltage on their ICD.[28] Should the electrophysiology team determine that the ICD device requires replacement, an anticoagulation and procedure coverage plan needs to be defined. After discharge, patients should reestablish contact with their electrophysiologist and/or resume home monitoring of their ICD or pacemakers.[4]

Outpatient Schedules

Laboratory values, such as complete blood count, chemistries, liver function test, international normalized ratio (INR), lactate dehydrogenase (LDH), and urinalysis, should be performed on a routine basis to assist in the assessment for pump thrombosis, infection, mucosal blood loss, and adequate anticoagulation. Serial periodic laboratory values are an important monitoring strategy for predicting pump thrombosis, as elevated LDH may be detectable months before clinical symptoms.[29] Although there are no defined guidelines for follow-up care, having a structured follow-up schedule is prudent (**Table 1**).

MANAGEMENT OF PATIENTS WITH A VENTRICULAR ASSIST DEVICE IN THE AMBULATORY SETTING
Blood Pressure

Cerebral vascular events are a devastating complication of VAD support and are the major cause of death between 6 months and 4 years post implant.[18] Blood pressure management is critical in the outpatient setting to decrease the risk of strokes. High blood pressure has 2 deleterious effects on patients with a VAD. As VAD pumps are afterload sensitive, hypertension hampers forward flow leading to stagnation of blood in the pump and thrombus formation. Thrombus formation can result in embolic strokes. CF combined

---

Table 1
Comprehensive VAD visit schedule

Office Visit/ Testing	Weeks						Months After Implantation										
	1	2	3	4	6	8	3	4	5	6	7	8	9	10	11	12	Thereafter
Office visit	X	X	X	X	X	X	X	X	X	X	—	—	X	—	—	X	q3 months, monthly if 1A
Routine laboratory tests																	
PT/INR	X	X	X	X	X	X	X	X	X	X	X	X	X	X	X	X	q1 mo
LDH	X	X	X	X	X	X	X	X	X	X	X	X	X	X	X	X	q3 mo
CBC	X	X	X	X	X	X	X	X	X	X	X	X	X	X	X	X	q3 mo
BMP, Mag	X	X	X	X	X	X	X	X	X	X	X	X	X	X	X	X	q3 mo
LFTs	X	X	X	X	X	X	X	X	X	X	X	X	X	X	X	X	q3 mo
PRA	—	—	—	—	—	—	B	—	—	B	—	—	—	—	—	B	q6 mo or upgrade in status
Drug monitoring																	
Digoxin	—	—	—	—	—	—	X	—	—	X	—	—	X	—	—	X	q3 mo
Other testing																	
ECHO	—	—	—	—	—	—	X	—	—	X	—	—	—	—	—	X	q6 mo
6MWT	—	—	—	—	—	—	—	—	—	X	—	—	—	—	—	X	—
Quality of life	—	—	—	—	—	—	X	—	—	X	—	—	—	—	—	X	q6 months, yearly after 2 y
Frailty testing	—	—	—	—	—	—	—	—	—	X	—	—	—	—	—	X	—
Right heart catheterization	—	—	—	—	—	—	X	—	—	—	—	—	—	—	—	—	BTT yearly, DT PRN
Noncontrast chest CT	—	—	—	—	—	—	B	—	—	—	—	—	—	—	—	—	PRN

Abbreviations: —, not needed at this time; 6MWT, 6-minute walk test; B, bridge to transplant patients; BMP, basic metabolic panel; CBC, complete blood count; CT, computed tomography; DT, destination therapy; ECHO, echocardiogram; LDH, lactate dehydrogenase; LFT, liver function test; Mag, magnesium; PRA, panel of reactive antibodies; PRN, as needed; PT/INR, prothrombin time/international normalized ratio; q, every; VAD, ventricular assist device; X, due.

with hypertension is contributory to hemorrhagic strokes.[30] The HVAD investigators performed a subanalysis on risk factors for neurologic events. These data revealed that the prevalence of hemorrhagic strokes was decreased with formalized protocols to monitor and manage blood pressure.[31] They were able to determine that an MAP greater than 90 mm Hg was a risk factor for neurologic events. Endurance study investigators also identified an MAP of 90 mm Hg as the inflection point for mitigation of stroke risk.[6] Hypertension and anticoagulation predispose patients with a VAD to hemorrhagic strokes; therefore, careful monitoring of MAP and INR are paramount to improved outcomes.[10,30]

Measurement of Blood Pressure in Patients with a Ventricular Assist Device

CF physiology and the resulting narrow pulse pressure create a challenge in assessing and measuring vital signs, especially using traditional methods. Variability in native heart function may contribute to pulsatile flow that may result in a palpable pulse; however, if no pulse is found, this is considered a normal state for most patients with CF pumps.

Selecting a method to measure the blood pressure is the source of debate within the VAD community, as noninvasive methods are designed to measure systolic and diastolic pressures. The gold standard for measuring CF blood pressure is an arterial line,[32] but clearly not available in the outpatient setting. Studies seeking to determine a reliable noninvasive method found that most automatic and manual blood pressure measurements are not sensitive enough to detect such small differences in systolic and diastolic blood pressure. Using a Doppler has been adapted by VAD programs when the noninvasive blood pressure (NIBP) does not detect a pressure. NIBP may be used especially in patients that are pulsatile.[29] Obtaining a Doppler pressure is necessary if the NIBP device is unable to detect the MAP. It is commonly assumed that the first sound heard is approximately equivalent to the mean arterial pressure, yet studies show this may be closer to the systolic.[6] The artificial pulse in the HeartMate3 device results in noncontinuous pressure, which may lead to variability when measuring the MAP. It may require multiple sequential measurements to obtain a clinically accurate calculation of the MAP.[33]

In spite of the limitations in measuring the blood pressure in patients with a CF VAD, a MAP in the range of 70 to 90 mm Hg is considered normal. Ambulatory patients with a VAD may have access to blood pressure cuffs through participation in clinical trials or through a durable medical equipment company. They may also return to clinic for vital sign checks to ensure the blood pressure regimen maintains the MAP in the goal range.

Medications

Medication regimens in the outpatient setting are a continuation of the inpatient plan. Medications are used to mitigate potential adverse events such as stroke and pump thrombosis. Medications are also used to achieve euvolemia and treat right heart failure. Blood pressure management focuses on optimization of angiotensin-converting enzymes, angiotensin receptor blockers, and beta blockade to achieve MAPs lower than 90 mm Hg.[8,30]

Anticoagulation

Anticoagulation continues in the outpatient setting using warfarin and an antiplatelet agent.[10] Anticoagulation management in the ambulatory setting can be a delicate balance, as patients' nutrition and volume status improves over time. As fluid retention around the gut and nutrient absorption improves, monitoring and management of warfarin may need to intensify. Patients may obtain a home INR point-of-care monitoring system from a durable medical equipment with a qualifying diagnosis such as atrial fibrillation or vascular thrombosis. Patients also may have INR measured and managed by Coumadin clinics. The implanting center has ultimate responsibility for the overall management and should ensure that any Coumadin clinic algorithms are approved by the center.

As vitamin K can cause abrupt reversal of INR, most implanting centers discourage the use of vitamin K even with super therapeutic INR levels. Patients must be instructed to contact the implanting center when seeking care outside the facility to ensure all medications are compatible with VAD anticoagulation plan.

Diuretics

Achieving euvolemia is a moving target for patients with a VAD in the outpatient setting. A delicate balance exists between heart failure volume overload versus improved renal perfusion and vascular contraction.[8] Clear discharge instructions regarding diuretic use and dose along with recommended volume intake is necessary at each visit due to the dynamic nature of VAD patient volume status.

Documentation

VAD parameters and alarm history review must be documented every clinic visit. Condition of the

DLES is also captured. Some centers have the capability to take and store serial pictures of the DLES to track infections. Modified Rankin scores are tracked in the outpatient setting to quantify the degree of disability for all patients who have suffered strokes. INTERMACS and many of the device clinical trials require follow-up modified Rankin scores. It can be built into electronic medical record documentation as a reminder to capture this data point.

Education and documentation must continue in the outpatient setting. At least annually, patients and caregivers should review VAD alarm response to include demonstration of controller exchange on a mock loop. They must also receive stroke awareness education to ensure they know the signs and symptoms of stroke and who to call to facilitate emergent evaluation and treatment.

Cardiac Rehabilitation

Cardiac rehabilitation (CR) is an established resource in the community to foster exercise tolerance and nurture self-care. Exercise training was felt to be safe in a patient with a VAD; therefore, CR is recommended in appropriate patients.[9] Benefits of participation in CR include nutrition counseling, smoking cessation support, and strength training.[34] Kerrigan and colleagues[35] demonstrated in a randomized, single-blind trial that CR improves cardiorespiratory fitness (10%), muscle strength (17%), and Kansas City Cardiomyopathy Questionnaire scores (23%) in patients with CF VADs. CR facilities should be made aware of the special considerations for monitoring CF VAD during exercise. Training for the CR staff may be necessary.

Leaving the Home and Traveling

The goal for all patients with a VAD is return to normal daily functions including performing activities of daily living, work, driving, and traveling. Implanting institution and governing state laws determine if patients with a VAD are permitted to drive. If traveling by air, patients will need a Transportation Security Administration letter stating all VAD equipment must be stowed in a carry-on bag to avoid misplaced baggage and comply with regulations stating no lithium batteries in checked bags. When traveling, patients should be aware of the closest VAD center for emergencies.

PALLIATIVE CARE AND END OF LIFE

Conversations about advanced directive, palliative care, and end-of-life care should commence before VAD implantation, regardless of the intent of device placement.[12] Social workers and palliative care providers are exquisitely positioned to be patient advocates when talking about goals of care, advanced directives, and end-of-life wishes. Not to be confused with hospice or withdrawal of care, the focus of palliative care is to improve quality of life through the prevention and relief of suffering.[36] Palliative care providers are essential team members and required by the Joint Commission for all DT LVAD centers. VAD therapy is considered life sustaining; therefore, elective withdrawal of support may be appropriate when quality of life is deemed poor and continued support would in effect prolong suffering.[8] Without proper planning, staff may find themselves unprepared for events and responsibilities.[37]

Patients and families consider disabling the VAD and "letting nature take its course," when faced with devastating complications like stroke and multisystem organ failure or comorbid conditions like cancer.[38] Shepherding a family and hospice team through deactivation can assist patients in fulfilling final wishes, such as dying at home. Clearly defined plan of care, such as a documented do not resuscitate/do not intubate ensure that patients, families, and home providers have the same goals. Additionally, when a date and time are identified for deactivation, the plan of care must include ensuring comfort medications are available and routes of administration are considered. When the VAD is disabled, the medications will not be circulated, so careful pre-deactivation administration of anxiolytics and opioids is necessary to ensure patient comfort. Unique postmortem considerations include funeral plans and discussion around cremation, as ICDs are combustible. As many patients with a VAD also have an ICD, families need to be counseled to discuss this with decedent affairs and/or the funeral home director. Families and caregivers may want to return the VAD equipment and supplies to the implanting center. VAD teams need to work through how to manage returned equipment.

SUMMARY

A structured, an expert ambulatory management plan is paramount to facilitating positive outcomes for patients with a VAD and minimizing the risk for complications.

REFERENCES

1. Robbins R, Oyer P. Bridge to transplant with the Novacor left ventricular assist system. Ann Thorac Surg 1999;68:695–7.

2. MacIver J, Ross H. Quality of life and left ventricular assist device support. Circulation 2012;126:866–74.
3. Rose E, Gelijns A, Moskowitz A, et al. Long-term use of a left ventricular assist device for end-stage heart failure. N Engl J Med 2001;345:1435–43.
4. Pamboukian S. Mechanical circulatory support: we are halfway there. J Am Coll Cardiol 2011;57(12):1383–5.
5. Frazier O, Rose E, Macmanus Q, et al. Multicenter clinical evaluation of the HeartMate 1000 IP left ventricular assist device. Ann Thorac Surg 1992;53:1080–90.
6. Rogers J, Pagani F, Tatooles A, et al. Intrapericardial left ventricular assist device for advanced heart failure. N Engl J Med 2017;376:451–60.
7. Chapman E, Parameshwar J, Jenkins D, et al. Psychosocial issues for patients with ventricular assist devices: a qualitative pilot study. Am J Crit Care 2007;16:72–81.
8. Slaughter M, Pagani F, Rogers J, et al. Clinical management of continuous-flow left ventricular assist devices in advanced heart failure. J Heart Lung Transplant 2010;29:S1–39.
9. Feldman D, Pamboukian SV, Teuteburg JJ, et al. The 2013 International Society for Heart Lung Transplant guidelines for mechanical circulatory support; executive summary. J Heart Lung Transplan 2013;32:174–9.
10. Smith E, Franzwa J. Chronic outpatient management of patients with left ventricular assist device. J Thorac Dis 2015;12:2112–24.
11. DeVore A, Mentz R, Patel C. Medical management of patients with continuous-flow left ventricular assist devices. Curr Treat Options Cardiovasc Med 2014;16(2):283.
12. Feldman D, Pamboukian SV, Teuteberg JJ, et al. The 2013 International Society for Heart and Lung Transplantation guidelines for mechanical circulatory support: executive summary. J Heart Lung Transpl 2013;32:157–87.
13. Van de Bussche T, Edwards L, Elliott T, et al. Regionalized approach to emergency medical services training for the care of the patients with mechanical assist devices. Prog Transplant 2010;20(2):129–32.
14. Elliott T, Sweet L, Wolfe A. Mechanical circulatory support devices. In: Holleran R, Wolfe A, Frakes M, editors. Transport in patient transport principles and practice. St Louis (MO): Elsevier; 2018.
15. Peberdy M, Gluck J, Ornato C, et al. Cardiopulmonary resuscitation in adults and children with MCS: a scientific statement from the American Heart Association. Circulation 2017;135:e1115–34.
16. Ha F, Toukhsati S, Cameron J, et al. Association between the 6-minute walk test and exercise confidence in patients with heart failure: a prospective observational study. Heart Lung 2018;47(1):54–60.
17. Mehra M, Canter C, Hannan M, et al. The 2016 International Society for Heart Lung Transplant listing criteria for heart transplantation: a 10-year update. J Heart Lung Transplant 2016;35(1):1–23.
18. Kirklin JJ, Pagani F, Kormos R, et al. Eighth annual INTERMACS report: special focus on framing the impact of adverse events. J Heart Lung Transplant 2017;36:1080–6.
19. Houston R, Kalathiya R, Hsu S, et al. Right ventricular after load sensitivity dramatically increases after left ventricular assist device implantation: a multicenter hemodynamic analysis. J Heart Lung Transplant 2016;35(7):868–76.
20. Tehrani D, Grinstein J, Kalantari S, et al. Cardiac output assessment in patients supported with left ventricular assist device: discordance between thermodulation and indirect Fick cardiac output measurements. ASAIO J 2017;63:433–7.
21. Stainback R, Estep J, Agler D, et al. Echocardiography in the management of patients with left ventricular assist devices: recommendations from the American Society of Echocardiography. J Am Soc Echocardiogr 2015;28:853–909.
22. Jorde U, Uriel N, Nahumi N, et al. Prevalence, significance, and management of aortic insufficiency in continuous flow left ventricular assist device recipients. Circ Heart Fail 2014;7:310–9.
23. Kusne S, Mooney M, Danziger-Isakov L, et al. An ISHLT consensus document for prevention and management strategies for mechanical circulatory support infection. J Heart Lung Transplant 2017;36(10):1137–53.
24. Barber J, Leslie G. A simple education tool for ventricular assist device patients and their caregivers. J Cardiovasc Nurs 2015;30(3):E1–10.
25. Cannon A, Elliott T, Ballew C, et al. Variability in infection control measures for the percutaneous lead among programs implanting long-term ventricular assist devices in the United States. Prog Transplant 2012;22(4):351–9.
26. Hannan M, Husan S, Mattner F, et al. Working formulation for the standardization of definitions of infections in patients using ventricular assist devices. J Heart Lung Transplant 2011;30(4):361–74.
27. Kadado A, Akar J, Hummel JP. Arrhythmias after left ventricular assist device implantation: incidence and management. Trends Cardiovasc Med 2018;28(1):41–50.
28. Garan A, Iyer V, Whang W, et al. Catheter ablation of ventricular tachyarrhythmias in patients supported by continuous-flow left ventricular assist devices. ASAIO J 2014;60:311–6.
29. Starling R, Moazami N, Sivestry S, et al. Unexpected abrupt increase in left ventricular assist device thrombosis. N Engl J Med 2014;370(1):33–40.

30. Willey J, Boehme A, Castagna F, et al. Hypertension and stroke in patients with left ventricular assist devices. Curr Hypertens Rep 2016;18(2):12.

31. Teuteberg J, Slaughter M, Rogers J, et al. The HVAD left ventricular assist device: risk factors for neurological events and risk mitigation strategies. JACC Heart Fail 2015;3(10):818–28.

32. Lanier G, Orlanes K, Hayashi Y, et al. Validity and reliability of a novel slow cuff-deflation system for noninvasive blood pressure monitoring in patients with continuous-flow left ventricular assist device. Circ Heart Fail 2013;6:1005–12.

33. Castagna F, Stohr E, Pinsino A, et al. The unique blood pressures and pulsatility of LVAD patients: current challenges and future opportunities. Cur Hypertens Rep 2017;19:85.

34. Wilson S, Givertz M, Stewart G, et al. Cardiac rehabilitation of patients with ventricular assist device, an offer to improve strong collaborative relationships. JACC 2010;55(10):1053–4.

35. Kerrigan D, Williams C, Ehrman J, et al. Cardiac rehabilitation improves functional capacity and patient-reported health status in patients with continuous-flow left ventricular assist devices. JACC Heart Fail 2014;2(6):653–9.

36. Allen L, Stevenson L, Grady K, et al. Decision making in advanced heart failure: a scientific statement from the AHA. Circulation 2012;125:1928–52.

37. Schaefer K, Griffin L, Smith C, et al. An interdisciplinary checklist for left ventricular assist device deactivation. J Palliat Med 2014;17(1):4–5.

38. Panke J, Ruiz G, Elliott T, et al. Discontinuation of a left ventricular assist device in the home hospice setting. J Pain Symptom Manage 2016;52(2):313–7.

A Comprehensive Imaging Approach to Guide the Management of Patients with Continuous-Flow Left Ventricular Assist Devices

Bashar Hannawi, MD[a], Jerry D. Estep, MD[b,c],*

KEYWORDS

- Left ventricular assist device • Multimodality imaging • Computed tomography • Echocardiography

KEY POINTS

- Imaging is an integral part in the care of patients supported with left ventricular assist devices (LVADs).
- Echocardiography is a readily available modality that can be used to facilitate the most common LVAD complications.
- Echocardiography has been shown to predict underlying hemodynamics to define left and right ventricular unloading while on LVAD support.
- Cardiac computed tomography is an available modality to diagnose LVAD-related outflow cannula problems, and intracardiac and aortic root clot when echocardiography images are nondiagnostic.

INTRODUCTION

Recent advances in mechanical circulatory support have allowed patients with end-stage heart failure to be successfully bridged to heart transplantation or live for many years on continuous-flow left ventricular assist devices (CF-LVADs) as destination therapy. As survival and quality of life continue to improve and the number of patients supported by CF-LVADs continues to grow,[1,2] utilization of different imaging modalities in the care for these patients has become an integral part of many heart failure centers. In this article, we review the currently available imaging modalities, with a focus on echocardiography, that aid to diagnose and manage common adverse events associated with CF-LVADs that are approved by the US Food and Drug Administration, including persistent heart failure, continuous aortic regurgitation, inflow cannula malposition, low-flow alarms, thromboembolic complications, and suspected pump thrombosis.

IMAGING IN THE MANAGEMENT OF STABLE PATIENTS SUPPORTED WITH CONTINUOUS-FLOW LEFT VENTRICULAR ASSIST DEVICES
Continuous-Flow Left Ventricular Assist Device Monitoring and Surveillance Protocols

For a comprehensive approach to the performance and interpretation of LVAD surveillance protocol, we refer readers to the recently

Disclosure Statement: Dr J.D. Estep serves as a consultant and medical advisor for Abbott and Medtronic Inc.
[a] Department of Cardiology, Houston Methodist Hospital, 6550 Fannin Street, Suite 18-209, Houston, TX 77030, USA; [b] Department of Cardiovascular Medicine, Cleveland Clinic, 9500 Euclid Avenue, Desk J3-4, Cleveland, OH 44195, USA; [c] Heart and Vascular Institute, Kaufman Center for Heart Failure, Cleveland Clinic, 9500 Euclid Avenue, Cleveland, OH 44195, USA
* Corresponding author. Department of Cardiovascular Medicine, Cleveland Clinic, 9500 Euclid Avenue, Desk J3-4, Cleveland, OH 44195.
E-mail address: estepj@ccf.org

published American Society of Echocardiography document on management of patients with LVADs.[3] Although these protocols are center specific, they provide essential information in the monitoring of device function and optimization in addition to detection of device-related complications. In general, most centers perform CF-LVAD surveillance protocols at set time intervals unless clinically recognized complications arise, then problems-focused protocols are performed. CF-LVAD surveillance protocols provide important information to assess (1) underlying hemodynamics to define the degree of left ventricle (LV) unloading provided by the CF-LVAD, (2) right ventricular (RV) function as a surrogate for right heart failure, (3) valvular function with focus on the aortic valve opening status and degree of mitral regurgitation, and (4) CF-LVAD–specific parameters, such as assessment of inflow and outflow cannula flow profiles and the inflow cannula position. After appropriate 2-dimensional (2D) color and spectral Doppler imaging acquisition, a comprehensive echocardiography report can be generated to guide heart failure providers who care for patients supported by CF-LVADs (**Table 1**).

The degree of LV unloading should be assessed during each CF-LVAD surveillance protocol examination. Clues associated with adequate LV unloading consist of a reduction in LV size relative to pre-implant measurements and reduced secondary mitral regurgitation. Other useful parameters include the position of the interventricular and interatrial septum, which reflects the pressure gradient between the LV and RV, and the left atrium (LA) and right atrium (RA), respectively. Adequate LV unloading in the absence of RV failure is associated with a neutral interventricular and interatrial position. A ventricular septum that is deviated to the right or left might indicate inadequate or excessive LV unloading. Similar to imaging patients with congestive heart failure without a CF-LVAD, a combination of Doppler-derived mitral inflow velocities, early mitral annular tissue Doppler, LA size, and pulmonary artery systolic pressure can objectively estimate left-sided and right-sided filling pressures with high accuracy.[4]

Although a closed aortic valve (AV) or intermittent opening of the AV typically reflects a properly functioning CF-LVAD and LV unloading, setting the pump speed to maintain AV opening is a secondary aim to minimize AV fusion and curb the development of continuous aortic regurgitation. A pump speed that is set too low (eg, HeartMate [HM] II pump speed <8600 rpm) may increase the risk of pump thrombosis. The low end of speed for each patient is usually determined during Echo ramp studies, which is the speed that allows at least intermittent AV opening without signs of heart failure.[5] AV opening is best assessed from the parasternal long axis view using 2D and M-mode imaging for at least 3 to 5 consecutive cycles and can be classified as closed, intermittent opening or noted as opening with every cardiac cycle after ventricular systole.

Standard echocardiographic criteria can be used to assess RV function in patients supported with CF-LVADs.[6,7] However, it is important to note that parameters, such as a qualitative assessment of RV systolic function, RV fractional area change, and tricuspid annular plane systolic excursion, are only surrogates for RV failure. Patients may have a reduction in these measurements with underlying normal right-sided filling pressures, normal cardiac output, and absent clinical heart failure symptoms and signs.

Valvular abnormalities should be measured and reported in accord with the latest American Society of Echocardiography guidelines.[8] Although significant mitral regurgitation can be a clue for inadequate LV unloading, significant tricuspid regurgitation can be due to inadequate or excessive LV unloading in addition to primary RV failure.

Normal inflow and outflow cannula flow profiles are defined as continuous and slightly pulsatile due to native LV contraction with a defined peak noted after ventricular systole. Normal peak inflow cannula velocities are between 1 and 2 m/s (typically <1.5 m/s).[3] An increased peak velocity may indicate inlet obstruction and can be due to thrombus, vegetation, LV trabeculae, or inflow cannula malposition and interaction with the endocardium (septum or LV free wall).

Based on a more recent report, peak outflow cannula velocities maybe higher than inflow cannula peak velocities. Based on one study, the average outflow velocity for the HM II was 1.86 m/s (range 0.98–2.73 m/s), whereas the average outflow velocity for the HVAD was 2.36 m/s (range 1.3–3.42 m/s).[9] This study suggests a difference in normal outflow cannula velocities between the 2 most commonly used CF-LVADs. Increased outflow cannula velocities can occur due to partial kinking and internal obstruction by a thrombus or a vegetation when the Doppler sample volume is in proximity to the obstruction. In comparison, outflow cannula velocities are decreased in pump (rotor) thrombosis associated with pump malfunction (decreased diastolic flow velocity), pump stoppage, and intrinsic obstruction when the Doppler sample volume is away from the site of obstruction.

Table 1
A sample echocardiographic report to guide management of patients with continuous-flow left ventricular assist devices (CF-LVAD)

Indication for Study	CF-LVAD Surveillance Echo
Procedures:	2-dimensional, color and spectral Doppler
Quality	If poor visualization of the endocardium, contrast can be used
Cardiac Surgery	CF-LVAD implantation date, type of LVAD (HM II, HVAD, HM3) and pump speed (eg, 9200 rpm, 2600 rpm, 5400 rpm)

Echocardiographic report

Noteworthy parameters and description recommendations		*Red flags (concerns)*
LV	LV size (LVEDD cm), inflow cannula position (toward the septum, MV, or lateral wall), nonturbulent or turbulent color Doppler, inflow pattern, peak systolic and diastolic inflow velocity (m/s), LVEF, wall motion	Small LVEDD (volume depletion vs excessive LV unloading due to high pump speed or underfilled LV due to RV failure or compression) Inflow cannula nonapical position or directed to the septum or posterior wall (malposition-associated adverse events) Inflow peak systolic velocity >2 m/s (inflow obstruction)
RV	RV size and systolic function (mild, moderate, severely depressed) or RVEF based on area change	Enlarged RV and depressed systolic RV function (RV failure sign)
Interventricular septum	Midline, deviated to the left, deviated to the right	Deviated to the left (Excessive LV unloading due to relative high pump speed and/or primary RV failure) Deviated to the right (left-sided HF sign)
LA	Mild (35–41), moderate (42–48), severe (>48) mL/m^2	LA volume index >33 mL/m^2 (left-sided HF sign)
RA	Enlarged (>33 for women, >39 for men) mL/m^2	Right-sided HF sign
Aorta	Aortic root size	Aortic root thrombus (thromboembolic risk)
Pericardium	Presence or absence, and size of pericardial effusion	Pericardial effusion with associated chamber collapse (cardiac tamponade)
Aortic valve	Leaflet structure; AV opening status (opens with every cardiac cycle, intermittent, or closed with every cardiac cycle with at least 3–5 cycles tested); presence or absence of regurgitation (present in systole, diastole, or both)	>Moderate AR regurgitation defined as vena contracta ≥0.3 cm and/or jet width/LVOT width >46% (clinical HF)
MV	Leaflet structure; presence or absence of regurgitation; severity of regurgitation	>Moderate MR (clinical HF)
Pulmonic valve	Leaflet structure; presence or absence of regurgitation	
Tricuspid valve	Leaflet structure (dilated annulus with or without poor leaflet coaptation); presence or absence of regurgitation; severity of regurgitation	>Moderate TR (inadequate LV unloading surrogate, excessive LV unloading leading to poor TV leaflet coaptation, or RV failure sign)

(continued on next page)

Table 1
(*continued*)

Diastology	Estimated LV filling pressure (normal or elevated)	Estep and colleagues. Algorithm: E/A >1 or ≤2 plus, any 2 of the following parameters or E/A >2 plus 1 of the following parameters: a. RAP >10 or sPAP >40 mm Hg b. LAVi >33 mL/m^2 c. E/e' >14 (clinical HF)
Other	Estimated sPAP based on TR jet Outflow cannula Doppler velocity	sPAP >40 mm Hg (partial LV unloading surrogate) Elevated peak outflow cannula velocity with sampling near obstruction site especially if combined with lack of RVOT SV and/or LV-dimension changes with ramp testing (outflow cannula kinking or obstruction) Outflow cannula systolic/diastolic ratio ≤5, diastolic acceleration ≥49 cm/s^2 (mild to moderate AR)

Abbreviations: A, late mitral diastolic flow velocity; AR, aortic regurgitation; AV, aortic valve; E, early mitral diastolic flow velocity; e', mitral annulus tissue Doppler early diastolic velocity; HF, heart failure; LA, left atrium; LAVi, left atrium volume indexed to body surface area; LV, left ventricle; LVEDD, left ventricle end-diastolic dimension; LVEF, left ventricular ejection fraction; LVOT, left ventricular outflow tract; MR, mitral regurgitation; MV, mitral valve; RAP, estimated right atrial pressure; RV, right ventricle; RVEF, right ventricle ejection fraction; RVOT SV, right ventricular outflow tract stroke volume; sPAP, estimated pulmonary artery systolic pressure; TR, tricuspid regurgitation; TV, tricuspid valve.

IMAGING IN THE MANAGEMENT OF CONTINUOUS-FLOW LEFT VENTRICULAR ASSIST DEVICE–RELATED COMPLICATIONS
Assessment of Heart Failure Post Left Ventricular Assist Device

Although the outcomes of patients undergoing CF-LVADs continue to improve, a sizable number of patients continue to experience readmissions for decompensated heart failure. Although the true incidence and long-term implications of persistent symptoms of heart failure while on CF-LVADs support are not known, based on the multicenter destination therapy trials results of the HM II, 23% to 24% of patients on CF-LVAD support have New York Heart Association (NYHA) class III/IV symptoms at 12-month follow-up.[10,11] Similar to these observations, single-center examinations using measured hemodynamics to help categorize and attribute high-grade symptoms to inadequate LV unloading defined by elevated pulmonary capillary wedge pressure (PCWP) report NYHA III/IV symptoms present in up to approximately 27% of patients on CF-LVADs.[4,12,13] In addition, 2 reports define the main causes of readmissions after CF-LVADs related to cardiac causes with up to 27% of the readmissions due to progression of cardiac disease with underlying right heart failure contributing to most of these cardiac causes.[14,15] Collectively, these observations highlight that

underlying abnormal hemodynamics (elevated ventricular filling pressures) may be present in a significant number of patients with a CF-LVAD, and these findings have important clinical implications.

Patients with inadequate LV unloading while on CF-LVAD support can have an elevated PCWP with or without an elevated RA pressure (RAP), and these patients may present with persistent or acquired shortness of breath. In contrast, predominate RV failure during CF-LVAD support is a profile becoming increasingly recognized and is due to an underlying elevated RAP in the presence of a normal PCWP.[16,17] A detailed echocardiographic assessment of these patients is crucial, as certain interventions, such as increasing pump speed, may be helpful in the group with smoldering LV failure but deleterious in patients with an underfilled LV and predominately RV failure (see **Table 1**).

Echocardiographic variables associated with inadequate LV unloading (estimated LA pressure based on the interatrial septum position, early mitral valve [MV] inflow deceleration time <150 ms, and the ratio of the MV deceleration time to early MV inflow velocity <2 m/s) have been associated with worse 90-day outcomes (mortality, heart failure readmission, and NYHA class III/IV symptoms).[18] With adequate LV unloading, the following echocardiography parameters may reduce and/or approach normal to reflect near normalization of estimated LV filling pressures. At 6-month postimplant follow-up compared with pre-implant, LV end-diastolic dimension (LVEDD) typically reduces by 16% (from 6.8 to 5.7 cm) and up to 21% (from 6.6 to 5.2 cm),[19,20] Early mitral diastolic flow velocity/late mitral diastolic flow velocity (E/A) ratio typically reduces by 42% (from 2.8 to 1.6),[21] E/mitral annulus tissue Doppler early diastolic velocity (e') reduction by 35% (from 25 to 13) and up to 48% (from 23 to 12),[21] LA volume index reduction by 45% (from 46 to 25 mL/m²),[21] and the deceleration time (DT) is typically prolonged by 34 to 40 ms.[19–21]

We previously examined the correlation of multiple echocardiographic parameters with an elevated PCWP as measured by right heart catheterization. In our study, measured pulmonary artery systolic pressure, RA pressure, Doppler (E/e') and LA size indexed to body surface area was feasible in 75% of patients and using an algorithm incorporating these parameters

accurately identified 90% of patients with a wedge pressure more than 15 mm Hg.[4] It is important to note that in our study, estimated RAP as a single parameter was highly specific (93%) for an elevated wedge pressure; however, sensitivity was only 78%, highlighting that multiple parameters are needed to best estimate left-sided filling pressure in this patient population. As reported by our group[4] and Uriel and colleagues,[12] an elevated RAP on CF-LVAD support is a surrogate of left-sided heart failure possibly due to inadequate LV unloading, and these patients may benefit from a ramp speed optimization study. Echocardiography can be helpful to identify these different patients' profiles and might obviate the need for an invasive hemodynamic assessment in all patients (**Figs. 1–4**).

Aortic Regurgitation Assessment

The assessment of aortic regurgitation (AR) in patients supported with CF-LVAD starts with the use

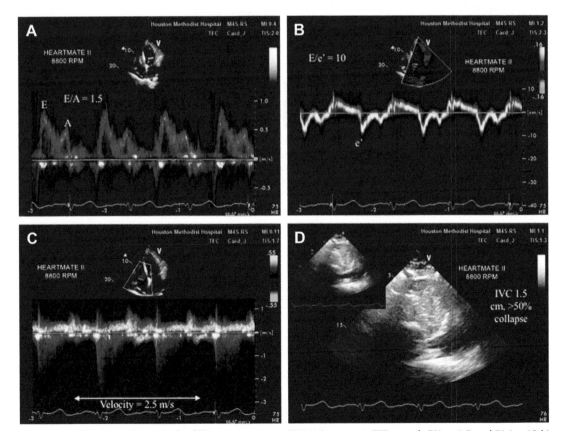

Fig. 1. Normal estimated ventricular filling pressures on CF-LVAD support. TTE reveals E/A = 1.5 and E/e' = 10 (*A, B*). sPAP is estimated at 30 mm Hg based on estimated RV systolic pressure $4v^2 = 25$ mm Hg (*C*) plus an estimated RAP of 5 mm Hg (*D*). Estimated PCWP is <15 mm Hg based on the algorithm of Estep and colleagues[4] with E/A<2 plus sPAP ≤40 mm Hg and E/e' ≤14. Findings were consistent with invasive hemodynamic assessments: RAP 6 mm Hg, PCWP 11 mm Hg, and sPAP 36 mm Hg. IVC, inferior vena cava; sPAP, systolic pulmonary artery pressure; V, velocity.

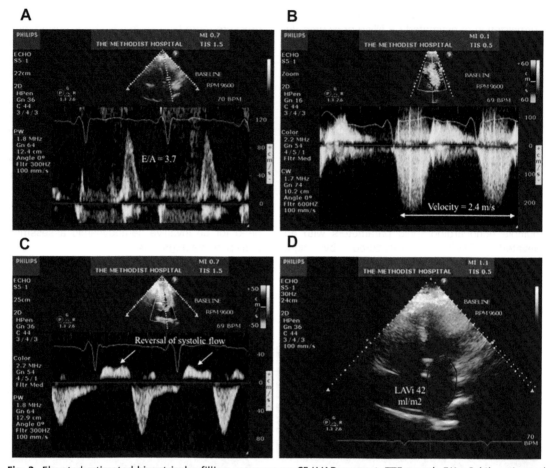

Fig. 2. Elevated estimated biventricular filling pressures on CF-LVAD support. TTE reveals E/A >2 (*A*), estimated sPAP of 43 mm Hg based on estimated RV systolic pressure $4v^2 = 23$ mm Hg (*B*) and RAP of 20 mm Hg (*C*), and a severely enlarged LA (*D*). Therefore, an estimated PCWP greater than 15 mm Hg. Findings correlated with invasive hemodynamic assessments: PCWP 22, systolic pulmonary artery pressure (sPAP) 38 mm Hg, and RAP 23, consistent with left-sided heart failure with secondary elevated right-sided filling pressures. LAVi, left atrium volume indexed to body surface area.

of transesophageal echocardiography in the operating room. It is possible that after CF-LVAD activation, undiagnosed AR will be unmasked due to the increase in diastolic aortic pressure and a reduction in LV pressure with LV unloading. Patients with more than mild AR noted intraoperatively should be considered for surgical repair given the anticipated progressive nature of AR and associated long-term adverse implications, including clinical heart failure.[22]

The true prevalence of clinically significant CF-LVAD–associated AR remains unknown. Based on detection using echocardiography, AR can occur in up to as many as two-thirds of patients.[23] Factors that are associated with development of AR include older age, female gender, persistent AV closure, and duration of CF-LVAD support.[23] AR in patients supported with CF-LVAD can be

predominately noted during diastole or seen during both diastole and systole (pancyclic and often referred to as continuous AR). Traditional echocardiographic parameters used to detect the severity of AR may underestimate the severity of AR in patients supported by CF-LVAD due to the eccentric jet nature in some patients and the presence of AR during systole and diastole in others. Two new CF-LVAD–specific Doppler parameters derived from examination of the outflow cannula were more recently studied and correlated highly and best with aortic regurgitant fraction compared with traditional measures. The novel measurements included the outflow cannula diastolic flow acceleration and systolic and end-diastolic flow velocities. These measurements were feasible in all patients in whom the outflow cannula was visualized (n = 18/20).[24] The 2 parameters reclassified

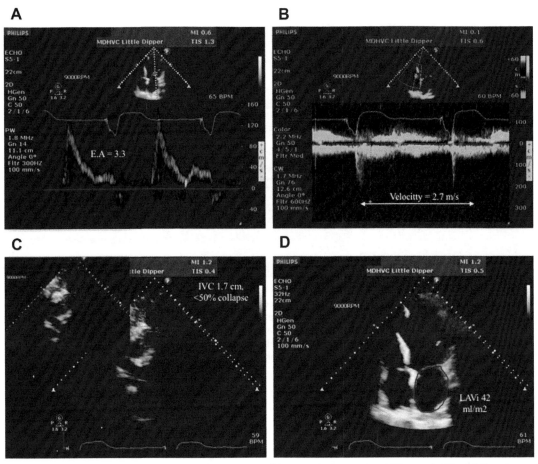

Fig. 3. Elevated LV filling pressure on CF-LVAD support with normal RA pressure. TTE reveals E/A >2 (*A*), estimated sPAP of 34 to 39 mm Hg based on estimated RV systolic pressure $4v^2 = 29$ mm Hg (*B*) plus estimated RAP of 5 to 10 mm Hg (*C*), and a severely enlarged LA (*D*). Therefore, an estimated PCWP greater than 15 mm Hg. Findings correlated with invasive hemodynamic assessments: PCWP 16, systolic pulmonary artery pressure (sPAP) 46 mm Hg, and RAP 10 mm Hg. LAVi, left atrium volume indexed to body surface area.

patients from trace/mild to at least moderate in up to one-third of patients and identified patients likely to experience the composite end point of death, AV intervention, urgent transplantation, and heart failure readmission.[24] Besides the frequency of AV opening,[23,25] the angle between outflow cannula and aorta measured on computed tomography (CT) was recently shown to correlate with the severity of AR. Patients who had a larger angle were more likely to develop more than mild AR (94° vs 77°; *P* = .021).[26]

Inflow Cannula Malposition

The ideal inflow cannula should be positioned in the LV apex directed toward the MV (**Figs. 5** and **6**). Although a precise imaging definition based on echocardiography or cardiac CT (CCT) of inflow cannula malposition has not be defined based on

examined association with adverse events related to malposition (eg, rotor thrombus, partial LV unloading, suction events, and/or LVAD-induced ventricular dysrhythmias), inflow cannula malposition using chest radiograph has been recently reported. In 27 patients supported with HVAD CF-LVADs, cannula coronal angle (relative to a horizontal line in the posteroanterior view) <65° was associated with a reduction in heart failure readmissions at 1-year follow-up (Harzard Ratio 10.33, *P* = .007).[27] In another study of 22 patients supported by HM II, an inflow cannula obstruction greater than 30% as assessed by CCT was associated with urgent listing for heart transplantation, urgent pump exchange, or death related to pump thrombosis.[28] Although inflow cannula malposition based on chest radiograph did not differentiate patients who developed adverse outcomes, it is possible that malposition is associated with a

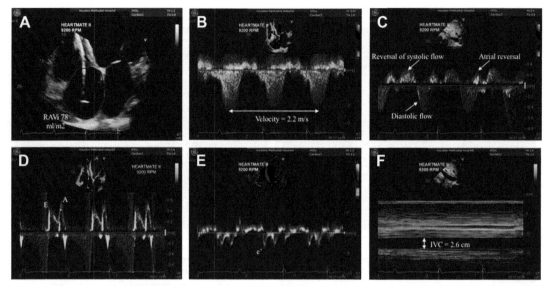

Fig. 4. Predominate late RV failure with normal estimated PCWP. TTE shows severely enlarged RA and intra-atrial septum bowing to the left indicating elevated right-sided filling pressure (*A*). Color and continuous wave Doppler shows low velocity, triangular tricuspid regurgitation jet (*B*), along with reversal of hepatic vein systolic flow (*C*) indicating severe tricuspid regurgitation. PCWP is estimated less than 15 mm Hg based on E/A ratio = 0.75 (*D*) and E/e' = 11 (*D, E*). RAP is estimated greater than 20 mm Hg (*C, F*). Clinically, patient presented in clinic with NYHA class I symptoms in setting of 1 to 2 plus lower extremity edema. IVC, inferior vena cava.

higher likelihood for inflow cannula obstruction. In all 6 patients who underwent surgery, cannula obstruction was caused by variable degree of pannus, thrombus, or myocardium. Interestingly, patients with adverse events were more likely to experience heart failure symptoms.[28] Incorporating CCT surveillance in patents supported by LVADs is evolving particularly for postimplant complications, including cannula malposition and to screen for pump and aortic root thrombosis in addition to detection of postsurgical complications like pericardial hematomas and effusions.[29] With new CT scanners (Dual Force), improved scanning protocols, and updated software to minimize metallic artifact, CCT imaging is a promising technique to improve visualization within the pump itself to more accurately document inflow cannula and/or rotor clot. **Fig. 7**.

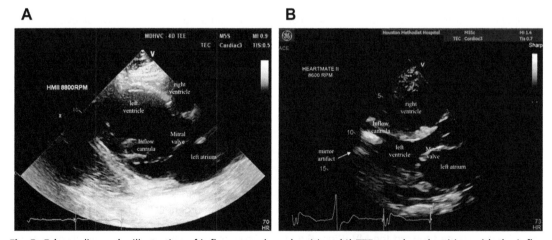

Fig. 5. Echocardiography illustration of inflow cannula malposition. (*A*) TTE reveals malposition with the inflow cannula positioned at the posterolateral wall of the LV. This patient had hemolysis and an episode of suspected pump thrombosis. (*B*) TTE reveals the inflow cannula positioned at the apex and pointing toward the apical anteroseptal wall of the LV. This patient had intermittent low-flow alarms.

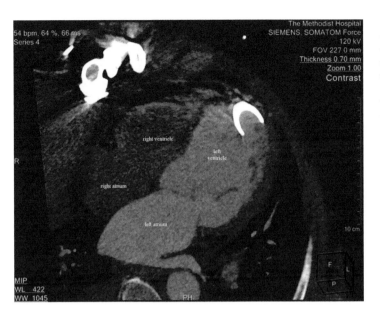

Fig. 6. CCT illustration of inflow cannula malposition. CCT angiogram reveals malposition of inflow cannula pointing toward and slightly abutting the distal anterolateral wall of the LV. Patient noted to have recurring CF-LVAD suction events.

Assessment of Continuous-Flow Left Ventricular Assist Device Alarms

Pump alarm review should be routinely performed during each outpatient follow-up and at any time when patients present with a change from their baseline status. CF-LVAD alarms are generally broken into 2 categories: low-flow and high-flow (high power) alarms. Low-flow alarms can be due to decrease in preload (hypovolemia), pericardial

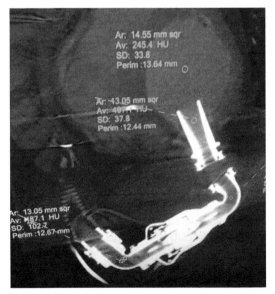

Fig. 7. CCT of a CF-LVAD. Newer CCT techniques are promising to improve visualization within the pump itself. See text. (*Courtesy of* Su Min Chang, MD, Houston, TX.)

tamponade, significant RV failure (**Fig. 8**), an increase in afterload (severe hypertension), mechanical complications (inflow malposition with associated obstruction or outflow obstruction), and arrhythmias (**Table 2**).

High-flow alarms along with high power can be due to peripheral vasodilation (sepsis, systemic inflammatory response syndrome), AR, and rotor thrombosis in the setting of hemolysis (pseudo high flow based on calculation due to an increase in power consumption). In this context, imaging modalities, specifically echocardiography and CCT, provide crucial information to differentiate the variety of underlying etiologies and aid in guiding treatment. Echocardiography can accurately differentiate high-flow alarms due to rotor thrombosis with pump malfunction versus patients with significant AR.

Detection of Pump Malfunction and Left Ventricular Assist Device Thrombosis

LVAD thrombus and subsequent pump malfunction can occur at any part of the device, including at the inlet of the inflow cannula, the rotor, and the outflow cannula. Several LVAD-specific echocardiography-derived parameters have been studied to aid diagnosis of pump thrombosis and pump malfunction. An increased systolic to diastolic velocity ratio at the inflow (mean 4.29) and outflow (mean 3.94) cannulas can be seen in patients with pump thrombosis compared with prethrombotic values of 2.40 and 2.63, respectively.[30]

In the original Columbia experience, of 17 patients tested for pump malfunction, 10 patients

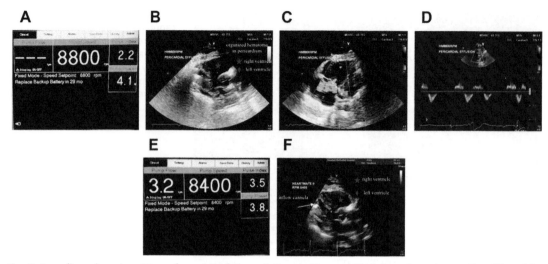

Fig. 8. Low-flow alarm in setting of overt RV failure. Patient with acute RV failure 1-week post HeartMate II implantation. (*A*) shows persistent low-flow alarms and reduced pulsatility (console—display) at 8800 rpm. TTE reveals an enlarged RV with severely depressed systolic function, and a small LV (*A, B*), severe tricuspid regurgitation (*C*), and systolic reversal of hepatic vein flow indicating a estimated RA pressure greater than 20 mm Hg (*D*). After reducing the pump speed to 8400 rpm and initiating inotropic support, pump flow improved to 3.2 liters per minute (*E*). Repeat echocardiogram reveals improved LV size indicating improved flow to the LV and CF-LVAD (*F*).

had minimal change in LVEDD. Of these patients, 9 underwent pump exchanges and were found to have evidence of pump outflow obstruction (8 pump thrombosis and 1 related to the outflow bend relief). The investigators found that all patients with pump malfunction and none without had LVEDD slope >−0.16. CF-LVADs are afterload dependent, and therefore, conditions associated with elevated afterload might affect the results of the ramp study. This was demonstrated in a recent study showing that 50% of the 18 abnormal studies determined by LVEDD slope were false positive.[31] These false-positive studies included 10 studies with significant (at least mild to moderate) AR and 6 studies in patients with uncontrolled hypertension (mean arterial pressure ≥85 mm Hg).[31] Moreover, the ramp testing to detect LV size reduction with speed enhancement is not accurate in patients supported by the HVAD due to a different LV morphology change with pump speed enhancement compared with the HVAD and therefore using echocardiography with ramp testing to screen for pump malfunction in the setting of hemolysis is not recommended in those patients supported by this device.[32,33]

Compared with the original ramp study, our group reported a simplified protocol with 95% specificity for detection of pump malfunction when 2 of the 3 tested echocardiographic parameters are met. Comparing parameters at pump speed of 8000 versus 11,000 rpm, patients with pump malfunction are expected to have a blunted change in LV size (LVEDD of <0.6 cm), persistent AV opening with a time duration difference of less than 80 ms, and a change in mitral inflow DT of less than 70 ms[34] (**Fig. 9**).

In addition to aiding in the diagnosis of pump thrombosis and malfunction, echocardiography can play a role in stratification of risk for future pump thrombosis. In patients with preoperative LVEDD greater than 6.0 cm, the risk of device thrombosis was higher in patients with axial (HM II) than patients with centrifugal-flow devices. This observation suggests that centrifugal devices (eg, HVAD) may be associated with a lower risk of device thrombosis in patients with a larger preoperative LV cavity.[35] Moreover, with adequate LV unloading, implantation of CF-LVAD leads to a 17% and 19% reduction in LVEDD and LV end-systolic diameter (LVESD) dimensions respectively at 1 month compared with measurements made before implantation.[19] Suboptimal LV unloading evident by inadequate LV dimensions decrement with optimal LVAD speed on predischarge ramp studies were found as risk a factor for late pump thrombosis. Among 64 patients supported with the HM II, LVEDD and LVESD decrement indices ≤15% were 83% sensitive for the development of pump thrombosis at 15-month follow-up.[36]

Thromboembolic Complications

Stroke is a devastating complication that can affect patients supported by CF-LVADs that can

Table 2
Continuous-flow left ventricular assist devices differential diagnosis and possible symptoms, signs, echocardiography, and cardiac computed tomography (CCT) findings

Alarm	Low-flow						
Symptoms/Signs	Heart failure symptoms, pre-syncope, syncope, palpitations						
Physical examination, Doppler BP, ECG, telemetry, PPM interrogation							
Additional possible signs	Mean BP >>90 mm Hg	VT, VF	Mean BP typically normal 65–85 mm Hg, ↑JVP		Mean BP <60 mm Hg, ↑JVP		Mean BP <60 mm Hg, ↓JVP
Echocardiogram	Nonspecific findings such as large LV, ↓AV opening ↑Outflow cannula peak velocity	Nonspecific findings, might occur including RV failure signs	Large LV, ↑AV opening ↑Outflow cannula peak velocity[b]	Normal or ↓inflow cannula peak velocity, and/or directed toward septal/inferior with or without abutting LV wall[a]	Small LV, large RV, depressed RV, minimal MR, significant TR, IVS bulges to left IAS bulges to left ↑Estimated RAP	Large pericardial effusion, chamber collapse, ↑Estimated ↑RAP	Small LV, no/mild MR, no/mild TR, normal estimated PCWP, ↓estimated RAP
CCT	CCT typically not needed, used to rule out other causes	CCT typically not needed, used to rule out other causes	OC kinking, thrombus, external compression, malposition	IC not entering from true apex and/or IC directed toward septal/inferior with or without abutting LV wall	Large RV, ↓RVEF, significant TR, reflux of contrast into IVC, dilated IVC	Large pericardial effusion, RV compression	CCT typically not needed, used to rule out other causes
Diagnosis	Malignant hypertension	Arrhythmias	Outflow cannula mechanical complications	Inflow cannula malposition	RV failure	Tamponade	Hypovolemia

Abbreviations: ↑, increased; ↓, decreased; AV, aortic valve; BP, blood pressure; ECG, electrocardiogram; IAS, intra-atrial septum; IC, inflow cannula; IVC, inferior vena cava; IVS, intra-ventricular septum; JVP, jugular venous pressure; LV, left ventricle; MR, mitral regurgitation; OC, outflow cannula; PCWP, estimated pulmonary capillary wedge pressure; PPM, permanent pacemaker; RV, right ventricle; RVEF, right ventricular ejection fraction; TR, tricuspid regurgitation; VF, ventricular fibrillation; VT, ventricular tachycardia.

[a] Depending on the degree of obstruction.

[b] Depending on the degree of obstruction and its location in relation to the Doppler sample volume (increased if in proximity to the sample volume).

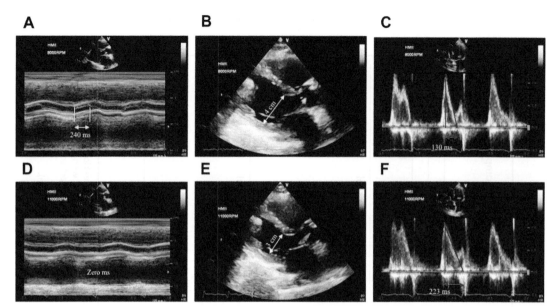

Fig. 9. Normal HeartMate II pump function using a simplified ramp study. Simplified ramp study reveals no evidence of pump malfunction. Three parameters are assessed at 8000 and 11,000 rpm: AV opening time difference (A, D) noted to be 240 ms, LVEDD (B, E) noted to be 1 cm, and MV-DT prolongation (C, F) noted to be 93 ms. Patients with no evidence of pump malfunction are expected to have a reduction of AV opening time by ≥80 ms, LV size reduction with LVEDD change ≥0.6 cm, and an increase in MV-DT ≥70 ms.

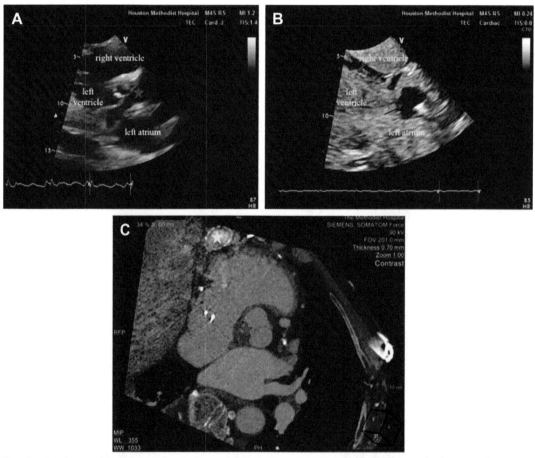

Fig. 10. ART detected by echocardiography and CCT. Patient 1: TTE, parasternal long axis view reveals a vague echo density in the aortic root noted by the red star (A). Micro bubble contrast was given to enhance visualization and confirmed the presence of a large ART, as noted by the red arrow (B). Patient 2: CCT angiogram reveals ART in the noncoronary cusp, as noted by the red star (C). Yellow star marks the outflow cannula.

significantly affect the long-term outcomes of these patients, including their eligibility for subsequent transplantation. In the Interagency Registry for Mechanically Assisted Circulatory Support registry, 10.57% of patients suffered from at least 1 stroke during a median follow-up of 9.79 months, more than half of them (51.38%) were categorized as ischemic.[37]

A thorough evaluation is necessary to identify the underlying cause of stroke in patients with a CF-LVAD with special attention to rule out thrombus related to the presence of mechanical support. This includes pump thrombus (inlet of the inflow cannula, inflow cannula itself, rotor, and the outflow cannula) and aortic root thrombus (ART), a recently recognized but increasingly encountered complication of CF-LVADs that can be detected in approximately 6% of patients.[38] Most cases occur within the first month postimplantation. A closed AV appears to be a risk factor for the development of ART.[39] Patients with ART might have a wide range of presentations from stroke and myocardial infarction with or without subsequent heart failure.

Transthoracic echocardiography (TTE) is the current imaging modality of choice for routine CF-LVAD surveillance. However, TTE can miss ART depending on the small size and location.[40] Microbubble contrast can be safely given to patients supported by CF-LVADs and can help to identify aortic root and LV clot (**Fig. 10**A, B).[41] In contrast to echocardiography, due to its high spatial resolution, CCT provides optimal visualization of the aortic root (**Fig. 10**C). In addition, CCT provides the ability to visualize the extent of the thrombus and can exclude involvement of the coronary arteries in patients presenting with ischemia or myocardial infarction. CCT, however, requires the use of iodinated contrast to permit visualization of the aortic root. In our experience, patients supported by CF-LVADs with a glomerular filtration rate greater than 60 mL/min per 1.73 m^2 tolerated CCT with contrast testing without significant nephrotoxicity.[42]

SUMMARY

Echocardiography plays an integral role in the detection of post device complications, including persistent or recurring heart failure, continuous AR, inflow cannula malposition, low-flow alarms, thromboembolic complications, and suspected pump thrombosis. CCT is a second-line imaging modality that permits better visualization of the inflow and outflow cannulas and aortic root compared with echocardiography, and is helpful to better understand adverse outcomes associated with inflow cannula malposition and outflow cannula kinking and to screen for intracardiac and ART in those patients with suspected thromboembolic complications. As the number of patients supported with CF-LVADs continues to grow, it is of utmost importance for providers who care for these patients to become familiar with the common complications and the diagnostic imaging approach to best guide management and prognosis.

REFERENCES

1. Kirklin JK, Pagani FD, Kormos RL, et al. Eighth annual INTERMACS report: special focus on framing the impact of adverse events. J Heart Lung Transplant 2017;36(10):1080–6.
2. Kirklin JK, Naftel DC, Pagani FD, et al. Seventh INTERMACS annual report: 15,000 patients and counting. J Heart Lung Transplant 2015;34(12):1495–504.
3. Stainback RF, Estep JD, Agler DA, et al. Echocardiography in the management of patients with left ventricular assist devices: recommendations from the American Society of Echocardiography. J Am Soc Echocardiogr 2015;28(8):853–909.
4. Estep JD, Vivo RP, Krim SR, et al. Echocardiographic evaluation of hemodynamics in patients with systolic heart failure supported by a continuous-flow LVAD. J Am Coll Cardiol 2014;64(12):1231–41.
5. Maltais S, Kilic A, Nathan S, et al. PREVENtion of HeartMate II pump thrombosis through clinical management: the PREVENT multi-center study. J Heart Lung Transplant 2017;36(1):1–12.
6. Rudski LG, Lai WW, Afilalo J, et al. Guidelines for the echocardiographic assessment of the right heart in adults: a report from the American Society of Echocardiography endorsed by the European Association of Echocardiography, a registered branch of the European Society of Cardiology, and the Canadian Society of Echocardiography. J Am Soc Echocardiogr 2010;23(7):685–713 [quiz: 786–8].
7. Lang RM. Recommendations for cardiac chamber quantification by echocardiography in adults: an update from the American Society of Echocardiography and the European Association of Cardiovascular Imaging. J Am Soc Echocardiogr 2015;28(1):1–39. e14.
8. Zoghbi WA, Adams D, Bonow RO, et al. Recommendations for noninvasive evaluation of native valvular regurgitation: a report from the American Society of Echocardiography developed in collaboration with the Society for Cardiovascular Magnetic Resonance. J Am Soc Echocardiogr 2017;30(4):303–71.
9. Grinstein J, Kruse E, Collins K, et al. Screening for outflow cannula malfunction of left ventricular assist

devices (LVADs) with the use of Doppler echocardiography: new LVAD-specific reference values for contemporary devices. J Card Fail 2016;22(10):808–14.

10. Slaughter MS, Rogers JG, Milano CA, et al. Advanced heart failure treated with continuous-flow left ventricular assist device. N Engl J Med 2009;361(23):2241–51.

11. Estep JD, Starling RC, Horstmanshof DA, et al. Risk assessment and comparative effectiveness of left ventricular assist device and medical management in ambulatory heart failure patients: results from the ROADMAP study. J Am Coll Cardiol 2015;66(16):1747–61.

12. Uriel N, Sayer G, Addetia K, et al. Hemodynamic ramp tests in patients with left ventricular assist devices. JACC Heart Fail 2016;4(3):208–17.

13. Shah P, Badoe N, Phillips S, et al. Unrecognized left heart failure in LVAD recipients: the role of routine invasive hemodynamic testing. ASAIO J 2018;64(2):183–90.

14. Smedira NG, Hoercher KJ, Lima B, et al. Unplanned hospital readmissions after HeartMate II implantation: frequency, risk factors, and impact on resource use and survival. JACC Heart Fail 2013;1(1):31–9.

15. Hasin T, Marmor Y, Kremers W, et al. Readmissions after implantation of axial flow left ventricular assist device. J Am Coll Cardiol 2013;61(2):153–63.

16. Takeda K, Takayama H, Colombo PC, et al. Late right heart failure during support with continuous-flow left ventricular assist devices adversely affects post-transplant outcome. J Heart Lung Transplant 2015;34(5):667–74.

17. Rich JD, Gosev I, Patel CB, et al. The incidence, risk factors, and outcomes associated with late right-sided heart failure in patients supported with an axial-flow left ventricular assist device. J Heart Lung Transplant 2017;36(1):50–8.

18. Topilsky Y, Hasin T, Oh JK, et al. Echocardiographic variables after left ventricular assist device implantation associated with adverse outcome. Circ Cardiovasc Imaging 2011;4(6):648–61.

19. Lam KM, Ennis S, O'Driscoll G, et al. Observations from non-invasive measures of right heart hemodynamics in left ventricular assist device patients. J Am Soc Echocardiogr 2009;22(9):1055–62.

20. Topilsky Y, Oh JK, Atchison FW, et al. Echocardiographic findings in stable outpatients with properly functioning HeartMate II left ventricular assist devices. J Am Soc Echocardiogr 2011;24(2):157–69.

21. Drakos SG, Wever-Pinzon O, Selzman CH, et al. Magnitude and time course of changes induced by continuous-flow left ventricular assist device unloading in chronic heart failure: insights into cardiac recovery. J Am Coll Cardiol 2013;61(19):1985–94.

22. Cowger J, Rao V, Massey T, et al. Comprehensive review and suggested strategies for the detection and management of aortic insufficiency in patients with a continuous-flow left ventricular assist device. J Heart Lung Transplant 2015;34(2):149–57.

23. Gasparovic H, Kopjar T, Saeed D, et al. De novo aortic regurgitation after continuous-flow left ventricular assist device implantation. Ann Thorac Surg 2017;104(2):704–11.

24. Grinstein J, Kruse E, Sayer G, et al. Novel echocardiographic parameters of aortic insufficiency in continuous-flow left ventricular assist devices and clinical outcome. J Heart Lung Transplant 2016;35(8):976–85.

25. Aggarwal A, Raghuvir R, Eryazici P, et al. The development of aortic insufficiency in continuous-flow left ventricular assist device-supported patients. Ann Thorac Surg 2013;95(2):493–8.

26. Iizuka K, Nishinaka T, Ichihara Y, et al. Outflow graft anastomosis site design could be correlated to aortic valve regurgitation under left ventricular assist device support. J Artif Organs 2018;21(2):150–5.

27. Imamura T, Adatya S, Chung B, et al. Cannula and pump positions are associated with left ventricular unloading and clinical outcome in patients with HeartWare left ventricular assist device. J Card Fail 2018;24(3):159–66.

28. Sacks J, Gonzalez-Stawinski GV, Hall S, et al. Utility of cardiac computed tomography for inflow cannula patency assessment and prediction of clinical outcome in patients with the HeartMate II left ventricular assist device. Interact Cardiovasc Thorac Surg 2015;21(5):590–3.

29. Vivo RP, Kassi M, Estep JD, et al. MDCT assessment of mechanical circulatory support device complications. JACC Cardiovasc Imaging 2015;8(1):100–2.

30. Jain A, Rohrer B, Gebhardt B, et al. Left ventricular assist device thrombosis is associated with an increase in the systolic-to-diastolic velocity ratio measured at the inflow and outflow cannulae. J Cardiothorac Vasc Anesth 2017;31(2):497–504.

31. Adatya S, Holley CT, Roy SS, et al. Echocardiographic ramp test for continuous-flow left ventricular assist devices: do loading conditions matter? JACC Heart Fail 2015;3(4):291–9.

32. Uriel N, Levin AP, Sayer GT, et al. Left ventricular decompression during speed optimization ramps in patients supported by continuous-flow left ventricular assist devices: device-specific performance characteristics and impact on diagnostic algorithms. J Card Fail 2015;21(10):785–91.

33. Sauer AJ, Meehan K, Gordon R, et al. Echocardiographic markers of left ventricular unloading using a centrifugal-flow rotary pump. J Heart Lung Transplant 2014;33(4):449–50.

34. Estep JD, Vivo RP, Cordero-Reyes AM, et al. A simplified echocardiographic technique for detecting continuous-flow left ventricular assist device malfunction due to pump thrombosis. J Heart Lung Transplant 2014;33(6):575–86.

35. Shah P, Birk S, Maltais S, et al. Left ventricular assist device outcomes based on flow configuration and pre-operative left ventricular dimension: an interagency registry for mechanically assisted circulatory support analysis. J Heart Lung Transplant 2017;36(6):640–9.

36. Joyce E, Stewart GC, Hickey M, et al. Left ventricular dimension decrement index early after axial flow assist device implantation: a novel risk marker for late pump thrombosis. J Heart Lung Transplant 2015;34(12):1561–9.

37. Acharya D, Loyaga-Rendon R, Morgan CJ, et al. INTERMACS analysis of stroke during support with continuous-flow left ventricular assist devices: risk factors and outcomes. JACC Heart Fail 2017;5(10): 703–11.

38. Fried J, Fukuhara S, Garan A, et al. Aortic root thrombus formation in patients with continuous-flow left ventricular assist devices (CF-LVADs). J Heart Lung Transplant 2016;35(4):S113.

39. Gulotta J, Morin DP, Krim SR. Letter to the editor: management of aortic root thrombosis after implantation of a continuous-flow left ventricular assist device: a real conundrum. Ochsner J 2017;17(4): 307–8.

40. Gupta SS, Pozo E, de Siqueira ME, et al. Asymptomatic large aortic root thrombus after left ventricular assist device implantation detected by cardiac computed tomography. J Cardiovasc Comput Tomogr 2017;11(1):72–3.

41. Fine NM, Abdelmoneim SS, Dichak A, et al. Safety and feasibility of contrast echocardiography for LVAD evaluation. JACC Cardiovasc Imaging 2014; 7(4):429–30.

42. Chang SM, Kassi M, Sharifeh T, et al. Diagnostic utility and safety of contrast enhanced gated multislices cardiac computed tomography (CT) for evaluation of patient s with left ventricular assist device (LVAD). Circulation 2012;126:A18981.

Right Ventricular Failure and Biventricular Support Strategies

Diyar Saeed, MD, PhD

KEYWORDS

- Circulatory support devices • Heart failure • Right ventricular failure • BVAD • Total artificial heart

KEY POINTS

- Adequate assessment of right ventricle (RV) before left ventricular assist device surgery is crucial.
- Perioperative management of RV dysfunction is imperative.
- Various temporary and permanent surgical options for RV support are discussed within this article.

INTRODUCTION

Left ventricular assist devices (LVADs) play a vital role in management of patients with end-stage heart failure. Some degree of right ventricular (RV) dysfunction can be observed in most patients with advanced heart failure assessed for LVAD implantation. It has been reported that RV failure (RVF) complicates 10% to 40% of LVAD implants.[1–5] The common working definition of RVF is described by Interagency Registry for Mechanically Assisted Circulatory Support (INTERMACS) as persistent signs and symptoms of RV dysfunction requiring placement of an RV assist device (RVAD), or the use of prolonged intravenous inotropic agents or nitric oxide after an LVAD (**Table 1**).[6] The development of RVF that requires RVAD support in LVAD recipients is associated with high mortality irrespective of the timing of device insertion.[6,7] As per the latest INTERMACS report, the need for RVAD support at the time of original operation is the foremost contributor to early mortality with nearly a fourfold increased risk of death.[8]

Two forms of RVF after LVAD implantation have been described: early and late RVF. The mechanism of early RVF in patients with an LVAD is multifactorial; increased venous return to the RV due to higher cardiac output from the LVAD, excessive leftward shift of the interventricular septum with continuous-flow (CF) LVADs, may also decrease septal contribution to RV contraction[9] leading to RVF.[10] Excessive perioperative volume resuscitation may also exacerbate RV dilation, and causes tricuspid valve incompetence and RVF.[11] Finally, atrial and ventricular tachyarrhythmias occur in more than 20% of patients with an LVAD and double the risk of RVF.[12,13]

The other form of RVF that is an increasingly recognized clinical phenomenon is late RVF (occurring >30 days after LVAD implantation). Recent studies have reported incidence rates of late right heart failure (RHF) of 8% to 11%, and have variably shown elevated central venous pressure/pulmonary artery pressure, HeartMate risk score, diabetes, and worse kidney function to be weakly associated with late RVF.[14,15] The pathophysiology of late RHF is controversial and remains poorly elucidated, but is associated with failure to thrive after LVAD implant.[7]

PERIOPERATIVE ASSESSMENT OF THE RIGHT VENTRICULAR FUNCTION

Important clues to assess RVF can be seen based on clinical examination, including the severity and

Disclosure: None.
Clinic for Cardiovascular Surgery, Heinrich-Heine University Düsseldorf, Moorenstraße 5, 40225 Düsseldorf, Germany
E-mail address: diyar.saeed@med.uni-duesseldorf.de

Table 1
Interagency registry for mechanically assisted circulatory support definition of right ventricular failure

RVF definition	Symptoms or findings of persistent RVF characterized by *both* of the following:
	• Elevated CVP documented by the following:
	  ○ Right atrial pressure >16 mm Hg on right heart catheterization
	  ○ Significantly dilated inferior vena cava with no inspiratory variation on echocardiography
	  ○ Elevated jugular venous pressure
	• Manifestations of elevated CVP characterized by the following:
	  ○ Peripheral edema (≥2+)
	  ○ Ascites or hepatomegaly on examination or diagnostic imaging
	  ○ Laboratory evidence of worsening hepatic (total bilirubin >2.0 mg/dL) or renal dysfunction (creatinine >2.0 mg/dL)

Severity scale	
Mild	Patient meets *both* criteria for RVF plus the following: • Postimplant inotropes, inhaled nitric oxide, or intravenous vasodilators not continued beyond postoperative day 7 after VAD implant AND • No inotropes continued beyond postoperative day 7 after VAD implant
Moderate	Patient meets *both* criteria for RVF plus the following: • Postimplant inotropes, inhaled nitric oxide, or intravenous vasodilators continued beyond postoperative day 7 and up to postoperative day 14 after VAD implant
Severe	Patient meets *both* criteria for RVF plus the following: • CVP or right atrial pressure >16 mm Hg AND • Prolonged postimplant inotropes, inhaled nitric oxide, or intravenous vasodilators continued beyond postoperative day 14 after VAD implant
Severe-acute	Patient meets *both* criteria for RVF plus the following: • CVP or right atrial pressure >16 mm Hg AND • Need for RVAD at any time after VAD implant OR • Death during VAD implants hospitalization with RVF as primary cause

Abbreviations: CVP, central venous pressure; RVAD, right ventricular assist device; RVF, right ventricular failure; VAD, ventricular assist device.

From Lampert BC, Teuteberg JJ. Right ventricular failure after left ventricular assist devices. J Heart Lung Transplant 2015;34(9):1124; with permission.

extent of lower extremity edema, ascites, hepatomegaly, liver enlargement, and scleral icterus. Further, laboratory and imaging studies to evaluate a patient before support with an LVAD include right heart catheterization, cardiac echocardiography, and blood tests. Blood tests include studies to determine nutritional status (serum protein, albumin and pre-albumin levels), renal function (serum blood urea nitrogen and creatinine levels) and hepatic function (prothrombin time/international normalized ratio (INR), total bilirubin, model of end-stage liver disease score, serum aspartate aminotransferase). A right atrial pressure (RAP) ≥18 mm Hg and a high RAP relative to the pulmonary capillary wedge pressure (PCWP, >0.63) are clues regarding the severity of RV impairment. Another important parameter is the RV stroke work index (RVSWI), which is a measurement of RV function: RVSWI = (mean PAP − mean RAP) × (Cardiac Index/Heart rate).[2,16,17] A low RVSWI has been associated with increased risk for severe RV failure requiring RVAD implantation.[18] Apart from the previously mentioned parameters, the main echocardiographic parameters that correlate with RVF after LVAD implantations are outlined in **Box 1**.[19]

Despite many publications, precise characterization of patients with significant RVF requiring biventricular support has not been described and continues to be center and physician specific. Multiple groups have identified preoperative risk factors and scores for post-LVAD RVF; however, no uniform predictors have yet been widely accepted. These risk scores typically were developed by small single-center studies with various definitions of RVF, leading to inconsistent predictors and no single model dependably forecasting RVF. Furthermore, most were developed in

Box 1
Echocardiographic parameters correlated with right ventricular failure after left ventricular assist device implantation

- Qualitative right ventricular dysfunction
- Tricuspid annular plane systolic excursion (TAPSE)
- Fractional area change
- Right ventricular index of myocardial performance
- Right ventricular systolic and diastolic longitudinal strain
- Right ventricle short-axis–to–long-axis ratio
- Right ventricle end-diastolic dimension-to-left ventricle end-diastolic dimension ratio
- Tricuspid annular dilation without significant tricuspid regurgitation
- Left ventricular ejection fraction
- Left ventricular end-diastolic dimension
- Tricuspid regurgitation duration corrected for heart rate
- Peak systolic (S′) velocity of the right ventricular free wall at the tricuspid annulus assessed with tissue Doppler
- Early diastolic (E′) velocity of the right ventricular free wall at the tricuspid annulus assessed with tissue Doppler
- Right ventricular E/E′ ratio
- TAPSE increase in response to dobutamine infusion
- Severity of tricuspid regurgitation
- 3-dimensional right ventricular end-systolic and end-diastolic volume index

From Neyer J, Arsanjani R, Moriguchi J, et al. Echocardiographic parameters associated with right ventricular failure after left ventricular assist device: a review. J Heart Lung Transplant 2016;35(3):286; with permission.

predominantly bridge-to-transplant patients with pulsatile devices, not reflecting the current LVAD population. Kalogeropoulos and colleagues[20] evaluated the performance of the 6 available prediction models (Michigan, Penn, Utah, Kormos, CRITT, Pittsburgh Decision Tree) in 116 patients and found that these scoring systems are all performing modestly. A recent meta-analysis of observational studies showed that among humoral markers, INR (even slightly increased over 1.1), N-terminal pro b-type natriuretic peptide, and white blood cell count may be helpful for the identification of patients at risk of RVF. Further, that meta-analysis confirms the importance of invasive hemodynamic assessment for RVF prediction, particularly RAP, RVSWI, and mean arterial pressure. Finally, qualitative assessment of RV performance, RV/left ventricular (LV) diameter ratio and RV free wall longitudinal 2-dimensional strain are crucial parameters to assess in routine echocardiographic evaluation of these patients.[21]

BIVENTRICULAR SUPPORT STRATEGIES

Patients with high risk for RVF despite hemodynamic optimization, need to be considered for planned biventricular support or a total artificial heart (TAH). There are several temporary or permanent biventricular assist device (BVAD) support strategies; the most common strategy is the implantation of a permanent CF-LVAD with a temporary RVAD. Other permanent BVAD support strategies include implanting 2 pulsatile extracorporeal pumps (Berlin Heart Excor), using a TAH, or implanting 2 permanent CF-LVADs.

TEMPORARY RIGHT VENTRICULAR ASSIST DEVICE SOLUTIONS

Earlier, many centers used to perform direct cannulation of the pulmonary artery and right atrium and left the chest open; however, this approach has been replaced with a better approach that allows chest closure. In the alternative approach, a Dacron graft is attached to the pulmonary artery passed through a subxiphoid or intercostal exit, where the RVAD outflow cannula is inserted. The inflow cannula is percutaneously cannulated in the femoral vein and the sternum is primarily closed (**Fig. 1**). It is common practice to use a centrifugal pump CentriMag (Abbott Inc., Abbott Park, IL) as an RVAD pump with or without oxygenator. On the day of RVAD explantation, the outflow graft of the RVAD is pulled, ligated, and the insertion site is secondarily closed. Meanwhile, the RVAD inflow cannula is removed and direct pressure is applied. The advantage of this technique is the feasibility of early extubation, the possibility of pulmonary support using an oxygenator attached to the circuit, and the possibility of RVAD explanation at bedside. The main disadvantage includes limitation of early and adequate mobilization. Using this approach, longer support durations are possible; at our institution, a patient was supported for 88 days using this approach and was fully mobilized on the intensive care unit floor without any complications.[22] This technique also can be used for temporary RVAD implantation in patients after minimally invasive LVAD implantation using the same J-Sternotomy approach.[22]

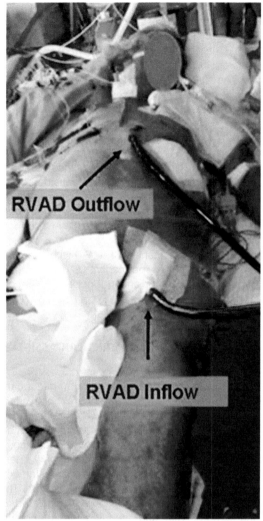

Fig. 1. A patient with simultaneous LVAD and RVAD support. The inflow cannula of the RVAD is inserted percutaneously into the right atrium through the left femoral vein. The outflow cannula is inserted into a graft that was attached to the pulmonary artery and exteriorized through the subxiphoid area. (*From* Saeed D, Maxhera B, Kamiya H, et al. Alternative right ventricular assist device implantation technique for patients with perioperative right ventricular failure. J Thor and Cardio Surg 2015;149(3):929; with permission.)

An alternative strategy includes direct cannulation of the right atrium and pulmonary artery (using Dacron graft) cannulation with chest closure. These patients can then ambulate in the intensive care unit.

Another temporary RVAD solution involves using the Protek Duo cannula (Cardiac Assist Inc, Pittsburgh, PA). The Protek Duo cannula has the advantage of full mobilization of the patient and

the cannula can be removed at bedside in the event of RV recovery. The RV circuit runs using an extracorporeal rotary pump, such as the Centri-Mag or TandemHeart (CardiacAssist Inc). The Protek Duo implant is challenging and the short cannula length may limit cannula usage in larger patients, as the outflow cannula may not reach the pulmonic circulation, leading to circulatory flow in the RV.

Another recent temporary percutaneous RVAD support strategy includes implanting the Impella RP (Abiomed Inc., Danvers, MA). The RECOVER RIGHT study evaluated the safety and efficacy of this novel percutaneous RVAD in a prospective, multicenter trial.[23] The main limitations of this device include mobilization issues related to femoral vein insertion site, inability to successfully place the device across the tricuspid valve and pulmonic valve in the right ventricle, and a flow rate of 4 L/min, which may not be sufficient for patients with a higher body mass index.

Finally, for patients who are on venoarterial extracorporeal membranous oxygenation (VA-ECMO) before LVAD implantation surgery or who develop postoperative RVF, some centers may consider keeping the patient for few days on VA-ECMO after LVAD implantation. Patients on VA-ECMO are high-risk patients with higher rate of postoperative RVF, morbidity, and mortality compared with other LVAD candidates.[24] Assessing RV in these patients on VA-ECMO is challenging. At our institution, one of the RV protective strategies to prevent postoperative RVF is performing the LVAD implantation on VA-ECMO without converting to cardiopulmonary bypass at the time of surgery. Our group has shown that postoperative bleeding complication and blood product requirements (and possibly RVF) can be significantly reduced when LVAD implantation is performed on VA-ECMO.[25,26] However, VA-ECMO, although suitable for cardiopulmonary support in some instances, has a higher rate of device-related complications (thromboembolism, hemolysis, ischemic leg complications, and bleeding) and limits a longer duration of support.

PERMANENT RIGHT VENTRICULAR ASSIST DEVICE SUPPORT SOLUTIONS
Biventricular Support Using Pulsatile Pumps

Berlin Heart Excor (Berlin Heart GmbH, Berlin Germany) is a pneumatically driven paracorporeal VAD introduced into clinical practice in 1992. The system is capable of providing short-term to long-term LV, RV, and biventricular assistance. The Berlin Heart Excor pumps come in 3 different sizes, 50, 60, and 80 mL, to suit various patient needs and have had satisfactory outcomes in pediatric patients.[27] With the exception of pediatric patients, only a few centers still use this device in adults.[28]

Biventricular Support Using Continuous-Flow Pumps

The lack of a reliable device designed specifically for RV support diminishes the treatment options for patients with biventricular failure or those with isolated RVF. Most devices are developed as an LVAD and only a few reports exist of continuous-flow experimental RVADs (eg, Dex-Aide RVAD).[29–32] However, no continuous-flow RVADs have made it to clinical trials. Due to the lack of a permanent RVAD solution, several clinicians started using CF-LVAD devices as RVAD.[33]

There are several limitations related to off-label use of CF-LVAD as RVAD that need to be addressed; anatomically, the RV is a complex 3-dimensional structure that appears triangular in sagittal section.[34] The RV forms a crescent-shaped chamber unlike the cone-shaped LV chamber,[35] comprising a sinus (body) and outflow tract, in contrast to the ellipsoidal concentric LV. Under normal baseline conditions, the unique anatomy, myocardial ultrastructure, and coronary physiology of the RV reflect characteristics of a high-volume/low-pressure pump.[36] Because of low pulmonary resistance, the RV pumps the same stroke volume as the LV but with approximately 25% of the stroke work.[34] There are several challenges encountered at the time of designing a proper RVAD pump, including pump dimensions and fitting issues within the chest cavity. Further, the following challenges for proper placement of RVAD are expected: protrusion of the inflow into the highly trabeculated RV, the relative proximity of the tricuspid chordae and distance of the inflow from the interventricular septum, and proper device inflow port orientation and fixation (right atrial placement).

Apart from the previously mentioned anatomic limitations of the RV and RVAD placement, there are several physiologic constraints for RVAD pumps. RVAD pumps operate at much lower afterloads (pulmonary arterial pressure) than LVADs and at significantly lower hydraulic loads and power consumption rates.[34] The pump flow and speed of the RVAD should be set at a lower level than pump flow and speed of the LVAD.[32] This is important from a technical standpoint during surgical procedures as well as for the management of both devices during long-term BVAD assistance to prevent pulmonary overflow and the development of pulmonary edema. To avoid such pulmonary overflow, either pump speed must be reduced to a very low speed or the outflow graft must be restricted to increase pump pressure rise. As a result, modifications are often necessary for current generation LVADs to be implanted as an RVAD. Intraoperative modifications include narrowing the outflow graft by up to 50% of its diameter or increasing the length to increase resistance to the flow, thereby allowing the RVAD to operate at a flow and speed similar to an LVAD. In the absence of this kind of modification, the only other option would be to run the RVAD at a lower speed, which adds the risk of pump thrombosis, which is still one of the main limiting factors of using LVAD pumps in the RVAD configuration.[37]

The use of 2 implantable CF-LVADs for biventricular support has been reported with the Jarvik pump (Jarvik 2000 FlowMaker; Jarvik Heart, Inc, New York, NY) for BVAD support in a young patient with worsening RVF.[38] Other groups consecutively reported on limited "off-label" clinical use of 2 LVADs using Dura Heart (Terumo Heart Inc, Ann Arbor, MI).[39] Further, the Methodist group in Texas reported a case of biventricular support using 2 HeartMate II pumps (Abbott, Abbott Park, IL) in a TAH configuration.[40] The same group reported recently a case of a HeartMate II LVAD patient with RVF, who was successively managed using the HVAD (Medtronic, Minneapolis, MN) as RVAD.[41] Most recently, the Berlin group reported 2 cases of biventricular support using the latest CF-VAD (2 HeartMate 3 pumps [Abbott] [Fig. 2]).[42] However, apart from the previously mentioned anecdotal case reports, the largest reported series of CF-LVADs for RVAD use are with the HVAD pump in a biventricular configuration.[33,43]

The operative details for an HVAD RVAD inflow cannula placement vary. The Berlin group has placed the RVAD inflow cannula in the anterior free wall of the RV just below the RV outflow tract. Importantly, this group interposes 5-mm silicone-coated rings between the apical fixation ring and the surface of the RV. This maneuver diminishes the chance of suction against the opposing wall of the RV.[44] Deuse and coworkers[45] reported the use of an HVAD for permanent RV support with no spacer rings. The patient who underwent implantation with an isolated RVAD was followed for 10 weeks and showed stable hemodynamics. The investigators suggested that diaphragmatic device implantation allows inflow orientation to be parallel to the septum and avoids the risk of suction. Recently, some centers reported right atrial cannulation as another implantation

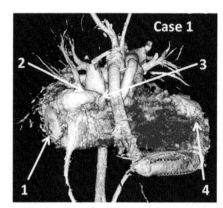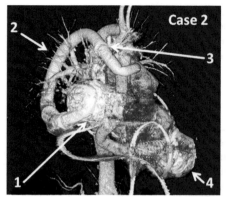

Fig. 2. Postoperative computed tomography scan reconstructions show the position of the RVAD pump and the outflow graft. 1, RVAD pump connected to the right atrium; 2, original pump prosthesis; 3, anastomosis between the original pump prosthesis and the 10-mm Hemashield prosthesis; and 4, LVAD pump connected to the apex of the LV. (*From* Potapov EV, Kukucka M, Falk V, et al. Biventricular support using 2 HeartMate 3 pumps. J Heart Lung Trans 2016;35(10):1270; with permission.)

technique.[46] Another approach is to completely excise the heart at the level of the atrioventricular junction and implant 2 HVAD pumps that are sutured to the tricuspid annulus or mitral annulus. In a case report from Strueber and associates,[47] a patient survived 14 weeks until cardiac transplantation with 2 HVADs that were implanted following removal of the patient's own heart. In another case series, Mulvihill and colleagues[48] reported 4 patients who were supported with 2 HVAD pumps in TAH configuration with an acceptable survival of 50%.

Unfortunately, the outcome of BVAD implantation remains also limited with 1-year survival of 50% to 60% and a high risk of pump thrombosis of the RVAD.[44] However, based on available literature, it appears that the right atrial implantation technique is superior to the RV implantation technique.[44,46] Medtronic is now working on regulatory approval for using the HVAD as an RVAD.

Biventricular Support Using Total Artificial Heart

The SynCardia TAH (Tucson, AZ) currently provides the most definitive option for patients with biventricular failure who are not candidates for isolated LVAD placement. The major complications of TAH implantation include stroke, infection, bleeding, thrombosis, renal failure, and chronic anemia.[49] The techniques for implantation are adaptable to almost all patients with advanced heart failure, including those with severe biventricular cardiomyopathy, complex congenital heart disease, failed LVADs, failed transplantations, and acquired structural heart defects that have failed or are not amenable to conventional surgical

treatment. Traditionally, a body surface area (BSA) less than 1.7 m² or a distance between the sternum and the anterior vertebral body of less than 10 cm were considered absolute contraindications to implant the SynCardia TAH.[50]

Recently there is a new, smaller 50-mL TAH that was designed to accommodate patients with a BSA as low as 1.2 m².[51] The 50-mL SynCardia is compatible with the Freedom Driver. Development of the portable Freedom Driver (approved by both CE Mark and the Food and Drug Administration) has enabled discharge of patients with artificial hearts while they await transplantation. To date, there have been more than 1400 TAH implants. Outcomes after TAH implantation vary across centers based on expertise with implantation and management of the device. The recently published results of the 50-mL TAH trial showed positive outcome in merely 50% of the patients.[51] Meanwhile, excellent single-center series have been published with a 1-year survival of 71%.[52] Although no head-to-head prospective randomized controlled trials have compared BVAD with TAH, 1 retrospective study from a multicenter French database showed no difference in mortality for patients implanted with a TAH compared with BVADs.[53] On the contrary, although the number of implants remains too small to draw conclusions, analysis of the latest INTERMACS registry (including data of 373 patients with TAH) has suggested improved 1-year and 2-year survival of patients implanted with a BVAD compared with TAH.[8] In conclusion, the TAH is an important and effective intervention for patients who are dying of biventricular heart failure. However, limited long-term outcomes, and relatively high complication rates compared with conventional LVADs limits its use to specific patient populations and its role in destination therapy remains unknown.

SUMMARY

Some degree of RV dysfunction can be observed in most patients with advanced heart failure being evaluated for LVAD implantation. Several pre-intraoperative and postoperative strategies have evolved to optimize RV function that focus on modifying the hemodynamic and/or laboratory abnormalities associated with RVF. Using the previously discussed measures, the risk of RVF may be minimized and the rate of post-LVAD RVF in recent years has been lowered. However, despite aggressive risk stratification and medical management, some patients still develop RVF requiring RVAD support. Needless to say, the requirement for an RVAD after LVAD implantation is associated with worse outcomes. The outcome is even worse when RVAD is implanted on an emergent basis. Therefore, a planned biventricular support or a TAH needs to be considered in patients at high risk for RVF.

Several biventricular support strategies are available. The most common approach is using a temporary RVAD with direct cannulation of the pulmonary artery, typically attached to a continuous-flow extracorporeal pump (CentriMag). The Protek Duo cannula and Impella RP are other promising approaches for temporary RV support.

Right-sided circulation, anatomy, and physiology impose specific restrictions on the ideal mechanical pump for RV support. Although major technologic and therapeutic advances have been achieved with chronic LVAD systems, progress in developing dedicated RVAD technology has been slow. The most common LVAD pump, which has been used off-label for RV support, is the HeartWare HVAD. At this time, the urgent need for effective and safe mechanical support therapy for RV support remains unmet. An ideal "future RVAD" pump is expected to be small in size, allows minimally invasive cannulation/replacement, has control algorithm to suit the patient's physiologic demand, is designed to promote long-term use (>1 years), has a low rate of thromboembolism, and has a robust and compact drive system to allow for patient mobility.

REFERENCES

1. Dang NC, Topkara VK, Mercando M, et al. Right heart failure after left ventricular assist device implantation in patients with chronic congestive heart failure. J Heart Lung Transplant 2006;25(1):1–6.

2. Kormos RL, Teuteberg JJ, Pagani FD, et al. Right ventricular failure in patients with the HeartMate II continuous-flow left ventricular assist device: incidence, risk factors, and effect on outcomes. J Thorac Cardiovasc Surg 2010;139(5):1316–24.

3. Matthews JC, Koelling TM, Pagani FD, et al. The right ventricular failure risk score a pre-operative tool for assessing the risk of right ventricular failure in left ventricular assist device candidates. J Am Coll Cardiol 2008;51(22):2163–72.

4. Patel ND, Weiss ES, Schaffer J, et al. Right heart dysfunction after left ventricular assist device implantation: a comparison of the pulsatile HeartMate I and axial-flow HeartMate II devices. Ann Thorac Surg 2008;86(3):832–40 [discussion: 832–40].

5. Saeed D, Maxhera B, Kamiya H, et al. Alternative right ventricular assist device implantation technique for patients with perioperative right ventricular failure. J Thorac Cardiovasc Surg 2015;149(3):927–32.

6. Lampert BC, Teuteberg JJ. Right ventricular failure after left ventricular assist devices. J Heart Lung Transplant 2015;34(9):1123–30.

7. Baumwol J, Macdonald PS, Keogh AM, et al. Right heart failure and "failure to thrive" after left ventricular assist device: clinical predictors and outcomes. The J Heart Lung Transplant 2011;30(8):888–95.

8. Kirklin JK, Pagani FD, Kormos RL, et al. Eighth annual INTERMACS report: special focus on framing the impact of adverse events. J Heart Lung Transplant 2017;36(10):1080–6.

9. Farrar DJ, Compton PG, Hershon JJ, et al. Right heart interaction with the mechanically assisted left heart. World J Surg 1985;9(1):89–102.

10. Moon MR, Bolger AF, DeAnda A, et al. Septal function during left ventricular unloading. Circulation 1997;95(5):1320–7.

11. Saeed D, Kidambi T, Shalli S, et al. Tricuspid valve repair with left ventricular assist device implantation: is it warranted? J Heart Lung Transplant 2011;30(5):530–5.

12. Brisco MA, Sundareswaran KS, Milano CA, et al. Incidence, risk, and consequences of atrial arrhythmias in patients with continuous-flow left ventricular assist devices. J Card Surg 2014;29(4):572–80.

13. Cantillon DJ, Saliba WI, Wazni OM, et al. Low cardiac output associated with ventricular tachyarrhythmias in continuous-flow LVAD recipients with a concomitant ICD (LoCo VT Study). J Heart Lung Transplant 2014;33(3):318–20.

14. Rich JD, Gosev I, Patel CB, et al. The incidence, risk factors, and outcomes associated with late right-sided heart failure in patients supported with an axial-flow left ventricular assist device. J Heart Lung Transplant 2017;36(1):50–8.

15. Takeda K, Takayama H, Colombo PC, et al. Incidence and clinical significance of late right heart failure during continuous-flow left ventricular assist

device support. J Heart Lung Transplant 2015;34(8): 1024–32.

16. Bonde P, Ku NC, Genovese EA, et al. Model for end-stage liver disease score predicts adverse events related to ventricular assist device therapy. Ann Thorac Surg 2012;93(5):1541–7 [discussion: 7–8].

17. Maxhera B, Albert A, Westenfeld R, et al. Minimally invasive right ventricular assist device implantation in a patient with Heartware left ventricular assist device. ASAIO J 2015;61(6):e42–3.

18. Ochiai Y, McCarthy PM, Smedira NG, et al. Predictors of severe right ventricular failure after implantable left ventricular assist device insertion: analysis of 245 patients. Circulation 2002;106(12 Suppl 1): I198–202.

19. Neyer J, Arsanjani R, Moriguchi J, et al. Echocardiographic parameters associated with right ventricular failure after left ventricular assist device: a review. J Heart Lung Transplant 2016;35(3): 283–93.

20. Kalogeropoulos AP, Kelkar A, Weinberger JF, et al. Validation of clinical scores for right ventricular failure prediction after implantation of continuous-flow left ventricular assist devices. J Heart Lung Transplant 2015;34(12):1595–603.

21. Bellavia D, Iacovoni A, Scardulla C, et al. Prediction of right ventricular failure after ventricular assist device implant: systematic review and meta-analysis of observational studies. Eur J Heart Fail 2017;19(7): 926–46.

22. Ortmann P, Saeed D, Lichtenberg A. Case report of extended "temporary" use of Levitronix CentriMag right ventricular assist device. Artif Organs 2012; 36(12):1072–3.

23. Anderson MB, Goldstein J, Milano C, et al. Benefits of a novel percutaneous ventricular assist device for right heart failure: the prospective RECOVER RIGHT study of the Impella RP device. J Heart Lung Transplant 2015;34(12):1549–60.

24. Maxhera B, Albert A, Ansari E, et al. Survival predictors in ventricular assist device patients with prior extracorporeal life support: selecting appropriate candidates. Artif organs 2014;38(9):727–32.

25. Abdeen MS, Albert A, Maxhera B, et al. Implanting permanent left ventricular assist devices in patients on veno-arterial extracorporeal membrane oxygenation support: do we really need a cardiopulmonary bypass machine? Eur J Cardiothorac Surg 2016; 50(3):542–7.

26. Saeed D, Assmann A, Abdeen M, et al. Implanting permanent left ventricular assist devices in patients on veno-arterial extracorporeal membrane oxygenation support. Multimed Man Cardiothorac Surg 2016;2017.

27. Hetzer R, Alexi-Meskishvili V, Weng Y, et al. Mechanical cardiac support in the young with the Berlin Heart EXCOR pulsatile ventricular assist device: 15 years' experience. Semin Thorac Cardiovasc Surg Pediatr Card Surg Annu 2006;9(1):99–108.

28. Schmid C, Tjan T, Etz C, et al. The Excor device—revival of an old system with excellent results. Thorac Cardiovasc surgeon 2006;54(6):393–9.

29. Fukamachi K, Saeed D, Massiello AL, et al. Development of DexAide right ventricular assist device: update II. ASAIO J 2008;54(6):589–93.

30. Saeed D, Arusoglu L, Gazzoli F, et al. Results of the European clinical trial of arrow CorAide left ventricular assist system. Artif organs 2013;37(2):121–7.

31. Saeed D, Massiello AL, Shalli S, et al. Introduction of fixed-flow mode in the DexAide right ventricular assist device. J Heart Lung Transplant 2010;29(1): 32–6.

32. Saeed D, Ootaki Y, Ootaki C, et al. Acute in vivo evaluation of an implantable continuous flow biventricular assist system. ASAIO J 2008;54(1):20–4.

33. Strueber M, Meyer AL, Malehsa D, et al. Successful use of the HeartWare HVAD rotary blood pump for biventricular support. J Thorac Cardiovasc Surg 2010;140(4):936–7.

34. Karimov JH, Sunagawa G, Horvath D, et al. Limitations to chronic right ventricular assist device support. Ann Thorac Surg 2016;102(2):651–8.

35. Ryan JJ, Archer SL. The right ventricle in pulmonary arterial hypertension: disorders of metabolism, angiogenesis and adrenergic signaling in right ventricular failure. Circ Res 2014;115(1):176–88.

36. Dell'Italia LJ. Anatomy and physiology of the right ventricle. Cardiol Clin 2012;30(2):167–87.

37. Krabatsch T, Potapov E, Stepanenko A, et al. Biventricular circulatory support with two miniaturized implantable assist devices. Circulation 2011; 124(11 Suppl):S179–86.

38. Frazier OH, Myers TJ, Gregoric I. Biventricular assistance with the Jarvik FlowMaker: a case report. J Thorac Cardiovasc Surg 2004;128(4):625–6.

39. Saito S, Sakaguchi T, Miyagawa S, et al. Biventricular support using implantable continuous-flow ventricular assist devices. J Heart Lung Transplant 2011;30(4):475–8.

40. Loebe M, Bruckner B, Reardon MJ, et al. Initial clinical experience of total cardiac replacement with dual HeartMate-II axial flow pumps for severe biventricular heart failure. Methodist DeBakey Cardiovasc J 2011;7(1):40–4.

41. Baldwin ACW, Sandoval E, Cohn WE, et al. Nonidentical continuous-flow devices for biventricular support. Tex Heart Inst J 2017;44(2):141–3.

42. Potapov EV, Kukucka M, Falk V, et al. Biventricular support using 2 HeartMate 3 pumps. J Heart Lung Transplant 2016;35(10):1268–70.

43. Hetzer R, Krabatsch T, Stepanenko A, et al. Long-term biventricular support with the HeartWare implantable continuous flow pump. J Heart Lung Transplant 2010;29(7):822–4.

44. Shehab S, Macdonald PS, Keogh AM, et al. Long-term biventricular HeartWare ventricular assist device support–case series of right atrial and right ventricular implantation outcomes. J Heart Lung Transplant 2016;35(4):466–73.

45. Deuse T, Schirmer J, Kubik M, et al. Isolated permanent right ventricular assistance using the HVAD continuous-flow pump. Ann Thorac Surg 2013; 95(4):1434–6.

46. Marasco SF, Stornebrink RK, Murphy DA, et al. Long-term right ventricular support with a centrifugal ventricular assist device placed in the right atrium. J Card Surg 2014;29(6):839–42.

47. Strueber M, Schmitto JD, Kutschka I, et al. Placement of 2 implantable centrifugal pumps to serve as a total artificial heart after cardiectomy. J Thorac Cardiovasc Surg 2012;143(2):507–9.

48. Mulvihill MS, Joseph JT, Daneshmand MA, et al. Usefulness of 2 centrifugal ventricular assist devices in a total artificial heart configuration: a preliminary report. J Heart Lung Transplant 2017;36(11):1266–8.

49. Cook JA, Shah KB, Quader MA, et al. The total artificial heart. J Thorac Dis 2015;7(12):2172–80.

50. Torregrossa G, Anyanwu A, Zucchetta F, et al. SynCardia: the total artificial heart. Ann Cardiothorac Surg 2014;3(6):612–20.

51. Wells D, Villa CR, Simon Morales DL. The 50/50 cc total artificial heart trial: extending the benefits of the total artificial heart to underserved populations. Semin Thorac Cardiovasc Surg Pediatr Card Surg Annu 2017;20:16–9.

52. Shah KB, Thanavaro KL, Tang DG, et al. Impact of INTERMACS profile on clinical outcomes for patients supported with the total artificial heart. J Card Fail 2016;22(11):913–20.

53. Kirsch M, Mazzucotelli JP, Roussel JC, et al. Survival after biventricular mechanical circulatory support: does the type of device matter? J Heart Lung Transplant 2012;31(5):501–8.

UNITED STATES POSTAL SERVICE ®

Statement of Ownership, Management, and Circulation
(All Periodicals Publications Except Requester Publications)

1. Publication Title	2. Publication Number	3. Filing Date
CARDIOLOGY CLINICS	000 – 701	9/18/2018

4. Issue Frequency	5. Number of Issues Published Annually	6. Annual Subscription Price
FEB, MAY, AUG, NOV	4	$339.00

7. Complete Mailing Address of Known Office of Publication (Not printer) (Street, city, county, state, and ZIP+4®)

ELSEVIER INC.
230 Park Avenue, Suite 800
New York, NY 10169

Contact Person
STEPHEN R. BUSHING
Telephone (Include area code)
215-239-3688

8. Complete Mailing Address of Headquarters or General Business Office of Publisher (Not printer)

ELSEVIER INC.
230 Park Avenue, Suite 800
New York, NY 10169

9. Full Names and Complete Mailing Addresses of Publisher, Editor, and Managing Editor (Do not leave blank)

Publisher (Name and complete mailing address)

TAYLOR E BALL, ELSEVIER INC.
1600 JOHN F KENNEDY BLVD. SUITE 1800
PHILADELPHIA, PA 19103-2899

Editor (Name and complete mailing address)

STACY EASTMAN, ELSEVIER INC.
1600 JOHN F KENNEDY BLVD. SUITE 1800
PHILADELPHIA, PA 19103-2899

Managing Editor (Name and complete mailing address)

PATRICK MANLEY, ELSEVIER INC.
1600 JOHN F KENNEDY BLVD. SUITE 1800
PHILADELPHIA, PA 19103-2899

10. Owner (Do not leave blank. If the publication is owned by a corporation, give the name and address of the corporation immediately followed by the names and addresses of all stockholders owning or holding 1 percent or more of the total amount of stock. If not owned by a corporation, give the names and addresses of the individual owners. If owned by a partnership or other unincorporated firm, give its name and address as well as those of each individual owner. If the publication is published by a nonprofit organization, give its name and address.)

Full Name	Complete Mailing Address
WHOLLY OWNED SUBSIDIARY OF REED/ELSEVIER, US HOLDINGS	1600 JOHN F KENNEDY BLVD, SUITE 1800 PHILADELPHIA, PA 19103-2899

11. Known Bondholders, Mortgagees, and Other Security Holders Owning or Holding 1 Percent or More of Total Amount of Bonds, Mortgages, or Other Securities. If none, check box ▶ ☐ None

Full Name	Complete Mailing Address
N/A	

12. Tax Status (For completion by nonprofit organizations authorized to mail at nonprofit rates) (Check one)
The purpose, function, and nonprofit status of this organization and the exempt status for federal income tax purposes:
☒ Has Not Changed During Preceding 12 Months
☐ Has Changed During Preceding 12 Months (Publisher must submit explanation of change with this statement)

PS Form **3526**, July 2014 [Page 1 of 4 (see instructions page 4)] PSN: 7530-01-000-9931 PRIVACY NOTICE: See our privacy policy on www.usps.com.

---

13. Publication Title	14. Issue Date for Circulation Data Below
CARDIOLOGY CLINICS	MAY 2018

15. Extent and Nature of Circulation			Average No. Copies Each Issue During Preceding 12 Months	No. Copies of Single Issue Published Nearest to Filing Date
a. Total Number of Copies (Net press run)			126	255
b. Paid Circulation (By Mail and Outside the Mail)	(1)	Mailed Outside-County Paid Subscriptions Stated on PS Form 3541 (Include paid distribution above nominal rate, advertiser's proof copies, and exchange copies)	59	111
	(2)	Mailed In-County Paid Subscriptions Stated on PS Form 3541 (Include paid distribution above nominal rate, advertiser's proof copies, and exchange copies)	0	0
	(3)	Paid Distribution Outside the Mails Including Sales Through Dealers and Carriers, Street Vendors, Counter Sales, and Other Paid Distribution Outside USPS®	26	52
	(4)	Paid Distribution by Other Classes of Mail Through the USPS (e.g., First-Class Mail®)	0	0
c. Total Paid Distribution (Sum of 15b (1), (2), (3), and (4))		▶	85	163
d. Free or Nominal Rate Distribution (By Mail and Outside the Mail)	(1)	Free or Nominal Rate Outside-County Copies included on PS Form 3541	34	76
	(2)	Free or Nominal Rate In-County Copies Included on PS Form 3541	0	0
	(3)	Free or Nominal Rate Copies Mailed at Other Classes Through the USPS (e.g., First-Class Mail)	0	0
	(4)	Free or Nominal Rate Distribution Outside the Mail (Carriers or other means)	0	0
e. Total Free or Nominal Rate Distribution (Sum of 15d (1), (2), (3) and (4))		▶	34	76
f. Total Distribution (Sum of 15c and 15e)		▶	119	239
g. Copies not Distributed (See Instructions to Publishers #4 (page #3))		▶	7	16
h. Total (Sum of 15f and g)		▶	126	255
i. Percent Paid (15c divided by 15f times 100)			71.43%	68.2%

* If you are claiming electronic copies, go to line 16 on page 3. If you are not claiming electronic copies, skip to line 17 on page 3.

16. Electronic Copy Circulation		Average No. Copies Each Issue During Preceding 12 Months	No. Copies of Single Issue Published Nearest to Filing Date
a. Paid Electronic Copies	▶	0	0
b. Total Paid Print Copies (Line 15c) + Paid Electronic Copies (Line 16a)	▶	85	163
c. Total Print Distribution (Line 15f) + Paid Electronic Copies (Line 16a)	▶	119	239
d. Percent Paid (Both Print & Electronic Copies) (16b divided by 16c × 100)	▶	71.43%	68.2%

☒ I certify that 50% of all my distributed copies (electronic and print) are paid above a nominal price.

17. Publication of Statement of Ownership

☒ If the publication is a general publication, publication of this statement is required. Will be printed
in the **NOVEMBER 2018** issue of this publication. ☐ Publication not required.

18. Signature and Title of Editor, Publisher, Business Manager, or Owner		Date
STEPHEN R. BUSHING - INVENTORY DISTRIBUTION CONTROL MANAGER	*Stephen R. Bushing*	9/18/2018

I certify that all information furnished on this form is true and complete. I understand that anyone who furnishes false or misleading information on this form or who omits material or information requested on the form may be subject to criminal sanctions (including fines and imprisonment) and/or civil sanctions (including civil penalties).

PS Form **3526**, July 2014 (Page 3 of 4) PRIVACY NOTICE: See our privacy policy on www.usps.com

Moving?

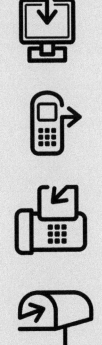

Make sure your subscription moves with you!

To notify us of your new address, find your **Clinics Account Number** (located on your mailing label above your name), and contact customer service at:

Email: journalscustomerservice-usa@elsevier.com

800-654-2452 (subscribers in the U.S. & Canada)
314-447-8871 (subscribers outside of the U.S. & Canada)

Fax number: 314-447-8029

Elsevier Health Sciences Division
Subscription Customer Service
3251 Riverport Lane
Maryland Heights, MO 63043

*To ensure uninterrupted delivery of your subscription, please notify us at least 4 weeks in advance of move.

Printed and bound by CPI Group (UK) Ltd, Croydon, CR0 4YY

03/10/2024

01040298-0019